Infant & Toddler Health Sourcebook

Infectious Diseases Sourcebook

Injury & Trauma Sourcebook

Learning Disabilities Sourcebook,
2nd Edition

Leukemia Sourcebook

Liver Disorders Sourcebook

Lung Disorders Sourcebook

Medical Tests Sourcebook, 2nd Edition

Men's Health Concerns Sourcebook,
2nd Edition

Mental Health Disorders Sourcebook,
3rd Edition

Mental Retardation Sourcebook

Movement Disorders Sourcebook

Muscular Dystrophy Sourcebook

Obesity Sourcebook

Osteoporosis Sourcebook

Pain Sourcebook, 2nd Edition

Pediatric Cancer Sourcebook

Physical & Mental Issues in Aging
Sourcebook

Podiatry Sourcebook, 2nd Edition

Pregnancy & Birth Sourcebook,
2nd Edition

Prostate Cancer Sourcebook

Prostate & Urological Disorders
Sourcebook

Public Health Sourcebook

Reconstructive & Cosmetic Surgery
Sourcebook

Rehabilitation Sourcebook

Respiratory Diseases & Disorders
Sourcebook

Sexually Transmitted Diseases
Sourcebook, 3rd Edition

Sleep Disorders Sourcebook,
2nd Edition

Smoking Concerns Sourcebook

Sports Injuries Sourcebook, 2nd Edition

Stress-Related Disorders Sourcebook

Stroke Sourcebook

Substance Abuse Sourcebook

Surgery Sourcebook

Thyroid Disorders Sourcebook

Transplantation Sourcebook

Traveler's Health Sourcebook

Urinary Tract & Kidney Diseases &
Disorders Sourcebook, 2nd Edition

Vegetarian Sourcebook

Women's Health Concerns Sourcebook,
2nd Edition

Workplace Health & Safety Sourcebook

Worldwide Health Sourcebook

Teen Health Series

Alcohol Information for Teens

Allergy Information for Teens

Asthma Information for Teens

Cancer Information for Teens

Complementary & Alternative
Medicine Information for
Teens

Diabetes Information for Teens

Diet Information for Teens,
2nd Edition

Drug Information for Teens,
2nd Edition

Eating Disorders Information
for Teens

Fitness Information for Teens

Learning Disabilities Information
for Teens

Mental Health Information for
Teens, 2nd Edition

Sexual Health Information for
Teens

Skin Health Information for
Teens

Sports Injuries Information
for Teens

Suicide Information for Teens

Tobacco Information for Teens

Fitness and Exercise
SOURCEBOOK

SOURCEBOOK

Third Edition

Health Reference Series

Third Edition

Fitness and Exercise SOURCEBOOK

*Basic Consumer Health Information about the
Physical and Mental Benefits of Fitness, Including
Cardiorespiratory Endurance, Muscular Strength,
Muscular Endurance, and Flexibility, with Facts about
Sports Nutrition and Exercise-Related Injuries and Tips
about Physical Activity and Exercises for People of
All Ages and for People with Health Concerns*

*Along with Advice on Selecting and Using Exercise
Equipment, Maintaining Exercise Motivation,
a Glossary of Related Terms, and a Directory of
Resources for More Help and Information*

Edited by
Amy L. Sutton

Omnigraphics

615 Griswold Street • Detroit, MI 48226

Bibliographic Note

Because this page cannot legibly accommodate all the copyright notices, the Bibliographic Note portion of the Preface constitutes an extension of the copyright notice.

Edited by Amy L. Sutton

Health Reference Series

Karen Bellenir, *Managing Editor*
David A. Cooke, M.D., *Medical Consultant*
Elizabeth Collins, *Permissions and Research Coordinator*
Laura Pleva Nielsen, *Index Editor*
Cherry Stockdale, *Permissions Assistant*
EdIndex, Services for Publishers, *Indexers*

* * *

Omnigraphics, Inc.

Matthew P. Barbour, *Senior Vice President*
Kay Gill, *Vice President—Directories*
Kevin Hayes, *Operations Manager*
David P. Bianco, *Marketing Director*

* * *

Peter E. Ruffner, *Publisher*
Frederick G. Ruffner, Jr., *Chairman*
Copyright © 2007 Omnigraphics, Inc.
ISBN 978-0-7808-0946-8

Library of Congress Cataloging-in-Publication Data

Fitness and exercise sourcebook : basic consumer health information about the physical and mental benefits of fitness, including cardiorespiratory endurance, muscular strength, muscular endurance, and flexibility, with facts about sports nutrition and exercise-related injuries and tips about physical activity and exercises for people of all ages and for people with health concerns; along with advice on selecting and using exercise equipment, maintaining exercise motivation, a glossary of related terms, and a directory of resources for more help and information / edited by Amy L. Sutton. -- 3rd ed.
    p. cm. -- (Health reference series)
    Summary: "Provides basic consumer health information about elements of physical fitness, including cardiorespiratory and muscular endurance, muscular strength, and flexibility. Includes index, glossary of related terms, and other resources"--Provided by publisher.
    Includes bibliographical references and index.
    ISBN 978-0-7808-0946-8 (hardcover : alk. paper) 1. Physical fitness--Handbooks, manuals, etc. 2. Exercise--Handbooks, manuals, etc. I. Sutton, Amy L. II. Title. III. Series.
    GV436.F53 2007
    613.7--dc22

                                                                    2006036852

∞

Printed in the United States

Table of Contents

Visit www.healthreferenceseries.com to view *A Contents Guide to the Health Reference Series*, a listing of more than 12,000 topics and the volumes in which they are covered.

Part III: Exercise Basics

Part IV: Fitness throughout Life

Part V: Physical Activity for People with Health Concerns

Part VI: Exercise-Related Injuries

Part VII: Maintaining Exercise Motivation

Part VIII: Additional Help and Information

Preface

About This Book

Regular physical activity offers exercisers a variety of health benefits, including a reduced risk of obesity, diabetes, high blood pressure, heart disease, stroke, dementia, and cancer. The advantages of exercise do not end there: Recent research has also shown that exercisers experience a mental boost from regular doses of physical activity.

Despite these and other positive effects of exercise, most Americans fail to make fitness a priority. According to the Centers for Disease Control and Prevention (CDC), more than 50% of U.S. adults do not exercise enough to reap health benefits, and 25% of Americans spend no time exercising at all.

For people who want to commit to a regular exercise program, however, there is good news. There is no need to spend hours toiling on the treadmill. In as few as 30 minutes a day several days a week, formerly inactive people of all ages can begin to experience the benefits of physical activity.

Fitness and Exercise Sourcebook, Third Edition provides updated information about the physical and mental benefits of exercise. It explains the basic components of physical fitness—including aerobic capacity, strength training, and flexibility—and discusses recent trends in fitness, including the growing popularity of yoga, Pilates, and balance training. Issues surrounding fitness in children, adolescents, pregnant women, and seniors are addressed, and the physical activity needs of people with common health conditions—such as asthma, high blood pressure, heart disease, and arthritis—are described. Readers will also find guidance on purchasing and using common exercise equipment, facts about preventing and treating sports injuries, suggestions for exercise activities, and tips for staying motivated. The volume concludes with a glossary of exercise-related terms and a directory of organizations that provide information about physical activity, fitness, and exercise.

How to Use This Book

This book is divided into parts and chapters. Parts focus on broad areas of interest. Chapters are devoted to single topics within a part.

Part I: The Physical and Mental Benefits of Fitness identifies the role of exercise in weight control, chronic disease prevention, metabolic regulation, and immune system function. It also discusses the positive mental health benefits of a regular exercise program, such as a reduced risk of stress and depression.

Part II: Sports Nutrition and Supplements provides tips on what to eat if you exercise, what to feed children and teens involved in sports, and guidance on maintaining adequate hydration levels. This part also describes popular sports nutrition supplements and the health risks of illegal products used to enhance athletic performance, such as steroids and androstenedione.

Part III: Exercise Basics offers guidance to both beginning and advanced exercisers who want to incorporate cardiovascular exercise, strength training, and flexibility and balance work into their personal physical activity program. This part also discusses the use of home exercise equipment, including treadmills, elliptical trainers, free weights, and pedometers. Information on exercise trends such as yoga and Pilates is provided, along with tips on hiring a personal trainer, choosing a health and fitness facility, and maintaining an exercise program away from home.

Part IV: Fitness throughout Life highlights the importance of physical activity for children, teens, pregnant women, and older adults. In addition to tips on helping children develop a lifelong love of fitness, this part offers information about the relationship between physical activity and academic achievement and the advisability of strength training for children and teens. This part also provides exercise suggestions for older adults who are just beginning to become physically active.

Part V: Physical Activity for People with Health Concerns describes exercise recommendations and considerations for people with conditions such as obesity, diabetes, asthma, high blood pressure, heart disease, stroke, arthritis and joint problems, chronic pain and fatigue, cancer, and HIV/AIDS.

Part VI: Exercise-Related Injuries includes information about both acute and chronic sports injuries and their treatment, including Achilles tendon disorders, knee problems, muscle soreness, shoulder problems, tennis elbow, shin splints, and strains and sprains. This part also offers tips on preventing common foot and skin problems that affect exercisers and discusses the physical and mental hazards of overtraining and exercise addiction.

Part VII: Maintaining Exercise Motivation offers tips on setting and achieving physical activity goals and details the value of enlisting the help of family members and friends for exercise support. This part also describes barriers that may make it difficult to exercise and provides strategies for overcoming them.

Part VIII: Additional Help and Information includes a glossary of important terms and a directory of government and private organizations that provide physical activity, fitness, and exercise information.

Bibliographic Note

This volume contains documents and excerpts from publications issued by the following U.S. government agencies: Centers for Disease Control and Prevention (CDC); Federal Trade Commission (FTC); National Cancer Institute (NCI); National Heart, Lung, and Blood Institute (NHLBI); National Institute of Arthritis and Musculoskeletal and Skin Diseases (NIAMS); National Institute on Aging (NIA); National Institute on Diabetes and Digestive and Kidney Diseases (NIDDK); National Institute on Drug Abuse (NIDA); National Institutes of Health (NIH); National Institutes of Health Division of Nutrition Research Coordination; National Institutes of Health Osteoporosis and Related Bone Diseases National Resource Center; National Women's Health Information Center (NWHIC); President's Council on Physical Fitness and Sports; U.S. Customs and Border Protection; U.S. Department of Health and Human Services (HHS); and the U.S. Food and Drug Administration (FDA).

In addition, this volume contains copyrighted documents from the following organizations: Action for Healthy Kids; Active Living by

Design; A.D.A.M., Inc.; AIDS InfoNet; American Academy of Dermatology; American Academy of Orthopaedic Surgeons; American College of Sports Medicine; American Council on Exercise; American Heart Association; American Physical Therapy Association; American Podiatric Medical Association; Anorexia Nervosa and Related Eating Disorders, Inc.; Better Health Channel; Cleveland Clinic Foundation; Cleveland Clinic Heart Center; Eat Right Montana; eMedicine.com, Inc.; Healthcommunities.com; IDEA Health & Fitness Association; Kansas State University Agricultural Experiment Station and Cooperative Extension Service; Medical College of Wisconsin; National Center on Physical Activity and Disability; National Fibromyalgia Association; National Jewish Medical and Research Center; National Stroke Association; Nemours Center for Children's Health Media/ TeensHealth.org; New York State Department of Health; Pedestrian and Bicycle Information Center; St. Francis Hospital and Health Centers; Trails and Greenways Clearinghouse; and the Wisconsin Governor's Challenge.

Full citation information is provided on the first page of each chapter or section. Every effort has been made to secure all necessary rights to reprint the copyrighted material. If any omissions have been made, please contact Omnigraphics to make corrections for future editions.

Acknowledgements

Thanks go to the many organizations, agencies, and individuals who have contributed materials for this *Sourcebook* and to medical consultant Dr. David Cooke and document engineer Bruce Bellenir. Special thanks go to managing editor Karen Bellenir and permissions and research coordinator Liz Collins for their help and support.

About the Health Reference Series

The *Health Reference Series* is designed to provide basic medical information for patients, families, caregivers, and the general public. Each volume takes a particular topic and provides comprehensive coverage. This is especially important for people who may be dealing with a newly diagnosed disease or a chronic disorder in themselves or in a family member. People looking for preventive guidance, information about disease warning signs, medical statistics, and risk factors for health problems will also find answers to their questions in the *Health Reference Series*. The *Series*, however, is not intended to serve as a tool for diagnosing illness, in prescribing treatments, or as a substitute for the physician/patient relationship. All people concerned about medical symptoms or the possibility of disease are encouraged to seek professional care from an appropriate health care provider.

Locating Information within the Health Reference Series

The *Health Reference Series* contains a wealth of information about a wide variety of medical topics. Ensuring easy access to all the fact sheets, research reports, in-depth discussions, and other material contained within the individual books of the *Series* remains one of our highest priorities. As the *Series* continues to grow in size and scope, however, locating the precise information needed by a reader may become more challenging.

A Contents Guide to the Health Reference Series was developed to direct readers to the specific volumes that address their concerns. It presents an extensive list of diseases, treatments, and other topics of general interest compiled from the Tables of Contents and major index headings. To access *A Contents Guide to the Health Reference Series*, visit www.healthreferenceseries.com.

Medical Consultant

Medical consultation services are provided to the *Health Reference Series* editors by David A. Cooke, M.D. Dr. Cooke is a graduate of Brandeis University, and he received his M.D. degree from the University of Michigan. He completed residency training at the University of Wisconsin Hospital and Clinics. He is board-certified in Internal Medicine. Dr. Cooke currently works as part of the University of Michigan Health System and practices in Ann Arbor, MI. In his free time, he enjoys writing, science fiction, and spending time with his family.

Our Advisory Board

We would like to thank the following board members for providing guidance to the development of this *Series*:

Dr. Lynda Baker,
Associate Professor of Library and Information Science,
Wayne State University, Detroit, MI

Nancy Bulgarelli,
William Beaumont Hospital Library, Royal Oak, MI

Karen Imarisio,
Bloomfield Township Public Library, Bloomfield Township, MI

Karen Morgan,
Mardigian Library, University of Michigan-Dearborn,
Dearborn, MI

Rosemary Orlando,
St. Clair Shores Public Library, St. Clair Shores, MI

Health Reference Series *Update Policy*

The inaugural book in the *Health Reference Series* was the first edition of *Cancer Sourcebook* published in 1989. Since then, the *Series* has been enthusiastically received by librarians and in the medical community. In order to maintain the standard of providing high-quality health information for the layperson the editorial staff at Omnigraphics felt it was necessary to implement a policy of updating volumes when warranted.

Medical researchers have been making tremendous strides, and it is the purpose of the *Health Reference Series* to stay current with the most recent advances. Each decision to update a volume is made on an individual basis. Some of the considerations include how much new information is available and the feedback we receive from people who use the books. If there is a topic you would like to see added to the update list, or an area of medical concern you feel has not been adequately addressed, please write to:

Editor
Health Reference Series
Omnigraphics, Inc.
615 Griswold Street
Detroit, MI 48226
E-mail: editorial@omnigraphics.com

Part One

The Physical and Mental Benefits of Fitness

Chapter 1

The Importance of Physical Activity

The evidence is growing and is more convincing than ever—people of all ages who are generally inactive can improve their health and well-being by becoming active at a moderate-intensity on a regular basis.

Regular physical activity substantially reduces the risk of dying of coronary heart disease, the nation's leading cause of death, and decreases the risk for stroke, colon cancer, diabetes, and high blood pressure. It also helps to control weight; contributes to healthy bones, muscles, and joints; reduces falls among older adults; helps to relieve the pain of arthritis; reduces symptoms of anxiety and depression; and is associated with fewer hospitalizations, physician visits, and medications. Moreover, physical activity need not be strenuous to be beneficial; people of all ages benefit from participating in regular, moderate-intensity physical activity, such as 30 minutes of brisk walking five or more times a week.

Despite the proven benefits of physical activity, more than 50% of American adults do not get enough physical activity to provide health benefits. Twenty-five percent of adults are not active at all in their leisure time. Activity decreases with age and is less common among women than men and among those with lower income and less education.

Excerpted from "Physical Activity for Everyone: The Importance of Physical Activity," by the Division of Nutrition and Physical Activity, National Center for Chronic Disease Prevention and Health Promotion, Centers for Disease Control and Prevention (CDC), March 30, 2006. For a complete list of references, see http://www.cdc.gov/nccdphp/dnpa.

Insufficient physical activity is not limited to adults. More than a third of young people in grades 9 through 12 do not regularly engage in vigorous-intensity physical activity. Daily participation in high school physical education classes dropped from 42% in 1991 to 32% in 2001.

Why should I be active?

Physical activity can bring you many health benefits. People who enjoy participating in moderate-intensity or vigorous-intensity physical activity on a regular basis benefit by lowering their risk of developing coronary heart disease, stroke, non-insulin-dependent (type 2) diabetes mellitus, high blood pressure, and colon cancer by 30% to 50% (USDHHS, 1996). Additionally, active people have lower premature death rates than people who are the least active.

Regular physical activity can improve health and reduce the risk of premature death in the following ways. It:

- reduces the risk of developing coronary heart disease (CHD) and the risk of dying from CHD;
- reduces the risk of stroke;
- reduces the risk of having a second heart attack in people who have already had one heart attack;
- lowers both total blood cholesterol and triglycerides and increases high-density lipoproteins (HDL or the "good" cholesterol);
- lowers the risk of developing high blood pressure;
- helps reduce blood pressure in people who already have hypertension;
- lowers the risk of developing non-insulin-dependent (type 2) diabetes mellitus;
- reduces the risk of developing colon cancer;
- helps people achieve and maintain a healthy body weight;
- reduces feelings of depression and anxiety;
- promotes psychological well-being and reduces feelings of stress;
- helps build and maintain healthy bones, muscles, and joints; and

- helps older adults become stronger and better able to move about without falling or becoming excessively fatigued.

Can a lack of physical activity hurt your health? Evidence shows that those who are not physically active are definitely not helping their health and may likely be hurting it. The closer we look at the health risks associated with a lack of physical activity, the more convincing it is that Americans who are not yet regularly physically active should become active.

Can everyone benefit from physical activity?

The good news about regular physical activity is that everyone can benefit from it.

- **Older adults.** No one is too old to enjoy the benefits of regular physical activity. Evidence indicates that muscle-strengthening exercises can reduce the risk of falling and fracturing bones and can improve the ability to live independently.

- **Parents and children.** Parents can help their children maintain a physically active lifestyle by providing encouragement and opportunities for physical activity. Families can plan outings and events that allow and encourage everyone in the family to be active.

- **Teenagers.** Regular physical activity improves strength, builds lean muscle, and decreases body fat. Activity can build stronger bones to last a lifetime.

- **People trying to manage their weight.** Regular physical activity burns calories while preserving lean muscle mass. Regular physical activity is a key component of any weight-loss or weight-management effort.

- **People with high blood pressure.** Regular physical activity helps lower blood pressure.

- **People with physical disabilities, including arthritis.** Regular physical activity can help people with chronic, disabling conditions improve their stamina and muscle strength. It also can improve psychological well-being and quality of life by increasing the ability to perform the activities of daily life.

- **Everyone under stress, including persons experiencing anxiety or depression.** Regular physical activity improves

5

one's mood, helps relieve depression, and increases feelings of well-being.

Chapter 2

Questions and Answers about Physical Activity and Exercise

How can physical activity improve my health?

An active lifestyle can help anyone. Being physically active can provide these benefits. It:

- reduces your risk of dying from heart disease or stroke;
- lowers your risk of getting heart disease, stroke, high blood pressure, colon cancer, and diabetes;
- lowers high blood pressure;
- helps keep your bones, muscles, and joints healthy;
- reduces anxiety and depression and improves your mood;
- helps you handle stress;
- helps control your weight;
- protects against falling and bone fractures in older adults;
- may help protect against breast cancer;
- helps control joint swelling and pain from arthritis;
- gives you more energy;
- helps you sleep better; and
- helps you look better.

Excerpted from "Physical Activity (Exercise)," by the National Women's Health Information Center (NWHIC), www.4woman.gov, January 2005.

Physical activity also is an important part of weight loss treatment. If you are overweight or obese, losing weight can lower your risk for many diseases. A growing number of women are overweight or obese. Being overweight or obese increases your risk of heart disease, type 2 diabetes, high blood pressure, stroke, breathing problems, arthritis, gallbladder disease, sleep apnea (breathing problems while sleeping), osteoarthritis, and some cancers. Obesity is measured with a body mass index (BMI). BMI shows the relationship of weight to height. Women with a BMI of 25 to 29.9 are considered overweight, whereas women with a BMI of 30 or more are considered obese. All adults (aged 18 years or older) who have a BMI of 25 or more are considered at risk for premature death and disability from being overweight or obese. These health risks increase as the BMI rises. Your health care provider can help you figure out your body mass, or you can go to www .cdc.gov/nccdphp/dnpa/bmi/calc-bmi.htm.

Not only are health care providers concerned about how much fat a person has, but also where the fat is located on the body. Women with a "pear" shape tend to store fat in their hips and buttocks. Women with an "apple" shape store fat around their waists. For most women, carrying extra weight around their waists or middle (with a waist larger than 35 inches) raises health risks (like heart disease, diabetes, or cancer) more than carrying extra weight around their hips or thighs.

How much physical activity should I do?

Engage in regular physical activity and reduce sedentary activities to promote health, psychological well-being, and a healthy body weight. To lower the risk of chronic disease, get at least 30 minutes of moderate-intensity physical activity, above usual activity, at work or home on most days of the week. Most people can get greater health benefits by engaging in physical activity of more vigorous intensity or longer duration. To help manage body weight and prevent gradual, unhealthy body weight gain, get about 60 minutes of moderate- to vigorous-intensity activity on most days of the week, while not exceeding caloric intake requirements. To keep weight loss off, get at least 60 to 90 minutes of daily moderate-intensity physical activity while not exceeding caloric intake requirements. Some people may need to consult with their doctor before participating in this level of activity. Achieve physical fitness by including cardiovascular conditioning, stretching exercises for flexibility, and resistance exercises or calisthenics for muscle strength and endurance.

How can I prevent injuries when I exercise?

If you're not active at all or have a medical problem, start your program with short sessions (5 to 10 minutes) of physical activity and build up to your goal. Before you start your activity, be sure to warm up for 5 to 10 minutes. Use the right equipment—whether it's walking shoes, running shoes, or knee pads—make sure it's in good condition and right for your skill level. Drink water before, during, and after exercise. At the end of your physical activity, cool down by decreasing the intensity of your activity so your heartbeat is normal. Be sure to stretch. If your chest feels tight or painful, or you feel faint or have trouble breathing at any time, stop the activity right away and talk to your health care provider.

Can I stay active if I have a disability?

One of the best things you can do for your health is to find an activity that gets your body moving and stick with it. You may be limited by a disability. This disability may make it harder, but it doesn't need to stop you from staying active. In most cases, people with disabilities can improve their heart, lungs, muscles, and bones—in addition to flexibility, mobility, and coordination—by becoming physically active. Talk to your health care provider about your personal needs.

What are some tips to help me get moving?

- Choose an activity that's fun.
- Change your activities, so you don't get bored.
- Doing housework may not be fun, but it does get you moving! So does gardening, yard work, and walking the dog.
- If you can't set aside one block of time, do short activities during the day, such as three, 10-minute walks.
- Create opportunities for activity, such as parking your car farther away, taking the stairs instead of the elevator, or walking down the hall to talk to a coworker instead of using e-mail.
- Don't let the cold weather keep you on the couch! You can still find activities to do in the winter like exercising to a workout video or joining a sports league. Or get a head start on your spring cleaning by choosing active indoor chores like window washing or reorganizing closets.

9

- Use different jogging, walking, or biking paths to vary your routine.
- Exercise with a friend or family member.
- If you have children, make time to play with them outside. Set a positive example!
- Make activities into social occasions—have dinner after you and a friend work out.
- Read books or magazines to inspire you.
- Set specific, short-term goals, and reward yourself when you achieve them.
- Don't feel badly if you don't notice body changes right away.
- Make your activity a regular part of your day, so it becomes a habit.
- Build a community group to form walking clubs, build walking trails, start exercise classes, and organize special events to promote physical activity.

Do I need to talk to my health care provider before I start?

Talk to your health care provider before you start any physical activity if you:

- have heart disease or had a stroke or are at high risk for them;
- have diabetes or are at high risk for it;
- are obese (body mass index of 30 or greater);
- have an injury (like a knee injury);
- are older than age 50; or
- are pregnant.

Chapter 3

Physical Activity Prevents Diseases and Infection

Chapter Contents

Section 3.1

Exercise Prevents Chronic Disease

"Physical Activity Fundamental to Preventing Disease" is by the
U.S. Department of Health and Human Services (HHS), June 20, 2002.
For a complete list of references, see http://aspe.hhs.gov.

Regular physical activity, fitness, and exercise are critically important for the health and well-being of people of all ages. Research has demonstrated that virtually all individuals can benefit from regular physical activity, whether they participate in vigorous exercise or some type of moderate health-enhancing physical activity. Even among frail and very old adults, mobility and functioning can be improved through physical activity. Therefore, physical fitness should be a priority for Americans of all ages.

Regular physical activity has been shown to reduce the morbidity and mortality from many chronic diseases. Millions of Americans suffer from chronic illnesses that can be prevented or improved through regular physical activity:

- 12.6 million people have coronary heart disease;

- 1.1 million people suffer from a heart attack in a given year;

- 17 million people have diabetes; about 90% to 95% of cases are type 2 diabetes, which is associated with obesity and physical inactivity (approximately 16 million people have pre diabetes);

- 107,000 people are newly diagnosed with colon cancer each year;

- 300,000 people suffer from hip fractures each year;

- 50 million people have high blood pressure; and

- nearly 50 million adults (between the ages of 20 and 74), or 27% of the adult population, are obese. Overall more than 108 million adults, or 61% of the adult population, are either obese or overweight.

In a 1993 study, 14 percent of all deaths in the United States were attributed to activity patterns and diet. Another study linked sedentary lifestyles to 23 percent of deaths from major chronic diseases. For example, physical activity has been shown to reduce the risk of developing or dying from heart disease, diabetes, colon cancer, and high blood pressure. On average, people who are physically active outlive those who are inactive.

Despite the well-known benefits of physical activity, most adults and many children lead a relatively sedentary lifestyle and are not active enough to achieve these health benefits. A sedentary lifestyle is defined as engaging in no leisure-time physical activity (exercises, sports, physically active hobbies) in a two-week period. Data from the National Health Interview Survey shows that in 1997 to 1998 nearly four in 10 (38.3 percent) adults reported no participation in leisure-time physical activity.

Approximately one third of persons age 65 or older lead a sedentary lifestyle. Older women are generally less physically active than older men. Fifty-four percent of men and 66 percent of women age 75 and older engage in no leisure-time physical activity. In general, African-American older adults are less active than white older adults. In the mid 1990s, 37 percent of white men age 75 and older reported no leisure-time physical activity, compared to 59 percent of African-American men age 75 and older; 47 percent of white women age 75 and older reported no leisure-time physical activity, compared to 60 percent of African-American women age 75 and older.

More than one third of young people in grades 9 to 12 do not regularly engage in vigorous physical activity. Furthermore, 43 percent of students in grades 9-12 watch television more than two hours per day. Physical activity declines dramatically over the course of adolescence, and girls are significantly less likely than boys to participate regularly in vigorous physical activity.

Economic Consequences of Inactivity

Physical inactivity and its associated health problems have substantial economic consequences for the U.S. health care system. In the long run, physical inactivity threatens to reverse the decades-long progress that has been made in reducing the morbidity and mortality associated with many chronic conditions such as cardiovascular disease. A physically inactive population is at both medical and financial risk for many chronic diseases and conditions including heart disease, stroke, colon cancer, diabetes, obesity, and osteoporosis.

The increasing prevalence of chronic medical conditions and diseases related to physical inactivity are associated with two types of

13

costs. First, there are health care costs for preventative, diagnostic, and treatment services related to these chronic conditions. These costs may include expenditures for physician visits, pharmaceuticals, ambulance services, rehabilitation services, and hospital and nursing home care. In addition, there are other costs associated with the value of lost wages by people unable to work because of illness and disability, as well as the value of future earnings lost by premature death. In 2000, the total cost of overweight and obesity was estimated to be $117 billion. In addition, the total estimated cost from chronic diseases is substantial.

Table 3.1. National Cost of Illness for Selected Diseases (in billions)

Disease	Cost
Heart Diseases	$183
Cancer	157
Diabetes	100
Arthritis	65

Source: National Institutes of Health, 2000.

Individuals suffering from chronic diseases bear a substantial portion of these medical costs. A recent study demonstrated that obese individuals spend approximately 36 percent more than the general population on health services and 77 percent more on medications. Furthermore, the study found that the effects of obesity on health spending were significantly larger than effects of current or past smoking.

The Medicare and Medicaid programs currently spend $84 billion annually on five major chronic conditions that could be significantly improved by increased physical activity, specifically diabetes, heart disease, depression, cancer, and arthritis.

- Medicare spent $10.4 billion on **diabetes treatment and services** in 2000 and is estimated to spend $12.7 billion in 2004.

- Medicare spending on **heart disease treatment and services** has grown from $21.1 billion in 1992 to $34.9 billion in 2000 and is expected to reach $42.8 billion in 2004.

- Medicare spending on **depression treatment and services** has grown from $1.3 billion in 1992 to $2.1 billion in 2000 and is estimated to increase to $2.5 billion in 2004.

- Medicare spending on **cancer treatment and services** has grown from $10.3 billion in 1992 to $15.2 billion in 2000 and is expected to increase to $18.5 billion in 2004.

- Medicare spending on **arthritis treatment and services** has grown from $3.4 billion in 1992 to $5.8 billion in 2000 and is estimated to be $7.1 billion in 2004.

Since regular physical activity helps prevent disease and promote health, it may actually decrease health care costs. A study performed by researchers at the Centers for Disease Control and Prevention found that physically active people had, on average, lower annual direct medical costs than did inactive people. The same study estimated that increasing regular moderate physical activity among the more than 88 million inactive Americans over the age of 15 years might reduce the annual national direct medical costs by as much as $76.6 billion in 2000 dollars. Further, it found that physically active people had fewer hospital stays and physician visits and used less medication than physically inactive people. The cost savings were consistent for men and women, for those with and without physical limitations, and even for smokers and nonsmokers. In this study, the biggest difference in direct medical costs was among women 55 and older, supporting the belief that the potential gain associated with physical activity is especially high for older women. The researchers concluded that adoption of a population-wide physical activity strategy might produce health care cost savings among most adult age groups.

Employers can benefit too. Workplace physical activity programs can reduce short-term sick leave by six to 32 percent, reduce health care costs by 20 to 55 percent, and increase productivity by 2 to 52 percent. In 1998, 93 percent of employers had programs that fostered employee health, up from 76 percent in 1992, according to Hewitt Associates. Such wellness programs typically offer help in smoking cessation, managing stress, prenatal care, nutrition, and fitness.

Physical Activity and Good Physical Health

Participation in regular physical activity—at least 30 minutes of moderate activity on at least five days per week, or 20 minutes of vigorous physical activity at least three times per week—is critical to sustaining good health. Youth should strive for at least one hour of exercise a day. Regular physical activity has beneficial effects on most (if not all) organ systems, and consequently it helps to prevent a broad range of health problems and diseases. People of all ages, both male and female, derive substantial health benefits from physical activity.

Regular physical activity reduces the risk of developing or dying from some of the leading causes of illness in the United States. Regular physical activity improves health in the following ways:

- reduces the risk of dying prematurely from heart disease and other conditions;
- reduces the risk of developing diabetes;
- reduces the risk of developing high blood pressure;
- reduces blood pressure in people who already have high blood pressure;
- reduces the risk of developing colon and breast cancer;
- helps to maintain a healthy weight;
- helps build and maintain healthy bones, muscles, and joints;
- helps older adults to become stronger and better able to move about without falling;
- reduces feelings of depression and anxiety; and
- promotes psychological well-being.

Regular physical activity is associated with lower mortality rates for both older and younger adults. Even those who are moderately active on a regular basis have lower mortality rates than those who are least active. Regular physical activity leads to cardiovascular fitness, which decreases the risk of cardiovascular disease mortality in general and coronary artery disease mortality in particular. High blood pressure is a major underlying cause of cardiovascular complications and mortality. Regular physical activity can prevent or delay the development of high blood pressure, and reduces blood pressure in persons with hypertension.

Regular physical activity is also important for maintaining muscle strength, joint structure, joint functioning, and bone health. Weight-bearing physical activity is essential for normal skeletal development during childhood and adolescence and for achieving and maintaining peak bone mass in young adults. Among postmenopausal women, exercise, especially muscle strengthening (resistance) activity, may protect against the rapid decline in bone mass. However, data on the effects of exercise on postmenopausal bone loss are not clear-cut and the timing of the intervention (e.g., stage of menopausal transition) can influence the response. Regardless, physical activity including muscle-strengthening exercise appears to protect against falling and fractures among the elderly, probably by increasing muscle strength and balance. In addition, physical activity may be beneficial for many people with arthritis.

Regular physical activity can help improve the lives of young people beyond its effects on physical health. Although research has not been conducted to conclusively demonstrate a direct link between physical activity and improved academic performance, such a link might be expected. Studies have found participation in physical activity increases adolescents' self-esteem and reduces anxiety and stress. Through its effects on mental health, physical activity may help increase students' capacity for learning. One study found that spending more time in physical education did not have harmful effects on the standardized academic achievement test scores of elementary school students; in fact, there was some evidence that participation in a two-year health-related physical education program had several significant favorable effects on academic achievement.

Participation in physical activity and sports can promote social well-being, as well as good physical and mental health, among young people. Research has shown that students who participate in interscholastic sports are less likely to be regular and heavy smokers or use drugs, and are more likely to stay in school and have good conduct and high academic achievement. Sports and physical activity programs can introduce young people to skills such as teamwork, self-discipline, sportsmanship, leadership, and socialization. Lack of recreational activity, on the other hand, may contribute to making young people more vulnerable to gangs, drugs, or violence.

Physical Activity and Good Mental Health

Regular physical activity reduces morbidity and mortality from mental health disorders. Mental health disorders pose a significant public health burden in the United States and they are a major cause of hospitalization and disability. Mental health disorders cost approximately $148 billion per year. Potentially, increasing physical activity levels in Americans could substantially reduce medical expenditures for mental health conditions.

In adults with affective disorders, physical activity has a beneficial effect on symptoms of depression and anxiety. Animal research suggests that exercise may stimulate the growth of new brain cells that enhance memory and learning—two functions hampered by depression. Clinical studies have demonstrated the feasibility and efficacy of exercise as a treatment for depression in older men and women. Currently, National Institute of Mental Health (NIMH) investigators are conducting research comparing the effectiveness of home-based and supervised aerobic exercise to the use of antidepressants in relieving depression in these groups, and reducing relapse rates. Other NIMH researchers are studying whether greater exercise levels result in more symptom improvement. Regular physical activity also appears to enhance well-being.

The preventive effects of physical activity on mental disorders are less well studied. Some studies suggest physical activity prevents depressive illness. Future research will clarify the extent to which physical activity may actually protect against the development of depression.

Regular physical activity may also reduce risk of cognitive decline in older adults, though more research is needed to clarify the mechanism of this possible effect. Among people who suffer from mental illness, physical activity appears to improve the ability to perform activities of daily living.

Physical Activity (Along with a Nutritious Diet) Is Key to Maintaining Energy Balance and a Healthy Weight

Regular physical activity along with a nutritious diet is key to maintaining a healthy weight. In order to maintain a healthy weight, there must be a balance between calories consumed and calories expended through metabolic and physical activity. Although overweight and obesity are caused by many factors, in most individuals, weight gain results from a combination of excess calorie consumption and inadequate physical activity.

Even though a large portion of a person's total caloric requirement is used for basal metabolism and processing food, an individual's various physical activities may account for as much as 15 to 40 percent of the calories he or she burns each day. While vigorous exercise uses calories at a higher rate, any physical activity will burn calories. For example, a 140-pound person can burn 175 calories in 30 minutes of moderate bicycling, and 322 calories in 30 minutes of moderate jogging. The same person can also burn 105 calories by vacuuming or raking leaves for the same amount of time.

The Epidemic of Overweight and Obesity

As a result of lifestyle and dietary changes, overweight and obesity have reached epidemic proportions in the United States. The Body Mass Index (BMI) is the most commonly used measure to define overweight and obesity. BMI is a measure of weight in relation to height. BMI is calculated as weight in pounds divided by the square of the height in inches, multiplied by 703.

According to the National Institutes of Health Clinical Guidelines, overweight in adults is defined as a BMI between 25 lbs/in^2 to 29.9 lbs/in^2; and obesity in adults is identified by a BMI of 30 lbs/in^2 or greater. These definitions are based on evidence that suggests that health risks are greater at or above a BMI of 25 lbs/in^2 compared to those at a BMI below that level. The risk of premature death increases with an increasing BMI. This increase in mortality tends to be modest until a BMI of 30 lbs/in^2 is reached.

Overweight and obesity are increasing in both genders and among all population groups. In 1999, an estimated 61 percent of adults in the U.S. were overweight or obese; this contrasts with the late 1970s, when an estimated 47 percent of adults were overweight or obese.

Among women, the prevalence of overweight and obesity generally is higher in women who are members of racial and ethnic minority populations than in non-Hispanic white women. Among men, Mexican Americans have a higher prevalence of overweight and obesity than non-Hispanic whites or non-Hispanic blacks. For non-Hispanic men, the prevalence of overweight and obesity among whites is slightly greater than among blacks.

Disparities in prevalence of overweight and obesity also exist based on socioeconomic status. For all racial and ethnic groups combined, women of lower socioeconomic status (income <130 percent of the poverty threshold) are approximately 50 percent more likely to be obese than those with higher socioeconomic status (income > 130 percent of the poverty threshold). Men are about equally likely to be obese whether they are in a low or high socioeconomic group.

The overweight and obesity epidemic is not limited to adults. What is particularly alarming is that the percentage of young people who are overweight has almost doubled in the last 20 years for children aged 6 to 11 and almost tripled for adolescents aged 12 to 19. In children and adolescents, overweight has been defined as a sex- and age-specific BMI at or above the 95th percentile for a reference population, based on Centers for Disease Control and Prevention (CDC) growth charts.

Associated Health Risks of Not Maintaining a Healthy Weight

Epidemiological studies show an increase in mortality associated with overweight and obesity. Approximately 300,000 deaths a year in this country are currently associated with overweight and obesity. Morbidity from obesity may be as great as from poverty, smoking, or problem drinking. Overweight and obesity are associated with an increased risk for developing various medical conditions including cardiovascular disease, certain cancers (endometrial, colon, postmenopausal breast, kidney, and esophageal), high blood pressure, arthritis-related disabilities, and type 2 diabetes.

Obesity is associated with an increased risk of:

- premature death;

- type 2 diabetes;

- heart disease;

- stroke;

- hypertension;

- gallbladder disease;

- osteoarthritis (degeneration of cartilage and bone in joints);

- sleep apnea;

- asthma;

- breathing problems;

- cancer (endometrial, colon, kidney, esophageal, and postmenopausal breast cancer);

- high blood cholesterol;

- complications of pregnancy;

- menstrual irregularities;

- hirsutism (presence of excess body and facial hair);

- stress incontinence (urine leakage caused by weak pelvic-floor muscles);

- increased surgical risk;

- psychological disorders such as depression; and

- psychological difficulties due to social stigmatization.

  [Source: Surgeon General's Call to Action to Prevent and Decrease Overweight and Obesity, 2001.]

It is also important for individuals who are currently at a healthy weight to strive to maintain it since both modest and large weight gains are associated with significantly increased risk of disease. For example, a weight gain of 11 to 18 pounds increases a person's risk for developing type 2 diabetes to twice that of individuals who have not gained weight, while those who gain 44 pounds or more have four times the risk of type 2 diabetes.

Recent research studies have shown that a gain of 10 to 20 pounds resulted in an increased risk of coronary heart disease (which can result in nonfatal heart attacks and death) of 1.25 times in women and 1.6 times in men. In these studies, weight increases of 22 pounds in men and 44 pounds in women resulted in an increased coronary heart disease risk of 1.75 and 2.65, respectively. In one study among women with a BMI of 34 or greater, the risk of developing endometrial cancer was increased by more than 6 times. Overweight and obesity are also known to exacerbate many chronic conditions such as hypertension and elevated cholesterol. Overweight and obese individuals also may suffer from social stigmatization, discrimination, and poor body image.

Although obesity-associated morbidities occur most frequently in adults, important consequences of excess weight as well as antecedents of adult disease occur in overweight children and adolescents. Overweight children and adolescents are more likely to become overweight or obese adults. As the prevalence of overweight and obesity increases in children and adolescents, type 2 diabetes, high blood lipids, and hypertension as well as early maturation and orthopedic problems are occurring with increased frequency. A common consequence of childhood overweight is psychosocial—specifically discrimination.

Call to Action

Because physical inactivity is a risk factor for many diseases and conditions, making physical activity an integral part of daily life is crucial. Physical activity need not be strenuous to be beneficial. People of all ages benefit from moderate physical activity, such as 30 minutes of walking five or more times a week. In addition, physical activity does not need to be sustained for long periods of time in order to provide health benefits. Repeated shorter bursts of moderate-intensity activity also yield health benefits. In other words, walking in two 15-minute segments or three 10-minute segments is beneficial.

There is a pressing need to encourage a more active lifestyle among the American people. Clearly, the goal of a more active population will be a challenge, requiring a commitment to change on the part of individuals, families, workplaces, and communities. Both the public and private sectors will need to band together to promote more healthy habits for those of all ages. Encouraging more activity can be as simple as establishing walking programs at schools, work sites, and in the community. Some communities have an existing infrastructure that supports physical activity, such as sidewalks and bicycle trails, and work sites, schools, and shopping areas in close proximity to residential areas. In many other areas, such community amenities need to be developed to foster walking, cycling, and other types of exercise as a regular part of daily activity. Schools provide many opportunities to engage children in physical activity as well as healthy eating. For adults, work sites provide opportunities to reinforce the adoption and maintenance of healthy lifestyle behaviors. Perhaps the most important change, however, is at the individual and family level. Each person must understand the value of physical activity for his or her health and well-being and commit to a lifestyle that is truly active.

Section 3.2

Exercise Benefits
Immune System Function

Sir William Osler, the famous Canadian medical doctor, once quipped, "There's only one way to treat the common cold—with contempt." And for good reason. The average adult has two to three respiratory infections each year. That number jumps to six or seven for young children.

Whether or not you get sick with a cold after being exposed to a virus depends on many factors that affect your immune system. Old age, cigarette smoking, mental stress, poor nutrition, and lack of sleep have all been associated with impaired immune function and increased risk of infection.

Keeping the Immune System in Good Shape

Can regular exercise help keep your immune system in good shape? Researchers are just now supplying some answers to this new and exciting question. Fitness enthusiasts have frequently reported that they experience less sickness than their sedentary peers. For example, a survey conducted during the 1980s revealed that 61 percent of 700 recreational runners reported fewer colds since they began running, while only 4 percent felt they had experienced more.

Further research has shown that during moderate exercise, several positive changes occur in the immune system. Various immune cells circulate through the body more quickly, and are better able to kill bacteria and viruses. Once the moderate exercise bout is over, the immune system returns to normal within a few hours.

In other words, every time you go for a brisk walk, your immune system receives a boost that should increase your chances of fighting off cold viruses over the long term.

Should You Exercise When Sick?

Fitness enthusiasts and endurance athletes alike are often uncertain of whether they should exercise or rest when sick. Although more research is needed, most sports medicine experts in this area recommend that if you have symptoms of a common cold with no fever (i.e., symptoms are above the neck), moderate exercise such as walking is probably safe.

Intensive exercise should be postponed until a few days after the symptoms have gone away. However, if there are symptoms or signs of the flu (i.e., fever, extreme tiredness, muscle aches, swollen lymph glands), then at least two weeks should probably be allowed before you resume intensive training.

Staying in Shape to Exercise

For athletes who are training intensely for competition, the following guidelines can help reduce their odds of getting sick.

1. **Eat a well-balanced diet.** The immune system depends on many vitamins and minerals for optimal function. However, at this time, there is no good data to support supplementation beyond 100 percent of the Recommended Dietary Allowances.

2. **Avoid rapid weight loss.** Low-calorie diets, long-term fasting, and rapid weight loss have been shown to impair immune function. Losing weight while training heavily is not good for the immune system.

3. **Obtain adequate sleep.** Major sleep disruption (e.g., three hours less than normal) has been linked to immune suppression.

4. **Avoid overtraining and chronic fatigue.** Space vigorous workouts and race events as far apart as possible. Keep "within yourself" and don't push beyond your ability to recover.

Chapter 4

Physical Activity and Weight Control

Chapter Contents

Section 4.1

How Does Physical Activity Help You Control Your Weight?

Excerpted from "Exercise and Weight Control," published by The President's Council on Physical Fitness and Sports (www.fitness.gov), October 15, 2004.

Just about everybody seems to be interested in weight control. Some of us weigh just the right amount, others need to gain a few pounds. Most of us "battle the bulge" at some time in our life. Whatever our goals, we should understand and take advantage of the important role of exercise in keeping our weight under control.

Carrying around too much body fat is a major nuisance. Yet excess body fat is common in modern-day living. Few of today's occupations require vigorous physical activity, and much of our leisure time is spent in sedentary pursuits.

Recent estimates indicate that 34 million adults are considered obese (20 percent above desirable weight). Also, there has been an increase in body fat levels in children and youth over the past 20 years. After infancy and early childhood, the earlier the onset of obesity, the greater the likelihood of remaining obese.

Excess body fat has been linked to such health problems as coronary heart disease, high blood pressure, osteoporosis, diabetes, arthritis, and certain forms of cancer. Some evidence now exists showing that obesity has a negative effect on both health and longevity.

Exercise is associated with the loss of body fat in both obese and normal weight persons. A regular program of exercise is an important component of any plan to help individuals lose, gain, or maintain their weight.

Overweight or Overfat?

Overweight and overfat do not always mean the same thing. Some people are quite muscular and weigh more than the average for their age and height. However, their body composition, the amount of fat versus lean body mass (muscle, bone, organs and tissue) is within a desirable range. This is true for many athletes. Others weigh an average amount yet carry around too much fat. In our society, however, over-weight often implies overfat because excess weight is commonly distributed as excess fat. The addition of exercise to a weight-control program helps control both body weight and body fat levels.

A certain amount of body fat is necessary for everyone. Experts say that percent body fat for women should be about 20 percent, 15 percent for men. Women with more than 30 percent fat and men with more than 25 percent fat are considered obese.

How much of your weight is fat can be assessed by a variety of methods including underwater (hydrostatic) weighing, skinfold thickness measurements, and circumference measurements. Each requires a specially trained person to administer the test and perform the correct calculations. From the numbers obtained, a body fat percentage is determined. Assessing body composition has an advantage over the standard height-weight tables because it can help distinguish between "overweight" and "overfat."

An easy self-test you can do is to pinch the thickness of the fat folds at your waist and abdomen. If you can pinch an inch or more of fat (make sure no muscle is included) chances are you have too much body fat.

People who exercise appropriately increase lean body mass while decreasing their overall fat level. Depending on the amount of fat loss, this can result in a loss of inches without a loss of weight, since muscle weighs more than fat. However, with the proper combination of diet and exercise, both body fat and overall weight can be reduced.

Energy Balance: A Weighty Concept

Losing weight, gaining weight, or maintaining your weight depends on the amount of calories you take in and use up during the day, otherwise referred to as energy balance. Learning how to balance energy intake (calories in food) with energy output (calories expended through physical activity) will help you achieve your desired weight.

Although the underlying causes and the treatments of obesity are complex, the concept of energy balance is relatively simple. If you eat more calories than your body needs to perform your day's activities, the extra calories are stored as fat. If you do not take in enough calories to meet your body's energy needs, your body will go to the stored fat to make up the difference. (Exercise helps ensure that stored fat, rather than muscle tissue, is used to meet your energy needs.) If you eat just about the same amount of calories to meet your body's energy needs, your weight will stay the same.

On the average, a person consumes between 800,000 and 900,000 calories each year. An active person needs more calories than a sedentary person, as physically active people require energy above and beyond the day's basic needs. All too often, people who want to lose weight concentrate on counting calorie intake while neglecting calorie output. The most powerful formula is the combination of dietary modification with exercise. By increasing your daily physical activity and decreasing your caloric input you can lose excess weight in the most efficient and healthful way.

Counting Calories

Each pound of fat your body stores represents 3,500 calories of unused energy. In order to lose one pound, you would have to create a calorie deficit of 3,500 calories by either taking in 3,500 less calories over a period of time than you need or doing 3,500 calories worth of exercise. It is recommended that no more than two pounds (7,000 calories) be lost per week for lasting weight loss.

Adding 15 minutes of moderate exercise, say walking one mile, to your daily schedule will use up 100 extra calories per day. (Your body uses approximately 100 calories of energy to walk one mile, depending on your body weight.) Maintaining this schedule would result in an extra 700 calories per week used up, or a loss of about 10 pounds in one year, assuming your food intake stays the same. To look at energy balance another way, just one extra slice of bread or one extra soft drink a day—or any other food that contains approximately 100 calories—can add up to ten extra pounds in a year if the amount of physical activity you do does not increase.

If you already have a lean figure and want to keep it, you should exercise regularly and eat a balanced diet that provides enough calories to make up for the energy you expend. If you wish to gain weight you should exercise regularly and increase the number of calories you consume until you reach your desired weight. Exercise will help ensure that the weight you gain will be lean muscle mass, not extra fat.

The Diet Connection

A balanced diet should be part of any weight-control plan. A diet high in complex carbohydrates and moderate in protein and fat will complement an exercise program. It should include enough calories to satisfy your daily nutrient requirements and include the proper number of servings per day from the basic four food groups: vegetables and fruits (4 servings), breads and cereals (4 servings), milk and milk products (2-4 depending on age) and meats and fish (2).

Experts recommend that your daily intake not fall below 1,200 calories unless you are under a doctor's supervision. Also, weekly weight loss should not exceed two pounds.

Remarkable claims have been made for a variety of crash diets and diet pills. And some of these very restricted diets do result in noticeable weight loss in a short time. Much of this loss is water and such a loss is quickly regained when normal food and liquid intake is resumed. These diet plans are often expensive and may be dangerous. Moreover, they do not emphasize lifestyle changes that will help you maintain your desired weight. Dieting alone will result in a loss of valuable body tissue such as muscle mass in addition to a loss in fat.

How Many Calories Are Burned?

The estimates for number of calories (energy) used during a physical activity are based on experiments that measure the amount of oxygen consumed during a specific bout of exercise for a certain body weight.

The energy costs of activities that require you to move your own body weight, such as walking or jogging, are greater for heavier people since they have more weight to move. For example, a person weighing 150 pounds would use more calories jogging one mile than a person jogging alongside who weighs 115 pounds. Always check to see what body weight is referred to in caloric expenditure charts you use.

Exercise and Modern Living

One thing is certain. Most people do not get enough exercise in their ordinary routines. All of the advances of modern technology—from electric can openers to power steering—have made life easier, more comfortable, and much less physically demanding. Yet our bodies need activity, especially if they are carrying around too much fat. Satisfying this need requires a definite plan, and a commitment. There are two main ways to increase the number of calories you expend:

1. Start a regular exercise program if you do not have one already.

2. Increase the amount of physical activity in your daily routine.

The best way to control your weight is a combination of the above. The sum total of calories used over time will help regulate your weight as well as keep you physically fit.

Table 4.1. Energy Expenditure for Sedentary, Moderate, and Vigorous Activities

Sedentary Activities	Energy Costs in Calories/Hour*
Lying down or sleeping	90
Sitting quietly	84
Sitting and writing, card playing, etc.	114
Moderate Activities	**(150-350)**
Bicycling (5 mph)	174
Canoeing (2.5 mph)	174
Dancing (ballroom)	210
Golf (twosome, carrying clubs)	324
Horseback riding (sitting to trot)	246
Light housework, cleaning, etc.	246
Swimming (crawl, 20 yards/min)	288
Tennis (recreational doubles)	312
Volleyball (recreational)	264
Walking (2 mph)	198
Vigorous Activities	**More than 350**
Aerobic dancing	546
Basketball (recreational)	450
Bicycling (13 mph)	612
Circuit weight training	756
Football (touch, vigorous)	498
Ice skating (9 mph)	384
Racquetball	588
Roller skating (9 mph)	384
Jogging (10-minute mile, 6 mph)	654
Scrubbing floors	440
Swimming (crawl, 45 yards/min)	522
Tennis (recreational singles)	450
Cross-country skiing (5 mph)	690

Note: Hourly estimates based on values calculated for calories burned per minute for a 150-pound (68-kilogram) person. Sources: William D. McArdle, Frank I. Katch, Victor L. Katch, *Exercise Physiology: Energy, Nutrition and Human Performance* (2nd edition), Lea & Febiger, Philadelphia, 1986; Melvin H. Williams, *Nutrition for Fitness and Sport*, William C. Brown Company Publishers, Dubuque, 1983.

Active Lifestyles

Before looking at what kind of regular exercise program is best, let's look at how you can increase the amount of physical activity in your daily routine to supplement your exercise program.

- Recreational pursuits such as gardening on weekends, bowling in the office league, family outings, an evening of social dancing, and many other activities provide added exercise. They are fun and can be considered an extra bonus in your weight-control campaign.

- Add more action to your day. Walk to the neighborhood grocery store instead of using the car. Park several blocks from the office and walk the rest of the way. Walk up the stairs instead of using the elevator; start with one flight of steps and gradually increase.

- Change your attitude toward movement. Instead of considering an extra little walk or trip to the files an annoyance, look upon it as an added fitness boost. Look for opportunities to use your body. Bend, stretch, reach, move, lift, and carry. Time-saving devices and gadgets eliminate drudgery and are a bonus to mankind, but when they substitute too often for physical activity they can demand a high cost in health, vigor, and fitness.

These little bits of action are cumulative in their effects. Alone, each does not burn a huge amount of calories. But when added together they can result in a sizable amount of energy used over the course of the day. And they will help improve your muscle tone and flexibility at the same time.

What Kind of Exercise?

Although any kind of physical movement requires energy (calories), the type of exercise that uses the most energy is aerobic exercise. The term aerobic is derived from the Greek word meaning "with oxygen." Jogging, brisk walking, swimming, biking, cross-country skiing, and aerobic dancing are some popular forms of aerobic exercise.

Aerobic exercises use the body's large muscle groups in continuous, rhythmic, sustained movement and require oxygen for the production of energy. When oxygen is combined with food (which can come from stored fat) energy is produced to power the body's musculature. The longer you move aerobically, the more energy needed and the more

ular aerobic exercise will improve your cardiores-
e, the ability of your heart, lungs, blood vessels, and
to use oxygen to produce energy needed for activ-
ealthier body while getting rid of excess body fat.
he aerobic exercise, supplement your program with
muscle strengthening and stretching exercises. The stronger your
muscles, the longer you will be able to keep going during aerobic activity, and the less chance of injury.

How Much? How Often?

Experts recommend that you do some form of aerobic exercise at
least three times a week for a minimum of 20 continuous minutes. Of
course, if that is too much, start with a shorter time span and gradually build up to the minimum. Then gradually progress until you are
able to work aerobically for 20 to 40 minutes. If you need to lose a
large amount of weight, you may want to do your aerobic workout five
times a week.

It is important to exercise at an intensity vigorous enough to cause
your heart rate and breathing to increase. How hard you should exercise depends to a certain degree on your age, and is determined by
measuring your heart rate in beats per minute.

The heart rate you should maintain is called your target heart rate,
and there are several ways you can arrive at this figure. The simplest
is to subtract your age from 220 and then calculate 60 to 80 percent
of that figure. Beginners should maintain the 60 percent level, more
advanced can work up to the 80 percent level. This is just a guide
however, and people with any medical limitations should discuss this
formula with their physicians.

You can do different types of aerobic activities, say walking one day,
riding a bike the next. Make sure you choose an activity that can be
done regularly, and is enjoyable for you. The important thing to remember is not to skip too many days between workouts or fitness
benefits will be lost. If you must lose a few days, gradually work back
into your routine.

The Benefits of Exercise in a Weight-Control Program

The benefits of exercise are many, from producing physically fit
bodies to providing an outlet for fun and socialization. When added
to a weight-control program these benefits take on increased significance.

We already have noted that proper exercise can help control weight by burning excess body fat. It also has two other body-trimming advantages 1) exercise builds muscle tissue and muscle uses calories up at a faster rate than body fat; and 2) exercise helps reduce inches and a firm, lean body looks slimmer even if your weight remains the same.

Remember, fat does not turn into muscle, as is often believed. Fat and muscle are two entirely different substances and one cannot become the other. However, muscle does use calories at a faster rate than fat, which directly affects your body's metabolic rate or energy requirement. Your basal metabolic rate (BMR) is the amount of energy required to sustain the body's functions at rest and it depends on your age, sex, body size, genes, and body composition. People with high levels of muscle tend to have higher BMRs and use more calories in the resting stage.

Some studies have even shown that your metabolic rate stays elevated for some time after vigorous exercise, causing you to use even more calories throughout your day. Additional benefits may be seen in how exercise affects appetite. A lean person in good shape may eat more following increased activity, but the regular exercise will burn up the extra calories consumed. On the other hand, vigorous exercise has been reported to suppress appetite. And physical activity can be used as a positive substitute for between-meal snacking.

Better Mental Health

The psychological benefits of exercise are equally important to the weight conscious person. Exercise decreases stress and relieves tensions that might otherwise lead to overeating. Exercise builds physical fitness which in turn builds self-confidence, enhanced self-image, and a positive outlook. When you start to feel good about yourself, you are more likely to want to make other positive changes in your lifestyle that will help keep your weight under control.

In addition, exercise can be fun, provide recreation, and offer opportunities for companionship. The exhilaration and emotional release of participating in sports or other activities are a boost to mental and physical health. Pent-up anxieties and frustrations seem to disappear when you're concentrating on returning a serve, sinking a putt, or going that extra mile.

Section 4.2

Even Moderate Physical Activity Promotes Weight Loss

From the press release "NHLBI Study Finds Moderate Physical Activity Promotes Weight Loss as well as Intense Exercise," by the National Institutes of Health, September 9, 2003.

Women trying to lose weight can benefit as much from moderate physical activity as from an intense workout, according to a study supported by the National Heart, Lung, and Blood Institute (NHLBI), part of the National Institutes of Health in Bethesda, Maryland.

Prior studies had focused on short-term weight loss. Data were lacking about the optimal degree and amount of physical activity for long-term weight loss.

The study—"Effect of Exercise Dose and Intensity on Weight Loss in Overweight, Sedentary Women: A Randomized Trial"—appears in the September 10, 2003, issue of the *Journal of the American Medical Association (JAMA)*.

The same issue of *JAMA* also includes an article on recreational physical activity and breast cancer risk. The study, based on data from the Women's Health Initiative's Observational Study, found that increased physical activity was associated with a reduced risk for breast cancer in postmenopausal women. Longer duration physical activity gave the most benefit but the physical activity did not need to be strenuous to reduce breast cancer risk.

The exercise dose and intensity trial involved 201 overweight but otherwise healthy women ages 21 to 45. All received reduced-calorie meals in addition to being randomly assigned to one of four physical activity regimens, which varied by intensity and duration. The regimens consisted of either a moderate- or vigorous-intensity physical activity performed for either a shorter (2 1/2 to 3 1/2 hours per week) or longer (3 1/2 to 5 hours per week) duration. The physical activity consisted primarily of brisk walking, and the regimens used about 1,000 or 2,000 kcal [kilocalories] per week.

Women in all four groups lost a significant amount of weight—about 13 to 20 pounds—and maintained their weight loss for a year. They also improved their cardiorespiratory fitness. However, the amount of weight lost or fitness improvement was not different among the four groups.

Section 4.3

Dieters Who Exercise More Lose More Weight over the Long Term

Excerpted from the Winter 2004 edition of *WIN Notes*, a quarterly newsletter produced by the Weight-control Information Network (WIN), a project of the National Institute of Diabetes and Digestive and Kidney Diseases (NIDDK) of the National Institutes of Health (NIH), U.S. Department of Health and Human Services (HHS).

Commonly, weight-control programs advise people to exercise for 30 minutes a day on most days of the week. A recent study, however, concludes that telling people to do more physical activity improves long-term weight loss.

In this study, 202 overweight men and women took part in an 18-month behavior therapy weight loss program. All participants sought to reduce their calorie intake to 1,000 to 1,500 calories a day and limit fat to 20 percent of calories. Half of participants set a physical activity goal of burning 1,000 calories a week (walking about 30 minutes a day). The other half set a goal of burning 2,500 calories a week (walking more than 75 minutes a day).

To meet the higher physical activity goal, high exercise group members were given extra support. They could ask friends or family to take part in the study with them and meet with an exercise coach. They were also given $3 a week when they met the goal of burning 2,500 calories.

After 18 months, participants who exercised more took off more weight. High exercisers weighed, on average, almost 15 pounds less than when the study began. Those exercising less lost about 9 pounds.

Both groups reported eating similar amounts of calories and fat, suggesting that the differences in weight loss were not due to differences in food intake. The study authors concluded that meeting high physical activity goals can improve long-term weight loss.

Results also come with two cautions from the study authors. First, the risk for exercise-related injuries may go up with increasing levels of physical activity. Participants doing more physical activity reported more exercise-related injuries and illnesses.

Second, even relatively heavy physical activity may not fully protect against weight regain. After 6 months of losing weight, all participants began to regain weight—although those doing more physical activity regained at a slower rate.

The full report, "Physical activity and weight loss: Does prescribing higher physical activity goals improve outcome?" appears in the October 2003 issue of the *American Journal of Clinical Nutrition*.

Section 4.4

Physical Fitness versus Body Mass Index: Which Has a Greater Effect on Health?

Excerpted from the Winter 2005 edition of *WIN Notes*, a quarterly newsletter produced by the Weight-control Information Network (WIN), a project of the National Institute of Diabetes and Digestive and Kidney Diseases (NIDDK) of the National Institutes of Health (NIH), U.S. Department of Health and Human Services (HHS).

Physical inactivity and a body mass index (BMI) greater than 25 can each lead to increased health risks such as heart disease, stroke, and type 2 diabetes. But when they are considered together, which presents the greater risk? Two recent studies examining the combined effect of BMI and physical activity on health reached different conclusions.

A prospective study of 37,878 healthy women enrolled in the Women's Health Study (WHS) looked at the association between BMI, physical activity, and the development of type 2 diabetes. Each year for 7 years, researchers gathered information on the women's BMI and physical activity levels, and whether they had been diagnosed with type 2 diabetes in the last year. They divided study participants into six groups based on BMI and activity levels: normal-weight active, normal-weight inactive, overweight active, overweight inactive, obese active, and obese inactive.

As expected, when the researchers looked at BMI and physical activity levels separately, they found that women who were overweight or obese had a higher risk of developing type 2 diabetes than normal-weight women, and inactive women had a higher risk than active women. However, when they examined the effects of BMI and physical activity together, increased activity within the same BMI group—normal-weight, overweight, or obese—offered a negligible reduction in the risk of developing type 2 diabetes, but increased BMI, regardless of activity level, led to a significantly higher risk.

A second study that examined the relationship of BMI and physical fitness to the development of cardiovascular disease in women found the opposite effect. Researchers assessed BMI and fitness among 906 women with suspected coronary artery disease (CAD) who were enrolled in the Women's Ischemia Syndrome Evaluation for diagnostic testing.

The women completed two questionnaires, one to assess fitness based on self-reported ability to perform various activities that correlate with treadmill test results, and one to assess average physical activity levels at home, work, and leisure.

Both high BMI and low fitness and activity scores were associated with CAD risk factors such as hypertension, diabetes, and dyslipidemia. However, diagnostic tests showed no difference in the presence or severity of CAD across BMI categories. In contrast, women with low fitness scores were significantly more likely to have obstructive and severe CAD. Follow-up over the course of 4 years revealed that these women suffered more adverse events including stroke, congestive heart failure, and death, regardless of BMI.

In a commentary on the two studies, researchers from the Cooper Institute, a research and education center that focuses on physical activity and health, noted differences in the studies that could partially account for the divergent results. Each one measured different outcomes—development of type 2 diabetes versus adverse cardiovascular events. The diabetes study followed healthy women; the CAD study followed women with suspected heart disease. Each study used different measures of self-reported physical activity with potentially unequal levels of accuracy.

Regardless of the disparities in study methods and results, the Cooper Institute researchers conclude that physical activity is the common denominator in achieving both increased fitness and long-term weight management. Rather than focus on the "fit vs. fat" debate, they suggest that the medical community support physical activity to promote both health and weight control.

Both studies were supported by the National Institutes of Health. The full reports, "Relationship of physical activity vs. body mass index with type 2 diabetes in women" and "Relationship of physical fitness vs. body mass index with coronary artery disease and cardiovascular events in women," appear in the September 8, 2004 issue of the *Journal of the American Medical Association*, as does the commentary.

Chapter 5

The Effect of Exercise on Metabolism

It is rare these days to pick up a health or fitness magazine from a grocery store shelf without our attention being drawn to an article proclaiming to have the latest information on the best way to exercise in order to boost metabolism. With the high risk for obesity in America, it would seem foolish to pass up reading an exposé on newly discovered secrets about how to change our metabolism from a "warm glow" to a "raging fire." Unfortunately, we are often exposed to considerable misinformation that can leave us frustrated when our implementation of these latest "secrets" falls short of all the metabolic benefits promised.

Components of Energy Expenditure

Metabolism is a word that, for our purposes, describes the burning of calories necessary to supply the body with the energy it needs to function. There are three major ways we burn calories during the day: resting metabolic rate (RMR), the thermic effect of food (TEF), and physical activity energy expenditure (PAEE). RMR is the number of calories we burn to maintain our vital body processes in a resting state. It is usually determined by measuring your body's oxygen utilization (which is closely tied to calorie burning) while you lay or sit quietly in the early morning before breakfast after a restful night's

"Does Exercise Affect Resting Metabolism?" is from the ACSM Fit Society® Page, Summer 2004, p. 4. Reprinted with permission of the American College of Sports Medicine.

sleep. RMR typically accounts for about 65 to 75 percent of your total daily calorie expenditure. The TEF results from eating food, and is the increase in energy expended above your RMR that results from digestion, absorption, and storage of the food you eat. It typically accounts for about 5 to 10 percent of the total calories you burn in a day. The last component, PAEE, accounts for the remainder of your daily energy expenditure, and, as the name suggests, is the increase in our calorie burning above RMR resulting from any physical activity. Included in PAEE is the energy expended in exercise, the activities of daily living, and even fidgeting. PAEE can vary considerably depending on how much you move throughout the day. For example, your PAEE would be high on a day that you participate in several hours of vigorous sports competition or exercise, while the calories you burn in physical activity would be quite low the next day if you choose to rest and recover.

Your total daily energy expenditure is the sum of these three components—if it is less than your energy intake, you will store most of the surplus energy, especially as body fat. If it is more than your energy intake, you will burn some body stores of energy to provide the needed energy not available from your food.

Is My Metabolic Rate Elevated Following Exercise?

Your calorie expenditure obviously increases above your resting rate when you exercise, with the magnitude of this increase dependent on how long and hard you exercise. One frequently asked question is "Do we continue to burn 'extra' calories after we finish exercising?" In other words, does our energy expenditure remain elevated above RMR for a period of time after we stop the exercise, and if so, does it contribute significantly to our total energy expenditure on the day we exercise? Research has clearly shown that energy expenditure does not return to pre-exercise resting baseline levels immediately following exercise. The amount of this post-exercise elevation of energy expenditure depends primarily on how hard you exercise (i.e., intensity) and to a lesser degree on how long you exercise (i.e., duration).

Endurance Exercise: Exercise of the intensity and duration commonly performed by recreational exercisers (e.g., walking for 30 to 60 minutes or jogging at a pace of 8 to 10 minutes per mile for 20 to 30 minutes) typically results in a return to baseline of energy expenditure well within the first hour of recovery. The post-exercise calorie bonus for this type of exercise probably accounts for only about 10 to 30 additional calories burned beyond the exercise bout itself. In athletes performing high intensity, long duration exercise, the post-exercise energy expenditure may remain elevated for a longer period and could contribute significantly to total daily calorie burning. Ironically, such athletes are typically less concerned about this "extra" calorie burning and its implications for body weight regulation than are the recreational exercisers. The average person who does considerably less strenuous exercise will likely experience little meaningful contribution of this post-exercise bonus to their total daily calorie expenditure.

Weight Lifting Exercise: A number of recent studies suggest that vigorous weight lifting exercise may elevate calorie burning above usual resting values for several hours after exercise. However, the average person at the gym who rests for several minutes between sets of exercise will likely not experience a prolonged elevation of postexercise energy expenditure.

Does Exercise Training Increase My RMR?

Endurance Exercise: A number of studies have found endurance-trained athletes to exhibit higher RMR than non-athletes. It appears likely that the combination of high exercise energy expenditure and high energy intake in these athletes can temporarily, but not permanently, elevate their RMR when measured the next morning after exercise. However, there is little evidence that the amount of physical activity performed by recreational exercisers for the purpose of weight control and health promotion will produce any increases in RMR, with the possible exception of such exercise in older individuals. It is clear that for both athletes and non-athletes, young and old, the major impact of exercise on total daily energy expenditure occurs during the activity itself, and not from increases in RMR.

Weight Lifting Exercise: Some fitness enthusiasts have promoted the idea that because regular weight lifting can increase skeletal muscle mass, such exercise will dramatically increase RMR. However, it is estimated that each pound of muscle burns about 5 to 10 calories per day while at rest, so you would have to bulk up quite a bit to increase your RMR. Most people who lift weights for health rather than for bodybuilding will not increase their muscle mass enough to have a major effect on RMR.

Summary

Regular exercise has many benefits and plays an important role in increasing our daily energy expenditure. However, despite what we may read in many popular magazines, the increase in energy expenditure from exercise occurs primarily while we are exercising, rather than due to any sizable exercise-induced elevations in our resting energy expenditure.

Chapter 6

The Neurological Benefits of Exercise

Chapter Contents

Section 6.1

Exercise May Slow Development of Alzheimer's-Like Brain Changes

From the press release "Exercise Slows Development of Alzheimer's-Like Brain Changes in Mice, New Study Finds," by the National Institute on Aging (NIA), a part of the National Institutes on Health (NIH), April 27, 2005.

Physical activity appears to inhibit Alzheimer's-like brain changes in mice, slowing the development of a key feature of the disease, according to a study. The research demonstrated that long-term physical activity enhanced the learning ability of mice and decreased the level of plaque-forming beta-amyloid protein fragments—a hallmark characteristic of Alzheimer's disease (AD)—in their brains.

A number of population-based studies suggest that lifestyle interventions may help to slow the onset and progression of AD. Because of these studies, scientists are seeking to find out if and how physically or cognitively stimulating activity might delay the onset and progression of Alzheimer's disease. In this study, scientists have now shown in an animal model system that one simple behavioral intervention—exercise—could delay, or even prevent, development of AD-like pathology by decreasing beta-amyloid levels.

Results of this study, conducted by Paul A. Adlard, Ph.D., Carl W. Cotman, Ph.D., and colleagues at the University of California, Irvine, are published in the April 27, 2005, issue of the *Journal of Neuroscience*. The research was funded in part by the National Institute on Aging (NIA), a component of the National Institutes of Health, U.S. Department of Health and Human Services. Additional funding was provided by the Christopher Reeve Paralysis Foundation.

To directly test the possibility that exercise (in the form of voluntary running) may reduce the cognitive decline and brain pathology that characterizes AD, the study utilized a transgenic mouse model of AD rather than normal mice. The transgenic mice begin to develop AD-like amyloid plaques at around 3 months of age. Initially, young mice (6 weeks or 1 month of age) were placed in cages with or without running wheels for periods of either 1 month or 5 months, respectively.

Mice with access to running wheels had the opportunity to exercise any time, while those without the wheels were classified as "sedentary."

On 6 consecutive days after the exercise phase, the researchers placed each mouse in a Morris water maze to examine how fast it could learn the location of a hidden platform and how long it retained this information. (This water maze task involves a small pool of water with a submerged platform that the mouse must learn how to find.) The animals that exercised learned the task faster. Thus the mice that used the running wheels for 5 months took less time than the sedentary animals to find the escape platform. The exercised mice acquired maximal performance after only 2 days on the task, while it took more than 4 days for the sedentary mice to reach that same level of performance. This suggests that exercise may help to offset learning/cognitive deficits present in AD patients.

Next, the investigators examined tissues from the brains of mice that had exercised for 5 months. They compared the levels of plaques, beta-amyloid fragments, and amyloid precursor protein, a protein found throughout the body and from which the beta-amyloid peptide is derived. In AD, beta-amyloid fragments clump together to form plaques in the hippocampus and cerebral cortex, the brain regions used in memory, thinking, and decision making.

Compared to the sedentary animals, mice that had exercised for 5 months on the running wheels had significantly fewer plaques and fewer beta-amyloid fragments (peptides) in the cerebral cortex and hippocampus, approximately by 50 percent. Additional studies, of exercised animals at 10 weeks old, showed that the mechanism underlying this difference began within the first month of exercise.

"These results suggest that exercise—a simple behavioral strategy—in these mice may bring about a change in the way that amyloid precursor protein is metabolized," says D. Stephen Snyder, Ph.D., director of the etiology of Alzheimer's program in the NIA's Neuroscience and Neuropsychology of Aging Program. "From other research, it is known that in the aging human brain, deposits of beta-amyloid normally increase. This study tells us that development of those deposits can be reduced and possibly eliminated through exercise, at least in this mouse model."

These findings follow another recent report of a link between an enriched environment and Alzheimer's-like brain changes. That study, published Orly Lazarov, Ph.D., and colleagues in the March 11, 2005, issue of the journal *Cell*, found that beta-amyloid levels decreased in the brains of another kind of transgenic mice when they were housed in groups and in environments that were enriched with running wheels, colored tunnels, and toys.

"Both of these studies are exciting because they offer insight into one of the pathways through which exercise and environment might promote resistance to development of cognitive changes that come with aging and AD," Snyder notes. "It is as though exercise or environmental enrichment forces the metabolism of amyloid precursor protein through a pathway that is less harmful and might even be beneficial. Further research will help us to understand those mechanisms, to learn how much and what kind of exercise is best, and to see if these same effects occur in humans."

Section 6.2

Exercise Associated with Reduced Risk of Dementia in Older Adults

From the press release by the National Institute on Aging (NIA), part of the National Institutes of Health (NIH), January 16, 2006.

Older adults who exercised at least three times a week were much less likely to develop dementia than those who were less active, according to a new study. The study did not demonstrate directly that exercise reduces risk of dementia, but it joins a growing body of observational research pointing to an association between exercise and cognitive decline, say scientists at the National Institute on Aging (NIA), a component of the National Institutes of Health (NIH), U.S. Department of Health and Human Services, which funded the study.

The research, reported in the January 17, 2006, issue of the *Annals of Internal Medicine*, was conducted by Eric B. Larson, M.D., Ph.D., and colleagues at the Group Health Cooperative (GHC), the University of Washington, and the VA Puget Sound Health Care System in Seattle, WA. Larson and co-investigators followed 1,740 GHC members age 65 or older for an average of 6.2 years between 1994 and 2003. When the study began, the participants—all of whom were tested and found to be cognitively normal—reported the number of days per week they engaged in at least 15 minutes of physical activity, such as walking, hiking, bicycling, aerobics, or weight training. Their cognitive function was then assessed, and new cases of dementia were identified every 2 years. By the end of the study, the rate of developing dementia was significantly lower for those who exercised more—13.0 per 1,000 "person years" for those who exercised three or more times weekly, compared with 19.7 per 1,000 "person years" for those who exercised fewer than three times per week—a 32 percent reduction in risk.

"Physical activity has been shown to be beneficial for health and aging in a number of areas," says Dallas Anderson, Ph.D., program director for population studies in the Dementias of Aging Branch of NIA's Neuroscience and Neuropsychology of Aging Program. "This emerging association between exercise and cognitive health is increasingly important to understand." The NIA is beginning to support clinical trials which seek to test exercise for its direct effect on cognitive function. Such research, Anderson says, should help sort out whether exercise reduces risk of cognitive decline or whether other factors related to exercise, such as increased social interaction, play a role. Additional study also may provide information on the possible merits of varying types of exercise.

Chapter 7

Physical Activity Benefits Bone Health

Chapter Contents

Section 7.1

Exercise for Healthy Bones

From the fact sheet "Exercise for Your Bone Health," by the National Institutes of Health Osteoporosis and Related Bone Diseases National Resource Center (www.osteo.org), August 2005.

Vital at every age for healthy bones, exercise is important for treating and preventing osteoporosis. Not only does exercise improve your bone health, it also increases muscle strength, coordination, and balance, and leads to better overall health.

Why Exercise?

Like muscle, bone is living tissue that responds to exercise by becoming stronger. Young women and men who exercise regularly generally achieve greater peak bone mass (maximum bone density and strength) than those who do not. For most people, bone mass peaks during the third decade of life. After that time, we can begin to lose bone. Women and men older than age 20 can help prevent bone loss with regular exercise. Exercising allows us to maintain muscle strength, coordination, and balance, which in turn help to prevent falls and related fractures. This is especially important for older adults and people who have been diagnosed with osteoporosis.

The Best Bone Building Exercise

The best exercise for your bones is the weight-bearing kind, which forces you to work against gravity. Some examples of weight-bearing exercises include lifting weights, walking, hiking, jogging, climbing stairs, tennis, and dancing. Examples of exercises that are not weight bearing include swimming and bicycling. While these activities help build and maintain strong muscles and have excellent cardiovascular benefits, they are not the best way to exercise your bones.

Exercise Tips

If you have health problems—such as heart trouble, high blood pressure, diabetes, or obesity—or if you are over age 40, check with your doctor before you begin a regular exercise program. According to the Surgeon General, the optimal goal is at least 30 minutes of physical activity on most days, preferably daily.

Listen to your body. When starting an exercise routine, you may have some muscle soreness and discomfort at the beginning, but this should not be painful or last more than 48 hours. If it does, you may be working too hard and need to ease up. **Stop** exercising if you have any chest pain or discomfort, and see your doctor before your next exercise session.

If you have osteoporosis, ask your doctor which activities are safe for you. If you have low bone mass, experts recommend that you protect your spine by avoiding exercises or activities that flex, bend, or twist it. Furthermore, you should avoid high-impact exercise in order to lower the risk of breaking a bone. You also might want to consult with an exercise specialist to learn the proper progression of activity, how to stretch and strengthen muscles safely, and how to correct poor posture habits. An exercise specialist should have a degree in exercise physiology, physical education, physical therapy, or a similar specialty. Be sure to ask if he or she is familiar with the special needs of people with osteoporosis.

A Complete Osteoporosis Program

Remember, exercise is only one part of an osteoporosis prevention or treatment program. Like a diet rich in calcium and vitamin D, exercise helps strengthen bones at any age. But proper exercise and diet may not be enough to stop bone loss caused by medical conditions, menopause, or lifestyle choices such as tobacco use and excessive alcohol consumption. It is important to speak with your doctor about your bone health. Discuss when you might be a candidate for a bone mineral density test. If you are diagnosed with low bone mass, ask what medications might help keep your bones strong.

Section 7.2

Exercise Builds Bone Mass in Postmenopausal Women

From "Exercise Builds Bone Mass in Postmenopausal Women Whether or Not They Use Hormone Therapy," by the National Institute of Arthritis and Musculoskeletal and Skin Diseases (NIAMS), part of the National Institutes of Health, November 2003.

Aerobic, weight-bearing, and resistance exercise improves bone mineral density (BMD) in postmenopausal women whether or not they use hormone therapy, according to results from the Bone, Estrogen and Strength (BEST) study funded by the National Institute of Arthritis and Musculoskeletal and Skin Diseases (NIAMS), a part of the Department of Health and Human Services' National Institutes of Health.

Scott Going, Ph.D., Timothy Lohman, Ph.D., Linda Houtkooper, Ph.D., and their colleagues at the University of Arizona conducted a randomized clinical trial in 320 postmenopausal women between the ages of 45 and 65 to test the effect of a specific exercise regimen on bone mineral density. The women who were randomized to the exercise regimen—a combination of weight-bearing and resistance exercises—showed significant improvement (1 to 2 percent) in BMD after one year at the hip and spine, two important sites of fractures that may result from the bone-wasting disease osteoporosis. Notably, this benefit was found in both women taking postmenopausal hormone therapy and those who did not, although the women taking hormones had a somewhat greater response to exercise.

The exercises involved 20 to 25 minutes of resistance training using back extensions, leg presses, squats, pull downs, dumbbell presses, and rowing, and 7 to 10 minutes of cardiovascular weight-bearing activity, such as skipping, jogging, and jumping rope.

The study shows that specific strength training and resistance exercises can retard and even reverse bone loss in healthy postmenopausal women, and that estrogen replacement is not necessary to gain the benefit of the exercise. All women received calcium supplements, and adequate calcium may be a factor in optimizing the effect of exercise on bone in postmenopausal women. The finding may provide reassurance for women who no longer take hormone replacement therapy because of the recent Women's Health Initiative findings. Osteoporosis is a disease characterized by low bone mass, bone fragility and increased susceptibility to fractures of the hip, spine and wrist. Women can lose up to 20 percent of their bone mass in the five to seven years following menopause, making them more susceptible to osteoporosis. In the United States today, 10 million individuals already have osteoporosis, and 18 million more have low bone mass, placing them at increased risk for this disorder.

Source: Going S, et al. Effects of exercise on bone mineral density in calcium-replete postmenopausal women with and without hormone replacement therapy. *Osteoporosis International* 2003; 14:637–643.

Chapter 8

The Effect of Exercise on Mental Health

Chapter Contents

Section 8.1

Controlling Stress with Physical Activity

People who exercise regularly will tell you they feel better. Some will say it's because chemicals called neurotransmitters, produced in the brain, are stimulated during exercise. Since it's believed that neurotransmitters mediate our moods and emotions, they can make us feel better and less stressed.

While there's no scientific evidence to conclusively support the neurotransmitter theory, there is plenty to show that exercise provides stress-relieving benefits.

Four Ways Exercise Controls Stress

1. **Exercise can help you feel less anxious.** Exercise is being prescribed in clinical settings to help treat nervous tension. Following a session of exercise, clinicians have measured a decrease in electrical activity of tensed muscles. People have been less jittery and hyperactive after an exercise session.

2. **Exercise can relax you.** One exercise session generates 90 to 120 minutes of relaxation response. Some people call this post-exercise euphoria or endorphin response. We now know that many neurotransmitters, not just endorphins, are involved. The important thing though is not what they're called, but what they do: They improve your mood and leave you relaxed.

3. **Exercise can make you feel better about yourself.** Think about those times when you've been physically active. Haven't you felt better about yourself? That feeling of self-worth contributes to stress relief.

4. **Exercise can make you eat better.** People who exercise regularly tend to eat more nutritious food. And it's no secret that good nutrition helps your body manage stress better.

It's Time to Get Started

Now that you know exercise can make a big difference in controlling stress, make some time for regular physical activity. We'll help you get started by listing three activities you can choose from:

1. **Aerobic activity.** All it takes is 20 minutes' worth, six to seven days a week. Twenty minutes won't carve a big chunk out of your day, but it will improve your ability to control stress significantly.

2. **Yoga.** In yoga or yoga-type activities, your mind relaxes progressively as your body increases its amount of muscular work. Recent studies have shown that when large muscle groups repeatedly contract and relax, the brain receives a signal to release specific neurotransmitters, which in turn make you feel relaxed and more alert.

3. **Recreational sports.** Play tennis, racquetball, volleyball, or squash. These games require the kind of vigorous activity that rids your body of stress-causing adrenaline and other hormones.

Not Just Any Exercise Will Do

Don't try exercising in your office. Outdoors or away from the office is the best place to find a stress-free environment. Even a corporate fitness center can have too many work-related thoughts for some people.

Stay away from overcrowded classes. If you work surrounded by people, a big exercise class may be counterproductive. Solo exercise may be more relaxing for you. If, however, you work alone, you may enjoy the social benefit of exercising in a group. A lot depends on your personality and what causes stress for you.

Don't skip a chance to exercise. Take a break every 90 minutes and you'll be doing yourself a favor. Ninety-minute intervals are a natural work-break period. And four 10-minute exercise breaks at this time will burn about as many calories as a solid 40-minute session. Work-break exercises can be as simple as walking or climbing stairs, stretching, or doing calisthenics. Controlling stress comes down to making the time to exercise. You're worth it!

Section 8.2

How Does Exercise Improve Depression?

"How Does Exercise Improve Depression?" © 2003 The Cleveland Clinic Foundation, 9500 Euclid Avenue, Cleveland, OH 44195, www.cleveland clinic.org. Additional information is available from the Cleveland Clinic Health Information Center, 216-444-3771, toll-free 800-223-2273 extension 43771, or at http://www.clevelandclinic.org/health.

What are the benefits of exercise?

Regular exercise has been proven to:

- reduce stress, anxiety, and depression;
- boost self-esteem; and
- improve sleep.

Exercise also has these health benefits:

- strengthens the heart;
- makes the body better able to use oxygen;
- builds energy levels;
- lowers blood pressure;
- improves muscle tone and strength;
- strengthens and builds bones;
- helps reduce body fat; and
- makes you look fit and healthy.

Exercise and depression: What's the link?

Research has shown that exercise is an effective, but often under-used, treatment for mild to moderate depression.

What types of exercise treat depression?

It appears that any form of exercise can help treat depression.

Do I need to see my health care provider before starting an exercise program?

Most people can begin an exercise program without checking with their health care providers. However, people with medical conditions (such as diabetes or heart disease) and people who have not exercised much should check with their health care providers before starting any exercise program.

How can I begin planning my exercise routine?

Here are some questions you can think about before choosing a routine:

- What physical activities do I enjoy?
- Do I prefer group or individual activities?
- What programs best fit my schedule?
- Do I have physical conditions that limit my choice of exercise?
- What goals do I have in mind? (For example: weight loss, strengthening muscles, improving flexibility, or mood enhancement)

How often should I exercise?

To get the most benefit, you should exercise at least 20 to 30 minutes most days of the week. If you are a beginner, exercise for 20 minutes and build up to 30 minutes.

How do I get started?

When starting out, you should plan a routine that is easy to follow and maintain. As the program becomes more routine, you can vary your exercise times and activities.

- Choose an activity you enjoy. Exercising should be fun, not a chore.
- Schedule regular exercise into your daily routine. Add a variety of exercises so that you don't get bored. Look into scheduled exercise classes at your local community center.
- Exercise does not have to put a strain on your wallet. Avoid buying expensive equipment or health club memberships unless you are certain you will use them regularly.
- Stick with it. If you exercise regularly, it will soon become part of your lifestyle.

What should I do if I feel pain during exercise?

Never ignore pain. If you experience pain, rest. You may cause stress and damage to your joints and muscles if you continue exercising.

If you still feel pain two hours after exercising, you have done too much and need to decrease your activity level. Some mild soreness after exercise is normal. If pain persists or is severe or you suspect you have injured yourself, contact your doctor right away.

Part Two

Sports Nutrition and Supplements

Chapter 9

What Is a Healthy Diet?

Why should I try to have a healthy diet?

Having a healthy diet is one of the most important things you can do to help your overall health. Along with physical activity, your diet is the key factor that affects your weight. Having a healthy weight for your height is important. Being overweight or obese increases your risk of heart disease, type 2 diabetes, high blood pressure, stroke, breathing problems, arthritis, gallbladder disease, sleep apnea (breathing problems while sleeping), osteoarthritis, and some cancers. You can find out if you're overweight or obese by figuring out your body mass index (BMI). Women with a BMI of 25 to 29.9 are considered overweight, whereas women with a BMI of 30 or more are considered obese. All adults (aged 18 years or older) who have a BMI of 25 or more are considered at risk for premature death and disability from being overweight or obese. These health risks increase as the BMI rises. Your health care provider can help you figure out your body mass, or you can go to www.cdc.gov/nccdphp/dnpa/bmi/calc-bmi.htm.

Having a healthy diet is sometimes easier said than done. It is tempting to eat less healthy foods because they might be easier to get or prepare, or they satisfy a craving. Between family and work or school, you are probably balancing a hundred things at once. Taking time to buy the ingredients for and cooking a healthy meal sometimes

Excerpted from "A Healthy Diet," by the National Women's Health Information Center (www.4women.gov), part of the U.S. Department of Health and Human Services, January 2005.

and my
and my

Fitness and Exercise Sourcebook, Third Edition

falls last on your list. But you should know that it isn't hard to make simple changes to improve your diet. And you can make sense of the mounds of nutrition information out there. A little learning and planning can help you find a diet to fit your lifestyle, and maybe you can have some fun in the process!

How can I start planning a healthy diet for me and my family?

You can start planning a healthy diet by looking at the Dietary Guidelines for Americans 2005 (http://www.healthierus.gov/dietary guidelines) by the U.S. Department of Agriculture (USDA) and the Department of Health and Human Services (HHS). The best way to give your body the balanced nutrition it needs is by eating a variety of nutrient-packed foods every day. Just be sure to stay within your daily calorie needs.

Mix up your choices within each food group:

- **Focus on fruits.** Eat a variety of fruits—whether fresh, frozen, canned, or dried—rather than fruit juice for most of your fruit choices. For a 2,000 calorie diet, you will need 2 cups of fruit each day (for example, 1 small banana, 1 large orange, and 1/4 cup of dried apricots or peaches).

- **Vary your veggies.** Eat more dark green veggies, such as broccoli, kale, and other dark leafy greens; orange veggies, such as carrots, sweet potatoes, pumpkin, and winter squash; and beans and peas, such as pinto beans, kidney beans, black beans, garbanzo beans, split peas and lentils.

- **Get your calcium-rich foods.** Get 3 cups of low-fat or fat-free milk—or an equivalent amount of low-fat yogurt and/or low-fat cheese (1 1/2 ounces of cheese equals one cup of milk)—every day. For kids aged 2 to 8, it's 2 cups of milk. If you don't or can't consume milk, choose lactose-free milk products and/or calcium-fortified foods and beverages.

- **Make half your grains whole.** Eat at least 3 ounces of whole-grain cereals, breads, crackers, rice, or pasta every day. One ounce is about 1 slice of bread, 1 cup of breakfast cereal, or 1/2 cup of cooked rice or pasta. Look to see that grains such as wheat, rice, oats, or corn are referred to as 'whole' in the list of ingredients.

- **Go lean with protein.** Choose lean meats and poultry. Bake it, broil it, or grill it. And vary your protein choices—with more fish, beans, peas, nuts and seeds.

64

- **Know the limits on fats, salt, and sugars.** Read the Nutrition Facts label on foods. Look for foods low in saturated fats and trans fats. Choose and prepare foods and beverages with a little salt (sodium) and/or sugars (caloric sweeteners).

What are the most important steps to a healthy diet?

The basic steps to good nutrition come from a diet that:

- helps you either lose weight or keeps your BMI in the "healthy" range.
- is balanced overall, with foods from all food groups, with lots of delicious fruits, vegetables, whole-grains, and fat-free or low-fat milk and milk products.
- is low in saturated fat, trans fat, and cholesterol. Keep total fat intake between 20 to 35 percent of calories, with most fats coming from sources of polyunsaturated and monounsaturated fatty acids, such as fish, nuts, and vegetable oils.
- includes a variety of grains daily, especially whole grains, a good source of fiber.
- includes a variety of fruits and vegetables (two cups of fruit and 2 1/2 cups of vegetables per day are recommended for a 2,000 calorie diet).
- has a small number of calories from added sugars (like in candy, cookies, and cakes).
- has foods prepared with less sodium or salt (aim for no more than 2,300 milligrams of sodium per day, or about one teaspoon of salt per day).
- does not include more than one drink per day (two drinks per day for men) if you drink alcoholic beverages.

It's hard to know if my portions are too big or too small for a healthy diet. Do I have to measure everything I'm eating?

It can be hard to learn if your portions of food are putting you over amounts of things you're trying to control. It doesn't help that sizes for everything from bananas to soft drinks have gotten larger in the past 20 years. It's not enough to eat the right kinds of food to maintain a healthy weight or to lose weight. Eating the right amount of food at each meal is just as important. If you are a healthy eater, it is possible to sabotage your efforts by eating more than the recommended amount of food. A serving is a specific amount of food, and it might be smaller than you realize. Here are some examples:

- A serving of meat (boneless, cooked weight) is 2 to 3 ounces, or roughly the size of the palm of your hand, a deck of cards, or an audiocassette tape.

- A serving of chopped vegetables or fruit is 1/2 cup, or approximately half a baseball or a rounded handful.

- A serving of fresh fruit is one medium piece, or the size of a baseball.

- A serving of cooked pasta, rice, or cereal is 1/2 cup, or half a baseball or a rounded handful.

- A serving of cooked beans is 1/2 cup, or half a baseball or a rounded handful.

- A serving of nuts is 1/3 cup, or a level handful for an average adult.

- A serving of peanut butter is two tablespoons, about the size of a golf ball.

I'm confused by all of the labels I see on foods, like "fat free" and "low calorie." What do these terms mean?

Terms like these are on many food packages. Here are some definitions based on one serving of a food. If you eat more than one serving, you will go over these levels of calories, fat, cholesterol, and sodium.

- **Calorie-free:** fewer than 5 calories
- **Low calorie:** 40 calories or fewer
- **Reduced calorie:** at least 25% fewer calories than the regular food item has
- **Fat free:** less than 1/2 gram of fat
- **Low fat:** 3 grams of fat or fewer
- **Reduced fat:** at least 25% less fat than the regular food item has

- **Cholesterol free:** fewer than 2 milligrams cholesterol and no more than 2 grams of saturated fat
- **Low cholesterol:** 20 milligrams or fewer cholesterol and 2 grams or less saturated fat
- **Sodium free:** fewer than 5 milligrams sodium
- **Very low sodium:** fewer than 35 milligrams sodium
- **Low sodium:** fewer than 140 milligrams sodium
- **High fiber:** 5 grams or more fiber

Chapter 10

Frequently Asked Questions about What to Eat If You Exercise

What diet is best for athletes?

It's important that an athlete's diet provides the right amount of energy, the 50-plus nutrients the body needs, and adequate water. No single food or supplement can do this. A variety of foods are needed every day. But just as there is more than one way to achieve a goal, there is more than one way to follow a nutritious diet.

Do the nutritional needs of athletes differ from nonathletes?

Competitive athletes, sedentary individuals, and people who exercise for health and fitness all need the same nutrients. However, because of the intensity of their sport or training program, some athletes have higher calorie and fluid requirements. Eating a variety of foods to meet increased calorie needs helps to ensure that the athlete's diet contains appropriate amounts of carbohydrate, protein, vitamins, and minerals.

Are there certain dietary guidelines athletes should follow?

Health and nutrition professionals recommend that 55% to 60% of the calories in our diet come from carbohydrate, no more than 30%

"Questions Most Frequently Asked about Sports Nutrition" is from The President's Council on Physical Fitness and Sports (www.fitness.gov), October 15, 2004.

from fat, and the remaining 10% to 15% from protein. Although the exact percentages may vary slightly for some athletes based on their sport or training program, these guidelines will promote health and serve as the basis for a diet that will maximize performance.

How many calories do I need in a day?

This depends on your age, body size, sport, and training program. For example, a 250-pound weight lifter needs more calories than a 98-pound gymnast. Exercise or training may increase calorie needs by as much as 1,000 to 1,500 calories a day. The best way to determine if you're getting too few or too many calories is to monitor your weight. Keeping within your ideal competitive weight range means that you are getting the right amount of calories.

Which is better for replacing fluids—water or sports drinks?

Depending on how muscular you are, 55% to 70% of your body weight is water. Being "hydrated" means maintaining your body's fluid level. When you sweat, you lose water which must be replaced if you want to perform your best. You need to drink fluids before, during, and after all workouts and events.

Whether you drink water or a sports drink is a matter of choice. However, if your workout or event lasts for more than 90 minutes, you may benefit from the carbohydrates provided by sports drinks. A sports drink that contains 15 to 18 grams of carbohydrate in every 8 ounces of fluid should be used. Drinks with a higher carbohydrate content will delay the absorption of water and may cause dehydration, cramps, nausea, or diarrhea. There are a variety of sports drinks on the market. Be sure to experiment with sports drinks during practice instead of trying them for the first time the day of an event.

What are electrolytes?

Electrolytes are nutrients that affect fluid balance in the body and are necessary for our nerves and muscles to function. Sodium and potassium are the two electrolytes most often added to sports drinks. Generally, electrolyte replacement is not needed during short bursts of exercise since sweat is approximately 99% water and less than 1% electrolytes. Water, in combination with a well-balanced diet, will restore normal fluid and electrolyte levels in the body. However, replacing electrolytes may be beneficial during continuous activity of longer than 2 hours, especially in a hot environment.

What do muscles use for energy during exercise?

Most activities use a combination of fat and carbohydrate as energy sources. How hard and how long you work out, your level of fitness, and your diet will affect the type of fuel your body uses. For short-term, high-intensity activities like sprinting, athletes rely mostly on carbohydrate for energy. During low-intensity exercises like walking, the body uses more fat for energy.

What are carbohydrates?

Carbohydrates are sugars and starches found in foods like breads, cereals, fruits, vegetables, pasta, milk, honey, syrups, and table sugar. Carbohydrates are the preferred source of energy for your body. Regardless of origin, your body breaks down carbohydrates into glucose that your blood carries to cells to be used for energy. Carbohydrates provide 4 calories per gram, whereas fat provides 9 calories per gram. Your body cannot differentiate between glucose that comes from starches or sugars. Glucose from either source provides energy for working muscles.

Is it true that athletes should eat a lot of carbohydrates?

When you are training or competing, your muscles need energy to perform. One source of energy for working muscles is glycogen, which is made from carbohydrates and stored in your muscles. Every time you work out, you use some of your glycogen. If you don't consume enough carbohydrates, your glycogen stores become depleted, which can result in fatigue. Both sugars and starches are effective in replenishing glycogen stores.

When and what should I eat before I compete?

Performance depends largely on the foods consumed during the days and weeks leading up to an event. If you regularly eat a varied, carbohydrate-rich diet you are in good standing and probably have ample glycogen stores to fuel activity. The purpose of the precompetition meal is to prevent hunger and to provide the water and additional energy the athlete will need during competition. Most athletes eat 2 to 4 hours before their event. However, some athletes perform their best if they eat a small amount 30 minutes before competing, whereas others eat nothing for 6 hours beforehand. For many athletes, carbohydrate-rich foods serve as the basis of the meal. However, there is no magic pre-event diet. Simply choose foods and beverages that you enjoy and that don't bother your stomach. Experiment during the weeks before an event to see which foods work best for you.

Will eating sugary foods before an event hurt my performance?

In the past, athletes were warned that eating sugary foods before exercise could hurt performance by causing a drop in blood glucose levels. Recent studies, however, have shown that consuming sugar up to 30 minutes before an event does not diminish performance. In fact, evidence suggests that a sugar-containing precompetition beverage or snack may improve performance during endurance workouts and events.

What is carbohydrate loading?

Carbohydrate loading is a technique used to increase the amount of glycogen in muscles. For five to seven days before an event, the athlete eats 10 to 12 grams of carbohydrate per kilogram body weight and gradually reduces the intensity of the workouts. (To find out how much you weigh in kilograms, simply divide your weight in pounds by 2.2.) The day before the event, the athlete rests and eats the same high-carbohydrate diet. Although carbohydrate loading may be beneficial for athletes participating in endurance sports that require 90 minutes or more of nonstop effort, most athletes needn't worry about carbohydrate loading. Simply eating a diet that derives more than half of its calories from carbohydrates will do.

As an athlete, do I need to take extra vitamins and minerals?

Athletes need to eat about 1,800 calories a day to get the vitamins and minerals they need for good health and optimal performance. Since most athletes eat more than this amount, vitamin and mineral supplements are needed only in special situations. Athletes who follow vegetarian diets or who avoid an entire group of foods (for example, never drink milk) may need a supplement to make up for the vitamins and minerals not being supplied by food. A multivitamin/mineral pill that supplies 100% of the Recommended Dietary Allowance (RDA) will provide the nutrients needed. An athlete who frequently cuts back on calories, especially below the 1,800 calorie level, is not only at risk for inadequate vitamin and mineral intake, but also may not be getting enough carbohydrate. Since vitamins and minerals do not provide energy, they cannot replace the energy provided by carbohydrates.

Will extra protein help build muscle mass?

Many athletes, especially those on strength-training programs or who participate in power sports, are told that eating a ton of protein or taking protein supplements will help them gain muscle weight. However, the true secret to building muscle is training hard and consuming enough calories. While some extra protein is needed to build muscle, most American diets provide more than enough protein. Between 1.0 and 1.5 grams of protein per kilogram body weight per day is sufficient if your calorie intake is adequate and you're eating a variety of foods. For a 150-pound athlete, that represents 68 to 102 grams of protein a day.

Why is iron so important?

Hemoglobin, which contains iron, is the part of red blood cells that carries oxygen from the lungs to all parts of the body, including muscles. Since your muscles need oxygen to produce energy, if you have low iron levels in your blood, you may tire quickly. Symptoms of iron deficiency include fatigue, irritability, dizziness, headaches, and lack of appetite. Many times, however; there are no symptoms at all. A blood test is the best way to find out if your iron level is low. It is recommended that athletes have their hemoglobin levels checked once a year.

The RDA for iron is 15 milligrams a day for women and 10 milligrams a day for men. Red meat is the richest source of iron, but fish and poultry also are good sources. Fortified breakfast cereals, beans, and green leafy vegetables also contain iron. Our bodies absorb the iron found in animal products best.

Should I take an iron supplement?

Taking iron supplements will not improve performance unless an athlete is truly iron deficient. Too much iron can cause constipation, diarrhea, and nausea and may interfere with the absorption of other nutrients such as copper and zinc. Therefore, iron supplements should not be taken without proper medical supervision.

Why is calcium so important?

Calcium is needed for strong bones and proper muscle function. Dairy foods are the best source of calcium. However, studies show that many female athletes who are trying to lose weight cut back on dairy products. Female athletes who don't get enough calcium may be at risk for stress fractures and, when they're older, osteoporosis. Young women between the ages of 11 and 24 need about 1,200 milligrams of calcium a day. After age 25, the recommended intake is 800 milligrams. Low-fat dairy products are a rich source of calcium and also are low in fat and calories.

Chapter 11

Nutrition Concerns for Athletes

Chapter Contents

Section 11.1

Facts about Sports Nutrition

"Fast Facts about Sports Nutrition" is from
The President's Council on Physical Fitness and Sports
(www.fitness.gov), October 15, 2004.

Water, Water Everywhere

You can survive for a month without food, but only a few days without water.

- Water is the most important nutrient for active people.

- When you sweat, you lose water, which must be replaced. Drink fluids before, during, and after workouts.

- Water is a fine choice for most workouts. However, during continuous workouts of greater than 90 minutes, your body may benefit from a sports drink.

- Sports drinks have two very important ingredients—electrolytes and carbohydrates.

- Sports drinks replace electrolytes lost through sweat during workouts lasting several hours.

- Carbohydrates in sports drinks provide extra energy. The most effective sports drinks contain 15 to 18 grams of carbohydrate in every 8 ounces of fluid.

Rev up Your Engine with Carbohydrates

Carbohydrates are your body's main source of energy.

- Carbohydrates are sugars and starches, and they are found in foods such as breads, cereals, fruits, vegetables, pasta, milk, honey, syrups, and table sugar.

- Sugars and starches are broken down by your body into glucose, which is used by your muscles for energy.

- For health and peak performance, more than half your daily calories should come from carbohydrates.

- Sugars and starches have 4 calories per gram, while fat has 9 calories per gram. In other words, carbohydrates have less than half the calories of fat.

- If you regularly eat a carbohydrate-rich diet you probably have enough carbohydrate stored to fuel activity. Even so, be sure to eat a precompetition meal for fluid and additional energy. What you eat as well as when you eat your precompetition meal will be entirely individual.

Flexing Your Options to Build Bigger Muscles

It is a myth that eating lots of protein and/or taking protein supplements and exercising vigorously will definitely turn you into a big, muscular person.

- Building muscle depends on your genes, how hard you train, and whether you get enough calories.

- The average American diet has more than enough protein for muscle building. Extra protein is eliminated from the body or stored as fat.

Score with Vitamins and Minerals

Eating a varied diet will give you all the vitamins and minerals you need for health and peak performance.

- Exceptions include active people who follow strict vegetarian diets, avoid an entire group of foods, or eat less than 1,800 calories a day. If you fall into any of these categories, a multivitamin and mineral pill may provide the vitamins and minerals missing in your diet.

- Taking large doses of vitamins and minerals will not help your performance and may be bad for your health. Vitamins and minerals do not supply the body with energy and, therefore are not a substitute for carbohydrates.

Popeye and All That Spinach

Iron supplies working muscles with oxygen.

- If your iron level is low, you may tire easily and not have enough stamina for activity.

- The best sources of iron are animal products, but plant foods such as fortified breads, cereals, beans, and green leafy vegetables also contain iron.

- Iron supplements may have side effects, so take them only if your doctor tells you to.

No Bones About It, You Need Calcium Every Day

Many people do not get enough of the calcium needed for strong bones and proper muscle function.

- Lack of calcium can contribute to stress fractures and the bone disease osteoporosis.

- The best sources of calcium are dairy products, but many other foods such as salmon with bones, sardines, collard greens, and okra also contain calcium. Additionally, some brands of bread, tofu, and orange juice are fortified with calcium.

A Weighty Matter

Your calorie needs depend on your age, body size, sport, and training program.

- The best way to make sure you are not getting too many or too few calories is to check your weight from time to time.

- If you're keeping within your ideal weight range, you're probably getting the right amount of calories.

Section 11.2

Feeding Your Child Athlete

"Do You Know How to Feed Your Child Athlete?" was provided by KidsHealth, one of the largest resources online for medically reviewed health information written for parents, kids, and teens. For more articles like this one, visit www.KidsHealth.org, or www.TeensHealth.org. © 2005 The Nemours Foundation. This article was updated and reviewed by Steven Dowshen, M.D., and Jessica Donze Black, R.D., C.D.E., M.P.H., in May 2005.

All kids need to eat balanced meals and have a healthy diet. But should that balance change if your child is on a sports team or working out? Maybe. Your child needs to eat the right mix of foods to support that higher level of activity, but that mix might not be too different than what is considered a healthy diet. Eating for sports should be an extension of healthy eating for life.

There are many "sports" foods and drinks marketed to athletes, like energy bars and gels. In general, most young athletes do not need these products to meet their energy needs. These products don't have magic ingredients that will improve a child's sports performance, but they can come in handy if your child doesn't have time to prepare a healthy meal or snack.

Because athletic kids are particularly reliant on the nutrients that a balanced diet can provide, it's usually not a good idea for them to diet. In sports where weight is emphasized, such as wrestling, swimming, dance, or gymnastics, your child may feel pressure to lose weight. If a coach, gym teacher, or another teammate says that your child needs to go on a diet, talk to your doctor first. If your doctor thinks your child should diet, the doctor can work with your child or refer you to a nutritionist to develop a plan that allows your child to work on the weight in a safe and healthy way.

What Are the Nutritional Needs of Young Athletes?

If your child is eating healthy, well-balanced meals and snacks, your child is probably getting the nutrients that he or she needs to perform well in sports. The new food guide pyramid, called MyPyramid, can

79

provide guidance on what kinds of foods and drinks should be included in your child's well-balanced meals and snacks.

But kids who are involved in strenuous endurance sports like cross-country running or competitive swimming, which involve 1½ to 2 hours of activity at a time, may need to consume more food to keep up with their increased energy demands. Most athletic young people will naturally crave the amount of food their bodies need, but if you are concerned that your child is getting too much or too little food, you may want to check in with your child's doctor.

Because different foods have different combinations of these nutrients, it's important to vary your child's meals and snacks as much as possible. It's a good idea to make sure that your child is getting the following nutrients:

- **Vitamins and minerals:** Your child needs a variety of vitamins and minerals. Brightly colored foods such as spinach, carrots, squash, and peppers tend to be packed with them. It's especially important your child get plenty of calcium and iron. Calcium helps your child build healthy bones, which are important especially if your child breaks a bone or gets a stress fracture. Calcium-rich foods include dairy products like milk, yogurt, and cheese, as well as leafy green vegetables such as broccoli. Iron helps carry oxygen to all the different body parts that need it. Iron-rich foods include red meat, chicken, tuna, salmon, eggs, dried fruits, leafy green vegetables, and whole grains.

- **Protein:** Protein can help build your child's muscles, along with regular training and exercise. But there's no need to overload on protein because too much of it can lead to dehydration and calcium loss. Protein-rich foods include fish, lean red meat and poultry, dairy products, nuts, soy products, and peanut butter.

- **Carbohydrates:** Carbohydrates provide energy for the body. Some diet plans have urged weight-conscious adults to steer clear of carbohydrates or "carbs" as they're often called. But for a young athlete, carbohydrates are an important source of fuel. There's not any need for your child to do any "carb loading" or eat a lot of carbs in advance of a big game, but without some of these foods in your child's diet, he or she will be running on empty. When you're choosing carbohydrates, look for whole-grain foods that are less processed and high in fiber, like pasta, brown rice, whole-grain bread, and cereal. Fiber helps lower cholesterol and may help prevent diabetes and heart disease.

It's a good idea to pack your child's meals with natural foods as much as possible. Natural foods such as whole-wheat breads and baked potatoes are more wholesome choices than heavily processed foods, like white breads and potato chips. Usually the less processed the food, the more nutritious it is. Choose products with ingredients such as whole wheat or oats rather than white flour. Encourage your child to pick up a piece of fruit, rather than a fruit drink, which may have added sugar. Remember that sugar may be listed by another name such as sucrose or fructose.

Drink Up

It's important for young athletes to drink plenty of fluid to avoid any heat illness and dehydration, which can zap a child's strength, energy, and coordination and lead to other health problems.

It's a good idea for your child to drink water or other fluids throughout the day, but especially before, during, and after periods of extended physical activity. Experts recommend that kids drink approximately 1 cup (240 milliliters) of water or fluid every 20 to 30 minutes of physical activity, depending on the child. Shorter competitions may not require drinking during the activity, but it's important to drink water after the game or event to restore whatever fluid your child lost through sweat during the event.

Children often don't recognize or respond to feelings of thirst. So it's a good idea to encourage your child to drink before thirst sets in.

Although many sports drinks are available, usually plain water is sufficient to keep kids hydrated. Sports drinks are designed to provide energy and replace electrolytes—such as sodium and potassium—that athletes lose in sweat. But your child's body typically has enough carbohydrates to serve as energy for up to 90 minutes of exercise. And in most cases, any lost electrolytes can be replenished by a good meal after the activity.

If your child participates in endurance sports such as long-distance running and biking or high-intensity exercise such as soccer, basketball, or hockey, it's a good idea for your child to replenish his or her body throughout the event. This is because the body can use the sugar immediately as energy to make up for the depleted energy stores in the body. Soda and juice may not quench your child's fluid needs as well because many of them have too much sugar and can upset the stomach. If your child wants juice, it's a good idea to mix it with water to reduce the concentration of sugar.

Pressures Facing Athletes

Some school-age athletes face unique pressures involving nutrition and body weight. In some sports, it's common for kids to feel they need to radically increase or reduce their weight to reach peak performance.

Unhealthy eating habits, like crash dieting, can also leave your child with less strength, endurance, and poorer mental concentration. Similar performance issues can come up when kids try to increase their weight too fast. When a person overeats, the food the body can't immediately use gets stored as fat. As a result, kids who overeat may gain weight, but their physical fitness will be diminished.

If you are concerned about your child's eating habits, it's a good idea to talk to your child's doctor.

Game Day

It's important for your child to eat well on game days, but make sure your child eats at least 2 hours before the event—early enough to digest the food before game time. The meal itself should not be very different from what your child has been eating throughout training.

It should have plenty of carbohydrates and protein and be low in fat because fat is harder to digest and can cause an upset stomach.

After the game or event, it's a good idea to make sure your child gets a well-balanced meal. Your child's body will be rebuilding muscle tissue and restoring carbohydrates and fluids for up to 24 hours after the competition. So it's important that your child get plenty of protein, fat, and carbohydrates in the postgame hours.

And remember, when packing your child's bag for the big day, don't forget the water bottle or the sports drink.

Meal and Snack Suggestions

You can't make up for a poor diet on game day, so it's important to feed your child healthy meals and snacks on a consistent basis, even during the off-season. That will provide a solid foundation whenever your child heads out for a competition.

Breakfast might include low-fat yogurt with some granola or a banana. Lunch might include bean burritos with low-fat cheese, lettuce, and tomatoes. A turkey sandwich and fruit may also be a hit. Dinner might be grilled chicken breasts with steamed rice and vegetables or pasta with red sauce and lean ground beef, along with a salad. Snacks might be pretzels, raisins, and fruit.

Section 11.3

Fueling the Active Individual

Excerpted from "Nutrition and Physical Activity: Fueling the Active Individual," by Melinda M. Manore, Ph.D., R.D., from the March 2004 issue (Series 5, No. 1) of *Research Digest*, a publication of the President's Council on Physical Fitness and Sports. For a complete listing of references, see http://www.fitness.gov.

Introduction

There is no doubt that the type, amount, composition, and timing of food intake can dramatically affect exercise performance, recovery from exercise, body weight and composition, and health. When exercise or physical work increases to more than 1 hour per day, the importance of adequate energy and nutrient intakes becomes more critical. As the American public becomes more concerned with health and health issues, the interest in nutrition and physical activity has increased. This interest in health has also heightened the sale of supplements, herbal preparations, and weight-loss products, all aimed at improving health, preventing or curing disease, improving sport performance, and changing body composition and weight. Sorting through this supplement soup is difficult because supplement manufacturers frequently make unsubstantiated claims about their products, leaving the consumer to sort the fact from the fiction. As stated in the 2000 Position Statement on Nutrition and Athletic Performance, published by the American Dietetic Association (ADA), Dietitians of Canada, and the American College of Sports Medicine (ACSM), any active individual "who wants to optimize health and exercise performance needs to follow good nutrition and hydration practices, use supplements and ergogenic aids carefully, minimize severe weight loss practices, and eat a variety of foods in adequate amounts."

Recently, the Food and Nutrition Board (FNB) of the Institute of Medicine (IOM) published new dietary reference intake (DRIs) for energy and macronutrients (protein, fat, and carbohydrate). They have also published new DRIs for micronutrients (vitamins and minerals) and related compounds. These DRIs are a set of reference values for

83

energy and specific nutrients designed to be used as guidelines for making dietary recommendations to individuals or groups of individuals. For the first time, the specific needs of active individuals were considered for energy and some nutrients. The dietary recommendations summarized in this chapter are based on extensive research in the area of nutrition and physical activity, and four current national and international publications related to the nutritional needs of active individuals. These four publications are the Position Statement on Nutrition and Athletic Performance mentioned above, the IOM's report for energy, macronutrients, the 2003 International Olympic Committee's (IOC) Consensus Statement on Sport Nutrition, and the accompanying research articles recently published in the *Journal of Sport Science* in 2004. These recommendations are general in nature, since energy and nutrient needs can vary greatly depending on the age, gender, exercise training intensity and duration, health issues, and the sport in which one participates. This chapter will address the current energy, macronutrient and fluid needs of active individuals, while briefly addressing micronutrients and supplements and specific nutrition and fluid recommendations for before, during, and after exercise.

Energy Needs

Active individuals need more energy (calories) each day than their sedentary counterparts—assuming individuals are the same age, body size, and participate in similar non-physically active daily activities. Exercise requires energy to fuel and repair the muscles, thus, meeting one's energy needs to maintain body weight should be a priority for any athlete or active individual. Energy balance is achieved when the energy consumed (sum of energy from food, supplements, and fluids) equals energy expenditure (sum of all the energy expended by the body in movement or to maintain body functions). Knowing whether one is in energy balance is simple: weight is maintained. If energy intake does not cover the costs of energy expenditure, then weight and muscle mass are lost, and the ability to perform strenuous exercise typically declines. Although weight loss is the goal of many Americans, weight loss in an active individual who is currently at a healthy body weight can decrease exercise performance and the health benefits associated with exercise training. When energy intake is restricted, fat and muscle mass will be utilized for energy to fuel the body, and the loss of muscle mass will result in the loss of strength and endurance. Additionally, chronically low energy intake usually results in poor nutrient intakes, including carbohydrate, protein, vitamins, and minerals.

84

Exactly how much energy an active individual needs each day will depend on a number of factors, including age, gender, body size, level and intensity of physical activity, and activities of daily living. The Food and Nutrition Board of the IOM reviewed the energy needs of active and very active individuals and provided some general recommendations based on age and body size. In general, active individuals walk between ~6–10 miles per day, while very active individuals walk greater than 10 miles per day at 2–4 mph. For example, for a 30-year old male weighing 72.2 kg (160 pounds) and having a body mass index (BMI) of 24.99 (kg per m^2), the estimated energy needs are 2,959 and 3,434 kcal per day for active and very active individuals, respectively. For a 30-year old women weighing 68 kg (150 pounds) and having a BMI of 24.99 (kg per m^2), the estimated energy needs are 2,477 and 2,807 kcal per day for active and very active individuals, respectively. Thus, the first goal of an active individual is to maintain adequate energy intake to assure that a healthy body weight is maintained. Although this seems like a simple task, there are many active individuals who find this difficult to do. For these individuals, a dietary plan that assures meals and snacks are not skipped will improve energy intake and help maintain weight. Finally, energy needs typically decrease with age, so even if activity levels do not change, the amount of energy required to maintain body weight will decrease. For this reason, body weight typically increases with age, even if activity levels remain constant.

Eating to Achieve or Maintain a Healthy Body Weight and Body Composition

Although active individuals typically have body weights that are within normal ranges for their height (BMI 19–25 kg per m^2), it is not unusual for them to want to change their body weight (e.g., either increase or decrease) to meet the demands of their sport or their own perception of an "ideal weight." Weight change should be accomplished slowly during a period when the individual is not participating in competitive events. If weight gain is desired, this can be accomplished by adding ~500–1000 kcal per day into the diet per day, while participating in strength training exercises to assure that the extra energy consumed is contributing to muscle mass and not fat gain. Increases in muscle mass usually occur slowly and depend on a number of factors, including one's genetic makeup, degree of positive energy balance that has occurred, amount of rest received, and the type of exercise training program being used.

Any diet for weight loss should result in a gradual decrease in weight (~1–2 pound per week or 0.5–1.0 kg per week) and maximize fat loss, while preserving lean tissues. If energy restriction is too severe, the nutritional quality of the diet is compromised, lean tissue is lost, and the ability to exercise decreases. In addition, severe energy restriction can lead to preoccupation with food, loss of motivation, and the inability to stay on the diet. In order to remain physically active while dieting, the diet needs to provide adequate carbohydrate for glycogen replacement and enough protein for the maintenance and repair of lean tissue. For these reasons, experts do not recommend fad diets that restrict energy too severely (typically less than 1800 kcal per day for women; less than 2000 kcal per day for men) or eliminate food groups (e.g., little or no carbohydrate; restricted to eating only certain foods) for active individuals.

Before beginning a weight-loss diet, an active individual needs to identify what constitutes a realistic healthy body weight for his or her activity level. This decision should be made based on past dieting experiences, type of activity engaged in, the social setting around work and home, genetics (family size and shape), health risk factors, and psychological issues. A healthy weight is one that can be realistically maintained, allows for positive advances in exercise performance, minimizes the risk of injury or illness, is consistent with long-term good health, and reduces the risk factors for chronic disease. If an unrealistic weight goal is set, there is a high probability of failure, which has a number of emotional and psychological outcomes. Unfortunately, failure to meet weight-loss goals in some sports can result in severe consequences, such as being cut from the team, restricted participation, or elimination from competition. These situations can result in active individuals chronically dieting to maintain a lower than healthy body weight, which can lead to disordered eating and in severe cases a clinical eating disorder.

Dieting for weight loss in active women and girls can be especially problematic, especially if weight is already within medical norms. Low energy intake combined with high energy output contributes to the development of menstrual dysfunction in women, which is characterized by a significant decrease in reproductive hormones and disruption of the normal menstrual cycle. The decrease in reproductive hormones, especially estrogen, can lead to loss of (or failure to gain) bone mass in young female athletes and active adult women. This pattern of low energy intake can put them at risk for one or more of the disorders in the female athlete triad (amenorrhea, disordered eating, osteoporosis).

Macronutrient Requirements for Exercise

Carbohydrate, protein, and fat are important nutrients for active individuals, but the amounts of these macronutrients needed will depend on an individual's exercise intensity, duration and frequency, the type of exercise engaged in, and their health, body size, age, and gender. Macronutrient recommendations for those engaged in daily physical activity are given below and in Table 11.1.

Carbohydrate Needs

The mix of fuel (protein, fat, carbohydrate) burned during exercise depends primarily on the intensity and duration of the exercise performed, one's level of fitness, and prior nutritional status. All other conditions being equal, as exercise intensity increases the use of carbohydrate for energy will also increase. The duration of exercise also changes substrates use. As duration of exercise increases (e.g., from

Table 11.1. Dietary Reference Intakes (DRIs) for Macronutrients and Recommendations for Active Individuals

Nutrient	New Guidelines (2002)	Old Guidelines (1989)	Guidelines for Active Individuals
Carbohydrate	45–65% of total energy	greater than or equal to 50% of total energy	The amount of carbohydrate required for moderate intensity exercise is 5–7 g per kg body weight; 7–12 g per kg body weight for high intensity endurance activities.
Protein	10–35% of total energy; 0.8 g per kg of body weight	10–15% of total energy; 0.8 g per kg of body weight	Protein requirements are typically higher in active individuals. Recommendations range from 1.2–1.7 g of protein per kg body weight. This level of protein typically represents 15% of total energy.
Fat	20–35% of total energy	less than or equal to 30% of total energy	Fat intakes between 20–35%. Carbohydrate and protein needs should met first.

60 to 120 min), muscle glycogen becomes depleted, causing the body to draw on circulating blood glucose as a source of carbohydrate. If blood glucose cannot be maintained within physiological range during exercise, the ability to perform intense exercise will decrease. Fat can be used as a source of energy over a wide range of exercise intensities; however, the proportion of energy contributed by fat decreases as exercise intensity increases. In these circumstances, carbohydrate becomes the dominant fuel source while the contribution from fat decreases. Protein can also be used for energy at rest and during exercise; however, in well-fed individuals it probably provides less than 5% of the energy expended. As the duration of exercise increases, the energy contribution of protein may increase to maintain blood glucose. The amount of carbohydrate, fat, and protein used for energy during exercise will also depend on when exercise occurs relative to the last meal and the level exercise intensity performed. For example, when subjects are tested after an overnight fast, the contribution of fat to the energy pool is greater than when these same individuals are tested after a meal. In both situations, the exercise performed was moderate (~50% of VO_2max). For higher intensity exercise (greater than 65% of VO_2max) neither prior feeding nor exercise training significantly altered fuel used.

Currently there is no research available suggesting that active healthy individuals need significantly different proportions of energy from carbohydrate, protein and fat than those proposed in the 2002 IOM report (45–65% of energy from carbohydrate, 10–35% of energy from protein, and 20–35% of energy from fat). This report determined an Acceptable Macronutrient Distribution Range (AMDR), which is defined as a range of intakes that are associated with reduced risk of chronic disease, while providing adequate intakes of essential nutrients. These new AMDRs for the macronutrients are very broad and allow for developing flexible dietary recommendations across a variety of activity levels, body sizes, food preferences, and health-related dietary issues.

Although high carbohydrate diets (greater than 65% of energy intake) have been advocated in the past for endurance athletes, the use of proportions in making dietary recommendations for active individuals is generally not practical. It is more helpful to make macronutrient recommendations for protein and carbohydrate based on body size (e.g., gram per kg body weight). For example, if energy intake is 5,000 kcal per day for an active adult male, even a diet containing 50% of the energy from carbohydrate will provide 625 g of carbohydrate. This level of carbohydrate is adequate to maintain muscle glycogen stores for a highly active individual. Similarly, if protein intakes in this diet were as low as 10% of energy intake, absolute protein intake (125 g per day; 1.8 g per kg) would easily meet the protein recommendations for athletes (1.2–1.7 g per day or 84–119 g in a 70 kg body weight person, see protein section below). Conversely, when energy intakes are low (less than or equal to 1800 kcal per day) even a diet providing 60% of the energy from carbohydrate may not maintain optimal carbohydrate stores (less than or equal to 5 g per kg in a 55-kg body weight person) in an active individual. In general, it is recommended that active individuals doing moderate duration/low-intensity physical activity consume 5–7 g per kg of carbohydrate per day. If exercise is intense and heavy endurance training is being done, then 7–12 g per kg of carbohydrate per day is recommended. Thus, dietary carbohydrate recommendations for the active individual will depend on the level of physical activity being performed.

Protein Needs

Active individuals often think that they need to consume high protein diets to cover the building and repair of their muscle tissue. Although not reflected in the new IOM report on energy and macronutrients, exercise physiologists and sport nutritionists generally agree that exercise increases the need for protein (g per kg body weight). Exercise may increase the need for protein in three ways: 1) increased need for protein to repair exercise-induced damage to muscle fibers; 2) support gains in muscle mass that occur with exercise; and 3) provide energy source during exercise. How much additional protein is needed may depend on the type of exercise performed (endurance vs. resistance), the intensity and duration of the activity, body composition (e.g., kg of lean tissue mass), and whether weight loss is being attempted.

Researchers examined the research on the protein needs of athletes and recommends 1.2–1.4 g per kg body weight per day for individuals participating in endurance sports and 1.6–1.8 g per kg body weight per day for those involved in resistance or speed exercise. The higher protein recommendations for individuals participating in resistance training allows for the accumulation and maintenance of lean tissue. Although these recommendations are higher than the current RDA for protein (0.8 g per kg body weight), they do not typically exceed the habitual protein intakes of most active individuals. As illustrated earlier, if energy intake is 3,000–5,000 kcal per day for a 70 kg active male, a diet providing 10% of energy from protein would contain 75–115 g of protein per day or 1.1–1.8 g per kg of protein for this individual. In reality, this individual would probably consume closer to 15% of energy from protein. Thus, there is usually little need to recommend that active individuals consume more protein. Increasing protein intakes beyond the recommended level is unlikely to result in additional increases in lean tissue, since there is a limit to the rate at which protein tissue can be accrued. Those individuals at greatest risk for low protein intakes are active individuals who restrict energy intake for weight loss or follow vegetarian diets, especially active women.

Fat Needs

Over the years the amounts and types of fat recommended for good health have changed, which is frustrating and confusing for the consumer. Dietary recommendations for active individuals have typically focused on getting adequate intakes of carbohydrate and protein, and keeping fat intake to 25–30% of energy intake, which is within the new AMDR for fat (20–35% of energy). Although fat is seen by many individuals as something to avoid, fat is a necessary component of a normal diet. Fat provides energy and essential elements for cell membranes, and is associated with the intakes of the fat-soluble vitamins E, A, and D. However, the type of fat consumed is important since the long-term negative effects of high saturated fat diets on health are well known. In addition, low fat intakes (less than 15–17% of energy) are generally not recommended for active individuals, since they are reported to decrease energy and nutrient intakes and exercise performance. Currently, there appear to be no health benefits to consuming a very low fat diet (less than 15% of energy from fat) in healthy individuals compared to more moderate fat intakes. Thus, unless there is some medical reason for restricting fat, dietary intakes should be within the AMDR for fat.

The new IOM report for macronutrients also gives recommendations for the types of fat to be included in the diet. These recommendations apply to all individuals, regardless of activity level. Diets should be low in saturated and trans fats, while providing adequate amounts of essential fatty acids (linoleic and a-linolenic acids). The essential fatty acids are required to make a number of potent biological compounds within the body that help regulate blood clotting, blood pressure, heart rate, and the immune response. Linoleic acid is found in vegetable and nut oils (e.g., sunflower, safflower, corn, soy, peanut oil) and it is recommended that adult men consume 14–17 g per day and adult women consume 11–12 g per day. Americans appear to get adequate amounts of linoleic acid, due to the high amount of salad dressings, salad oils, margarine, and mayonnaise-based foods they consume. The second essential fatty acid, a-linolenic acid, is found primarily in leafy green vegetables, walnuts, soy oil and foods, canola oil, and fish products and fish oils. Americans are most likely to have low intakes of this essential fatty acid. The recommended intakes for a-linolenic is 1.6 g per day for adult men and 1.1 g per day for adult women. If active individuals consume very low fat diets (less than 15% of energy), getting adequate amounts of the essential fatty acids can be a problem. Research has also examined the impact of high fat diets (40–70% of energy intake) on fat utilization during exercise and athletic performance. It was hypothesized that consuming a high fat diet would enhance fat oxidation and utilization during exercise. Unfortunately, most individuals cannot tolerate these high fat levels for long, nor can health professionals recommend them for long-term health; thus, there is little support for recommending these diets to active individuals.

Hydration

It is well-documented in the research literature that exercise performance is optimal when athletes and active individuals maintain fluid balance during exercise. Conversely, exercise performance is impaired with progressive dehydration, which can eventually lead to potentially life-threatening heat injury if action is not taken. Thus, it is imperative that all active individuals attempt to remain well hydrated. The ACSM and the National Athletic Trainers' Association (NATA) have position statements that provide comprehensive overviews of the research and recommendations on maintaining hydration before, during, and after exercise. Active individuals exercising in special environmental conditions (heat, cold, altitude) need to take extra precautions to remain hydrated.

Maintaining Water and Electrolyte Balance

Maintaining fluid and electrolyte balance means that active individuals need to replace the water and electrolytes lost in sweat. This requires that active individuals, regardless of age, strive to hydrate well before exercise, drink fluids throughout exercise, and rehydrate once exercise is over. As outlined by ACSM and NATA, generous amounts of fluids should be consumed 24-h before exercise and 400–600 mL of fluid should be consumed 2-h before exercise. During exercise, active individuals should attempt to drink ~150–350 mL (6–12 oz) of fluid every 15–20 minutes. If exercise is of long duration (usually greater than 1 h) or occurs in a hot environment, sport drinks containing carbohydrate and sodium should be used. When exercise is over most active individuals have some level of dehydration. Drinking enough fluids to cover 150% of the weight lost during exercise may be needed to replace fluids lost in sweat and urine. This fluid can be part of the post-exercise meal, which should also contain sodium, either in the food or beverages, since diuresis occurs when only plain water is ingested. Sodium helps the rehydration process by maintaining plasma osmolality and the desire to drink.

Micronutrient Requirements for Exercise

Micronutrients, such as vitamins and minerals, play an important role in maintaining the health of the active individual. They are involved in energy production, synthesis of hemoglobin for the production of red blood cells, maintenance of bone health, adequate immune function, building and repair of muscle tissue, and the protection of body tissues from oxidative damage. There are a number of ways that exercise is hypothesized to alter the need for vitamins and minerals. For example, exercise stresses many of the metabolic pathways in which these micronutrients are required, while exercise training may cause muscle biochemical adaptations that increase micronutrient needs. Exercise may also increase the turnover and loss of micronutrients from the body, and the need for these micronutrients to repair and maintain the higher lean tissue mass of the active individual. It is assumed that the current DRIs are appropriate for athletes and active individuals, unless otherwise stated. Those individuals at the greatest risk of poor micronutrient status are those individuals who restrict energy intake or use severe weight loss practices, eliminate one or more of the food groups from their diet, or who restrict or eliminate one or more food groups from the diet (e.g., no or little carbohydrate or fat). Individuals participating in these types of eating behaviors may need to use a multivitamin or mineral supplement to improve overall micronutrient status.

Eating for Good Health and Exercise Performance

Compared to their sedentary counterparts, the diet of an active individual requires additional fluid to cover sweat losses, energy to fuel physical activity, protein for building and repair of muscle tissue, and carbohydrate for the replacement of muscle glycogen. In some cases the need for other nutrients also increases (e.g., B-complex, antioxidant vitamins, iron). As more energy is consumed to cover the cost of exercise, it is assumed the intake of these other nutrients will also increase. Thus, as energy requirements increase, the first goal should be to consume nutrient-dense carbohydrate-based food groups (e.g., whole grain breads and cereals, vegetables, and fruits) and lean protein sources (e.g., lean meats, fish, poultry, dairy, legumes). The aim should be to increase energy intake to maintain weight using nutrient-dense foods that will also provide vitamins and minerals, instead of meeting additional energy needs with high-fat and sugar foods. This is especially true for active individuals who are small (low BMIs) or have lower energy needs.

Timing of food intake is also important for active individuals. Eating sensibly before exercise assures that there is enough energy to fuel the exercise event, while eating after exercise will help refuel the body. We know that being well fed before exercise can improve performance, and that the post-exercise meal helps replace muscle glycogen and repair muscle tissue damage. Depending on the sport, eating or using a sport drink during exercise can also improve performance and delay time to fatigue. Active individuals, who exercise more than once per day, may need to time eating around exercise, use sport drinks during exercise, and make sure that meals are not skipped.

Supplements

Nearly 25% of Americans use dietary supplements daily and ~35–40% use them occasionally. For individuals engaged in physical activity, the estimates are as high as 50–100%. This high use of supplements has created a 14 billion-dollar industry, which constantly bombards consumers with advertisements for their products. It is not surprising that the American consumer is very confused about whether they should use vitamin or mineral supplements, how much to take, and which product to buy. Unfortunately, there is no governmental body that regulates dietary supplements and verifies that what is on the label is also in the bottle. In addition, there is little or no regulation as to the claims made on the bottle. The Dietary Supplement Health and Education Act of 1994 allows supplement manufacturers to make claims regarding the effect of products on the structure and function of the body, as long as they do not claim to "diagnose, mitigate, treat, cure, or prevent" a specific disease. This allows supplement manufacturers to make a "broad" range of health statements for their supplements, which may or may not be accurate and substantiated by clinical research. Thus, the consumer is left with the task of evaluating the product and the claims of the product.

How does the consumer know which supplement to buy or recommend? Listed below are some general guidelines an active individual can follow when selecting a supplement.

- Use a multivitamin/mineral supplement that contains micronutrients in amounts close to recommended amounts (e.g., one-a-day type supplements). This approach helps avoid nutrient-nutrient interactions or reaching toxic levels of any one nutrient. However, most multivitamin/mineral supplements do not contain the recommended amount for some minerals, such as calcium. For individuals who avoid or cannot use dairy products, a major source of calcium in the U.S. diet, calcium supplements or calcium-fortified foods may need to be used. Look for supplements that provide ~50–100% of the Daily Value (DV) or Recommended Dietary Allowance (RDA), and avoid those that provide many times the recommended amounts.

- Use individual supplements sparingly unless warranted due to a health problem or a lack of the nutrient in the diet. Individuals should avoid the 5–10 pill/day routine. Using large doses of vitamins and minerals will increase the risk of nutrient-nutrient interactions and may lead to toxic effects. Some supplements can also interfere with prescription and over-the-counter medications, so keeping closer to the RDA or DV will help avoid these pitfalls.

- Select supplements from a reputable, well-established company and look for supplements that carry the U.S. Pharmacopoeia (USP) or National Formulary (NF) notation. These notations mean that the manufacturer has voluntarily complied with a strict set of standards regarding product purity, strength, packaging, labeling and weight variation. The Food and Drug Association (FDA) does not inspect vitamin and mineral supplements, so using supplements from a reputable company will help assure that you get what is listed on the label.

Chapter 12

Water Intake and Exercise

Chapter Contents

Section 12.1

How Much Water Should You Drink during Exercise?

"American College of Sports Medicine Clarifies Indicators for Fluid Replacement," American College of Sports Medicine, News Release, February 12, 2004.

Avoid Relying on Thirst Alone to Gauge Body's Fluid Replacement Needs

The American College of Sports Medicine (ACSM) is pleased the recent Institute of Medicine (IOM) report, which set dietary intake levels for water, salt, and potassium for the maintenance of health and well-being, also indicates athletes and other active people have higher fluid replacement needs. While much of the report focuses on daily fluid requirements for the public, ACSM's experts note that thirst is not the best indicator of how much these individuals should replace in terms of fluid and sodium losses following prolonged physical activity and/or heat exposure. Fluids before, during, and after exercise are an important part of regulating body temperature and replacing body fluids lost through sweat.

"This report is important because it debunks some common misconceptions about fluid and electrolyte intake. However, it is important to clarify the report's use of the phrase 'on a daily basis.' Daily fluid intake is governed mostly by behavioral factors, such as eating meals or even walking past a water fountain. Thirst is important during and after physical activity, especially in hot environmental conditions," said ACSM President W. Larry Kenney, Ph.D. "However, the clear and important health message should be that thirst alone is not the best indicator of dehydration or the body's fluid needs."

Dehydration resulting from the failure to adequately replace fluids during exercise can lead to impaired heat dissipation, which can elevate body core temperature and increase strain on the cardiovascular system. Dehydration is a potential threat to all athletes, especially those who are not acclimatized for strenuous activity in hot environments.

To minimize the potential for heat exhaustion and other forms of heat illness, Kenney and other ACSM experts recommend water losses due to sweating during exercise be replaced at a rate close to or equal to the sweating rate. This can be accomplished by athletes weighing themselves before and after the exercise bout. This recommendation is based on sound scientific data and clinical experience dealing with athletes suffering from heat-related illness.

The report also makes mention of active people avoiding excessive fluid consumption which may, in the extreme, result in hyponatremia. While hyponatremia is a rare occurrence, it is a dangerous condition that may arise when athletes drink too much water, diluting the body's sodium levels. It is most often seen in prolonged endurance athletes, such as those participating in marathons and triathlons. ACSM's current hydration guidelines address this threat in addition to the more commonly occurring dehydration problem, and provide recommendations that can help prevent both health hazards for the athlete. Generally, persons participating in prolonged or strenuous physical activity (including both exercise and occupational settings) should continue to heed current hydration guidelines. Water and sports drinks are not dangerous to athletes when consumed as recommended—in volumes approximating sweat losses. Water in particular quenches the sensation of thirst before body fluid replacement is achieved, so thirst should not be the only determinant of how much fluid is consumed under such conditions.

"Relying on thirst to determine an active individual's fluid replacement needs is inadequate, especially so in older exercisers. As we age, thirst becomes an even poorer indicator of the body's fluid needs," said Kenney.

In a similar vein, the IOM report's guidance on chronic sodium intake should not be confused with recommendations that athletes liberally salt their food and consume sports drinks when acclimatizing to, or exercising in, hot conditions. While cutting back on overall sodium in the diet is sound advice for the majority of the public, athletes have a special need to replenish lost sodium stores in the short term.

Section 12.2

Guidance for Athletes on Preventing Hyponatremia and Dehydration

"American College of Sports Medicine Offers Guidance to Athletes on Preventing Hyponatremia and Dehydration during Upcoming Races," American College of Sports Medicine, News Release, July 26, 2005.

A report, which appears in the June [2005] issue of *Current Sports Medicine Reports*, addresses key issues and reviews research findings on the topics of hyponatremia and dehydration for endurance athletes—a subject that has generated significant media attention this year. The published report, ACSM Roundtable Series: Hydration and Physical Activity, is based on findings from an international panel of hydration experts who conducted an evidence-based analysis on numerous past published studies.

Based on the findings of this report as well as previously published statements, ACSM is issuing the following guidelines to the endurance community.

Work to Minimize Risk of Both Hyponatremia and Dehydration

Hyponatremia is a dangerous condition that occurs when an athlete consumes too much fluid (either water or other fluids), diluting the body's sodium levels. Despite heightened media attention to this issue this year, the international ACSM panel concluded that exertional hyponatremia is relatively rare and appears to occur most often in slow-paced athletes (running events lasting longer than four hours or triathlons lasting longer than 9-13 hours). The incidence of symptomatic hyponatremia during endurance exercise events such as the marathon and triathlon is generally low (probably less than one in 1,000 finishers).

The panel also concluded that especially during hot-weather training, dehydration occurs more frequently and has severe consequences, increasing the risk of heat exhaustion and heat stroke during and immediately after activity. Fluid deficits in athletes can affect physical and mental performance, increase cardiovascular strain and decrease heat tolerance.

"While hyponatremia has gotten more attention lately, far more athletes are affected by dehydration," said W. Larry Kenney, Ph.D., FACSM, past president of ACSM and co-chair of the ACSM Roundtable. "However, there are dangers associated with both extremes of behavior—severe under-drinking and severe over-drinking. Not drinking at all is not a safe option for preventing hyponatremia. The key is 'drinking intelligently, not drinking maximally'," he added.

Drink to Match Fluid Loss and on a Schedule

The experts concluded that appropriate fluid intake (before, during and after exercise) is important to help regulate body temperature and replace fluids lost in sweat. Since fluid and electrolyte needs are widely variable based on the athlete's genetics and environmental conditions, athletes should know their body's hourly sweat rate (weight lost during exercise per hour + fluid consumed during exercise per hour = hourly sweat rate) and aim to replace the total amount lost during that time.

According to the previously published ACSM Exercise and Fluid Replacement Position Stand, athletes are encouraged to drink early and at regular intervals rather than rapid fluid replacement. It is noted that perception of thirst, an imperfect index of the magnitude of fluid deficit, cannot be used to provide complete restoration of water lost by sweating.

As such, individuals participating in prolonged intense exercise must rely on strategies such as monitoring body weight loss and ingesting volumes of fluid during exercise at a rate equal to that lost from sweating, to ensure complete fluid replacement. Drinking over a set period of time is more effective for complete rehydration as rapid replacement of fluid stimulates increased urine production, reducing body water retention. If athletes are not sweating heavily (such as slow runners) and are not thirsty, then their fluid replacement needs are probably modest.

Consume Salty Foods and Beverages

According to the published roundtable report, research shows foods and beverages with sodium help promote fluid retention and stimulate fluid intake. The report also notes that athletes performing prolonged exercise should ingest snacks or fluids containing sodium to help off-set the loss of salt in sweat, in an effort to prevent hyponatremia.

Chapter 13

All about Sports Supplements

You may read claims for sports supplements that say they can add muscle mass, make muscles work more efficiently, or improve athletic performance. Although some supplements may have these short-term benefits, they may also cause short- and long-term health problems. For many of these drugs, researchers don't yet know what the long-term risks are of these drugs. Read more about some of these drugs and the known and unknown risks of their use.

Anabolic Steroids

These are manmade drugs that mimic male sex hormones. Steroids can help the body make muscle tissue, reduce muscle damage after exercising, and enhance male features. In the past, steroids were only used only by athletes, but in recent years, steroid use by non-athletes has become more common. Now, an increasing number of anabolic steroid users simply want to "look good"—which to many people means being big and muscular. Although these drugs have medical uses, such as treating delayed puberty, some types of impotence, and wasting of the body caused by HIV infection or other diseases, when abused, anabolic steroids have these serious health consequences:

"Sports Supplements" is from the National Women's Health Information Center (NWHIC), www.4woman.gov, part of the U.S. Department of Health and Human Services, June 2005.

- Deepening of the voice, enlargement of the clitoris, hair loss, facial hair growth, and hormone problems in women
- Shrinkage of the testicles, problems with erections, lower sperm count, and increased breast size in men
- Mood swings and aggression
- Change in hair growth patterns
- Acne
- Change in a person's voice
- Tears in the muscles and tendons
- In adolescence, they can cause bones to stop growing
- Raised cholesterol levels
- Cardiovascular, kidney, and liver disease
- Clotting disorders
- Tumor growth
- Cancer
- Increased risk of HIV and hepatitis (from sharing needles)
- Suicidal depression

Creatine

Creatine is a substance made by the liver and also found in certain foods, like meat. It helps release energy into the muscles. Creatine may help athletes enhance their performance by providing quick energy during high-intensity exercise, like sprinting. It can also help athletes recover faster after these activities. However, creatine may cause these health problems:

- Diarrhea
- Nausea and vomiting
- Stomach and muscle cramps
- Weight gain
- Water retention
- Dehydration
- Kidney, muscle, heart, and liver damage

Safety information about taking creatine is lacking, and the long-term effects of creatine use are unknown. There is no government regulation of creatine. So there is no guarantee about the purity or safety of this drug.

Ephedra (Ma Huang)

Ephedra, also called Ma Huang, is a naturally occurring substance derived from botanicals. It is a stimulant has been promoted for boosting sports performance and energy. However, ephedra can cause rapid or irregular heartbeats, high blood pressure, nerve damage, stroke, and memory loss. It has also caused death. In addition, using ephedra with caffeine, even drinking soda, can worsen its medical risks.

It may be particularly dangerous for kids and adolescents, since ephedra can impair the body's ability to cool itself, and raise the risk for heat-related sickness during exercise. Young people don't sweat as much as adults, so they don't have the same ability to adjust their body temperatures while exercising.

On April 12, 2004, the Food and Drug Administration (FDA) banned the sale of dietary supplements containing ephedra. On April 14, 2005, a federal judge ruled against the FDA ban of ephedra. The judge said that ephedra is wrongly regulated by the FDA, because it is treated as a drug and not a food. With all drugs, the FDA requires the manufacturer prove the drug is safe. For other dietary supplements, which are regulated as foods, the FDA has to prove the drugs are harmful in order to ban them. Now, the FDA can't stop the manufacturer from selling supplements containing ephedra.

Caffeine

Caffeine is a stimulant found in soda, coffee, chocolate, and other foods. There are also pills and suppositories that are made of pure caffeine. Reports have suggested that a higher dose of pure caffeine (not from a drink) before exercising improves performance during prolonged endurance exercise and short-term intense exercise.

However, most studies of caffeine have taken place in laboratories, and not real-life sports events. Side effects of caffeine include anxiety, jitters, problems focusing, stomach problems, trouble sleeping, irritability, and in high doses, heart arrhythmias and mild hallucinations.

Vitamins and Minerals

Vitamin and mineral deficiencies among athletes are uncommon. For these athletes, there is no benefit to taking vitamin and mineral supplements—it will not improve athletic performance. Only athletes with a deficiency in a certain vitamin or mineral will benefit from taking a supplement. Athletes without a vitamin or mineral deficiency who take certain supplements may experience harmful health effects.

Protein and Amino Acids

Athletes can meet their protein requirements through diet alone, without taking protein or amino acid supplements. Foods such as fish, meat, eggs, and milk are rich in essential amino acids. Taking massive single doses of protein to accelerate muscle growth doesn't work. Foods such as milk, yogurt, or an energy bar with at least 10 grams of protein can help an athlete repair muscles after a hard workout. Excessive amounts of protein could cause dehydration, stomach upset, and kidney problems.

Androstenedione (Andro)

Andro is a hormone that naturally occurs in the body. The body converts it to testosterone, which builds muscles and creates male features. Athletes use andro in strength supports, like football. However, if the body has too much androgen, it shuts down its own production of testosterone. Also, it carries many of the same risks as steroids, including stunted growth in adolescents, high blood pressure, heart and liver problems, excess body hair, and shrunken testicles.

In March 2004, the FDA sent warning letters to 23 firms to stop their distribution of dietary supplements that contain androstenedione. FDA will determine whether further actions are necessary if firms refuse to stop distribution of these products. In addition, Congressional leaders are pursuing legislation to classify andro-containing products as a controlled substance. This legislation would enable the U.S. Drug Enforcement Agency (DEA) to regulate these types of products as anabolic steroids under the Controlled Substances Act.

Facts about Supplements

- **Supplements and drugs can interact.** For example, ginseng can increase the stimulant effects of caffeine, found in coffee, tea, and soda. It can also lower blood sugar levels, creating the possibility of problems when used with diabetes drugs.

- **"Natural" does not always mean safe or without harmful effects.** Some supplements come from natural sources but may not be safe. Supplements, like ephedra, come from natural sources but can cause medical problems.

- **The FDA regulates supplements as foods rather than drugs.** In general, the laws about putting foods (including supplements) on the market and keeping them on the market are less strict than the laws for drugs:
  - Research studies in people to prove a supplement's safety are not required before the supplement is marketed.
  - The manufacturer does not have to prove that the supplement is effective.
  - The manufacturer does not have to prove supplement quality.
  - If the FDA finds a supplement to be unsafe once it is on the market, only then can it take action against the manufacturer and/or distributor, by issuing a warning or requiring the product to be removed from the marketplace.

- **What's in the bottle doesn't always match what's on the label.** A supplement might not contain the ingredients on the label; contain higher or lower amounts of the active ingredient; or be contaminated.

If you decide to take supplements, follow these tips from the Gatorade Sports Science Institute on how to select supplements. The supplement should:

- **carry USP (United States Pharmacopeia) on the label.** USP means that the supplement passes tests for how well it dissolves, disintegration, potency, and purity. The manufacturer should also be able to demonstrate that the product passes tests for content potency, purity, and uniformity.

- **be made by nationally known food and drug manufacturers.** Reputable manufacturers follow strict quality control procedures. If the company does not answer questions or address complaints, do not use their product.

- **be supported by research.** Reputable companies should provide research from peer-reviewed journals to support claims.

- **make accurate and appropriate claims.** If statements are unclear or the label makes preposterous claims, it is unlikely the company follows good quality control procedures. If the claims sound too good to be true, be wary.

- **recommend that you talk with a doctor or pharmacist about dietary supplements.** These products may interact with prescription and over-the-counter medications as well as other supplements and cause potentially serious adverse effects. Read the product label, follow all directions, and heed warnings.

Chapter 14

The Health Risks of Anabolic Steroids

Anabolic-androgenic steroids are manmade substances related to male sex hormones. "Anabolic" refers to muscle building, and "androgenic" refers to increased masculine characteristics. "Steroids" refers to the class of drugs. These drugs are available legally only by prescription to treat conditions that occur when the body produces abnormally low amounts of testosterone, such as delayed puberty and some types of impotence. They are also prescribed to treat body wasting in patients with AIDS and other diseases that result in loss of lean muscle mass. Abuse of anabolic steroids, however, can lead to serious health problems, some of which are irreversible.

Today, athletes and others abuse anabolic steroids to enhance performance and also to improve physical appearance. Anabolic steroids are taken orally or injected, typically in cycles of weeks or months (referred to as "cycling"), rather than continuously. Cycling involves taking multiple doses of steroids over a specific period of time, stopping for a period, and starting again. In addition, users often combine several different types of steroids to maximize their effectiveness while minimizing negative effects (referred to as "stacking").

Health Hazards

The major side effects from abusing anabolic steroids can include liver tumors and cancer, jaundice (yellowish pigmentation of skin,

The InfoFacts publication "Steroids (Anabolic-Androgenic)" is from the National Institute of Drug Abuse (NIDA, www.drugabuse.gov), March 2005.

tissues, and body fluids), fluid retention, high blood pressure, increases in LDL (bad cholesterol), and decreases in HDL (good cholesterol). Other side effects include kidney tumors, severe acne, and trembling. In addition, there are some gender-specific side effects:

- For men—shrinking of the testicles, reduced sperm count, infertility, baldness, development of breasts, increased risk for prostate cancer.

- For women—growth of facial hair, male-pattern baldness, changes in or cessation of the menstrual cycle, enlargement of the clitoris, deepened voice.

- For adolescents—growth halted prematurely through premature skeletal maturation and accelerated puberty changes. This means that adolescents risk remaining short for the remainder of their lives if they take anabolic steroids before the typical adolescent growth spurt.

In addition, people who inject anabolic steroids run the added risk of contracting or transmitting HIV/AIDS or hepatitis, which causes serious damage to the liver.

Scientific research also shows that aggression and other psychiatric side effects may result from abuse of anabolic steroids. Many users report feeling good about themselves while on anabolic steroids, but researchers report that extreme mood swings also can occur, including manic-like symptoms leading to violence. Depression often is seen when the drugs are stopped and may contribute to dependence on anabolic steroids. Researchers report also that users may suffer from paranoid jealousy, extreme irritability, delusions, and impaired judgment stemming from feelings of invincibility.[1]

Research also indicates that some users might turn to other drugs to alleviate some of the negative effects of anabolic steroids. For example, a study of 227 men admitted in 1999 to a private treatment center for dependence on heroin or other opioids found that 9.3 percent had abused anabolic steroids before trying any other illicit drug. Of these 9.3 percent, 86 percent first used opioids to counteract insomnia and irritability resulting from the anabolic steroids.[2]

Extent of Use

The Monitoring the Future (MTF) Survey annually assesses drug use among the Nation's 8th-, 10th-, and 12th-grade students. These data are from the 2004 Monitoring the Future Survey, funded by the

National Institute on Drug Abuse, National Institutes of Health, Department of Health and Human Services, and conducted by the University of Michigan's Institute for Social Research. The survey has tracked 12th-graders' illicit drug use and related attitudes since 1975; in 1991, 8th- and 10th-graders were added to the survey. The latest data are online at http://www.drugabuse.gov.

"Lifetime" refers to use at least once during a respondent's lifetime. "Annual" refers to an individual's drug use at least once during the year preceding their response to the survey. "30-day" refers to an individual's drug use at least once during the month preceding their response to the survey.

Annual use of anabolic steroids remained stable at under 1.5 percent for students in 8th, 10th, and 12th grades in the early 1990s, then started to rise. Peak rates of annual use occurred in 2002 for 12th graders (2.5 percent), in 2000 and 2002 for 10th graders (2.2 percent), and in 1999 and 2000 for 8th graders (1.7 percent). Eighth graders reported significant decreases in lifetime and annual steroid use in 2004, as well as a decrease in perceived availability of these drugs. A significant decrease in lifetime use was also measured among 10th graders for 2004.

Most anabolic steroids users are male, and among male students, past year use of these substances was reported by 1.3 percent of 8th graders, 2.3 percent of 10th graders, and 3.3 percent of 12th graders in 2004.

Table 14.1. Anabolic Steroid Use by Students from the Year 2004 Monitoring the Future Survey

	8th Graders	10th Graders	12th Graders
Lifetime	1.9%	2.4%	3.4%
Annual	1.1	1.5	2.5
30-day	0.5	0.8	1.6

References

1. Pope, H.G., and Katz, D. L. Affective and psychotic symptoms associated with anabolic steroid use. *American Journal of Psychiatry* 145(4):487–490, 1988.

2. The *New England Journal of Medicine* 320:1532, 2000.

Chapter 15

The Dangers of Androstenedione (Andro) Products

Federal health officials say a crackdown on companies that manufacture, market, or distribute products containing androstenedione, or andro, is necessary due to concerns about the safety of the substance. Widely marketed to athletes and bodybuilders, androstenedione has been advertised to promote muscle growth, improve muscular strength, reduce fat, and slow aging. But androstenedione acts like a steroid once it is metabolized by the body, and can pose similar kinds of health risks as steroids.

"Young people, athletes, and other consumers should steer clear of andro because there are serious, substantial concerns about its safety," said former Health and Human Services (HHS) Secretary Tommy G. Thompson said in announcing the crackdown. "Young people should understand that there are no shortcuts to a stronger body and that the best way to get faster and stronger is through good diet, nutrition, and exercise."

"Athletics benefit young people's health and give them a lesson in the value of hard work," added John P. Walters, director of the White House Office of National Drug Control Policy. "Androstenedione and other performance-enhancing drugs undercut these benefits by endangering our children's healthy development and teaching them that cheating is an acceptable component of pursuing excellence."

From "Crackdown on 'Andro' Products," published in the May-June 2004 issue of *FDA Consumer* magazine (www.fda.gov/fdac), U.S. Food and Drug Administration.

As part of the crackdown, the Food and Drug Administration sent letters in March 2004 to 23 companies, asking them to stop distributing products sold as dietary supplements that contain androstenedione and warning them that they could face enforcement actions if they do not take appropriate actions.

About 1 out of 40 high school seniors reported that they had used andro in the past year, according to the HHS 2002 Monitoring the Future survey, which tracks drug use among students. The survey, conducted by the National Institute on Drug Abuse, also found that about 1 out of 50 10th graders had taken andro during the previous year.

People produce androstenedione naturally during the making of testosterone and estrogen. When people consume androstenedione, it is converted to testosterone and estrogen. Scientific evidence shows that when androstenedione is taken over time and in sufficient quantities, it may increase the risk of serious and life-threatening diseases.

Potential long-term consequences of the use of androstenedione products in men include decreased testicle size, impotence, and the development of female characteristics such as breast enlargement. Women who use these products may develop male characteristics such as male pattern baldness, deepening of the voice, and increased facial hair. In addition, women also may develop abnormal menstrual cycles, abnormal menstrual bleeding, and blood clots. Androstenedione use also increases the risks for breast cancer and endometrial cancer in women. Children who use these products are at risk for puberty beginning earlier and bone growth stopping prematurely.

The U.S. Food and Drug Administration (FDA) considers dietary supplements that contain androstenedione to be adulterated under the Federal Food, Drug, and Cosmetic Act (FD&C Act). Supplements containing new dietary ingredients have to meet certain requirements, and because these requirements have not been met for androstenedione, supplements containing the ingredient cannot be marketed legally.

Under the FD&C Act, the FDA is also responsible for taking action against any unsafe dietary supplement product after it reaches the market. The FDA also informed firms that it is aware of no history of use or other information establishing that a dietary supplement containing androstenedione is safe.

The National Collegiate Athletic Association, the National Football League, and the International Olympic Committee have all banned the use of androstenedione. The American Academy of Pediatrics, the Endocrine Society, the American Medical Association, and other health professional groups have cautioned against the use of certain steroids and their precursors, like androstenedione, because of their potential long-term adverse health consequences.

The FDA will determine whether further actions are necessary if firms refuse to stop distribution of androstenedione products. Such actions could include seizing illegal products as well as pursuing injunctions or seeking criminal sanctions against people who violate the law.

Part Three

Exercise Basics

Chapter 16

Guidelines for Developing a Personal Exercise Program

Making a Commitment

You have taken the important first step on the path to physical fitness by seeking information. The next step is to decide that you are going to be physically fit. This information is designed to help you reach that decision and your goal.

The decision to carry out a physical fitness program cannot be taken lightly. It requires a lifelong commitment of time and effort. Exercise must become one of those things that you do without question, like bathing and brushing your teeth. Unless you are convinced of the benefits of fitness and the risks of unfitness, you will not succeed.

Patience is essential. Don't try to do too much too soon and don't quit before you have a chance to experience the rewards of improved fitness. You can't regain in a few days or weeks what you have lost in years of sedentary living, but you can get it back if you persevere. And the prize is worth the price.

This chapter contains the basic information you need to begin and maintain a personal physical fitness program. These guidelines are intended for the average healthy adult. It tells you what your goals should be and how often, how long, and how hard you must exercise

Excerpted from the pamphlet "Fitness Fundamentals: Guidelines for Personal Exercise Programs," by The President's Council on Physical Fitness and Sports (www.fitness.gov), October 15, 2004.

to achieve them. It also includes information that will make your workouts easier, safer, and more satisfying. The rest is up to you.

Checking Your Health

If you're under 35 and in good health, you don't need to see a doctor before beginning an exercise program. But if you are over 35 and have been inactive for several years, you should consult your physician, who may or may not recommend a graded exercise test. Other conditions that indicate a need for medical clearance are:

- high blood pressure;
- heart trouble;
- family history of early stroke or heart attack deaths;
- frequent dizzy spells;
- extreme breathlessness after mild exertion;
- arthritis or other bone problems;
- severe muscular, ligament or tendon problems; and
- other known or suspected disease.

Vigorous exercise involves minimal health risks for persons in good health or those following a doctor's advice. Far greater risks are presented by habitual inactivity and obesity.

Knowing the Basics

Physical fitness is most easily understood by examining its components, or "parts." There is widespread agreement that these four components are basic:

- **Cardiorespiratory Endurance**—the ability to deliver oxygen and nutrients to tissues and to remove wastes over sustained periods of time. Long runs and swims are among the methods employed in measuring this component.

- **Muscular Strength**—the ability of a muscle to exert force for a brief period of time. Upper-body strength, for example, can be measured by various weight-lifting exercises.

- **Muscular Endurance**—the ability of a muscle, or a group of muscles, to sustain repeated contractions or to continue applying force against a fixed object. Push-ups are often used to test endurance of arm and shoulder muscles.

- **Flexibility**—the ability to move joints and use muscles through their full range of motion. The sit-and-reach test is a good measure of flexibility of the lower back and backs of the upper legs.

- **Body Composition** is often considered a component of fitness. It refers to the makeup of the body in terms of lean mass (muscle, bone, vital tissue, and organs) and fat mass. An optimal ratio of fat to lean mass is an indication of fitness, and the right types of exercises will help you decrease body fat and increase or maintain muscle mass.

A Workout Schedule

How often, how long, and how hard you exercise and what kinds of exercises you do should be determined by what you are trying to accomplish. Your goals, your present fitness level, age, health, skills, interest and convenience are among the factors you should consider. For example, an athlete training for high-level competition would follow a different program than a person whose goals are good health and the ability to meet work and recreational needs.

Your exercise program should include something from each of the four basic fitness components described previously. Each workout should begin with a warmup and end with a cooldown. As a general rule, space your workouts throughout the week and avoid consecutive days of hard exercise.

Here are the amounts of activity necessary for the average healthy person to maintain a minimum level of overall fitness. Included are some of the popular exercises for each category.

- **Warmup**—5-10 minutes of exercise such as walking, slow jogging, knee lifts, arm circles, or trunk rotations. Low intensity movements that simulate movements to be used in the activity can also be included in the warmup.

- **Muscular Strength**—a minimum of two 20-minute sessions per week that include exercises for all the major muscle groups. Lifting weights is the most effective way to increase strength.

- **Muscular Endurance**—at least three 30-minute sessions each week that include exercises such as calisthenics, push-ups, sit-ups, pull-ups, and weight training for all the major muscle groups.

119

- **Cardiorespiratory Endurance**—at least three 20-minute bouts of continuous aerobic (activity requiring oxygen) rhythmic exercise each week. Popular aerobic conditioning activities include brisk walking, jogging, swimming, cycling, rope-jumping, rowing, cross-country skiing, and some continuous action games like racquetball and handball.

- **Flexibility**—10-12 minutes of daily stretching exercises performed slowly, without a bouncing motion. This can be included after a warmup or during a cooldown.

- **Cooldown**—a minimum of 5-10 minutes of slow walking, low-level exercise, combined with stretching.

A Matter of Principle

The keys to selecting the right kinds of exercises for developing and maintaining each of the basic components of fitness are found in these principles:

- **Specificity**—pick the right kind of activities to affect each component. Strength training results in specific strength changes. Also, train for the specific activity you're interested in. For example, optimal swimming performance is best achieved when the muscles involved in swimming are trained for the movements required. It does not necessarily follow that a good runner is a good swimmer.

- **Overload**—work hard enough, at levels that are vigorous and long enough to overload your body above its resting level, to bring about improvement.

- **Regularity**—you can't hoard physical fitness. At least three balanced workouts a week are necessary to maintain a desirable level of fitness.

- **Progression**—increase the intensity, frequency, and/or duration of activity over periods of time in order to improve.

Some activities can be used to fulfill more than one of your basic exercise requirements. For example, in addition to increasing cardiorespiratory endurance, running builds muscular endurance in the legs, and swimming develops the arm, shoulder, and chest muscles. If you select the proper activities, it is possible to fit parts of your muscular endurance workout into your cardiorespiratory workout and save time.

Measuring Your Heart Rate

Heart rate is widely accepted as a good method for measuring intensity during running, swimming, cycling, and other aerobic activities. Exercise that doesn't raise your heart rate to a certain level and keep it there for 20 minutes won't contribute significantly to cardiovascular fitness.

The heart rate you should maintain is called your target heart rate. There are several ways of arriving at this figure. One of the simplest is: maximum heart rate (220 - age) x 70%. Thus, the target heart rate for a 40-year-old would be 126.

Some methods for figuring the target rate take individual differences into consideration. Here is one of them:

1. Subtract age from 220 to find maximum heart rate.

2. Subtract resting heart rate (see below) from maximum heart rate to determine heart rate reserve.

3. Take 70% of heart rate reserve to determine heart rate raise.

4. Add heart rate raise to resting heart rate to find target rate.

Resting heart rate should be determined by taking your pulse after sitting quietly for five minutes. When checking heart rate during a workout, take your pulse within five seconds after interrupting exercise because it starts to go down once you stop moving. Count pulse for 10 seconds and multiply by six to get the per-minute rate.

Clothing

All exercise clothing should be loose-fitting to permit freedom of movement and should make the wearer feel comfortable and self-assured.

As a general rule, you should wear lighter clothes than temperatures might indicate. Exercise generates great amounts of body heat. Light-colored clothing that reflects the sun's rays is cooler in the summer, and dark clothes are warmer in winter. When the weather is very cold, it's better to wear several layers of light clothing than one or two heavy layers. The extra layers help trap heat, and it's easy to shed one of them if you become too warm.

In cold weather, and in hot, sunny weather, it's a good idea to wear something on your head. Wool watch or ski caps are recommended for winter wear, and some form of tennis or sailor's hat that provides shade and can be soaked in water is good for summer.

Never wear rubberized or plastic clothing, such garments interfere with the evaporation of perspiration and can cause body temperature to rise to dangerous levels.

The most important item of equipment for the runner is a pair of sturdy, properly fitting running shoes. Training shoes with heavy, cushioned soles and arch supports are preferable to flimsy sneakers and light racing flats.

When to Exercise

The hour just before the evening meal is a popular time for exercise. The late afternoon workout provides a welcome change of pace at the end of the work day and helps dissolve the day's worries and tensions.

Another popular time to work out is early morning, before the work day begins. Advocates of the early start say it makes them more alert and energetic on the job.

Among the factors you should consider in developing your workout schedule are personal preference, job and family responsibilities, availability of exercise facilities, and weather. It's important to schedule your workouts for a time when there is little chance that you will have to cancel or interrupt them because of other demands on your time.

You should not exercise strenuously during extremely hot, humid weather or within two hours after eating. Heat and/or digestion both make heavy demands on the circulatory system, and in combination with exercise can be an overtaxing double load.

Chapter 17

Debunking Ten Common Exercise Myths

"Fitness Tips: 10 Exercise Myths" is reproduced with permission of IDEA Health & Fitness Association, (800) 999-IDEA, www.IDEAfit.com. © 2006 IDEA Health & Fitness Association.

Although some old fitness fictions, such as "no pain, no gain" and "spot reducing" are fading fast, plenty of popular exercise misconceptions still exist. Here are some of the most common myths as well as the not-so-common facts based on current exercise research.

1. You will burn more fat if you exercise longer at a lower intensity.

The most important focus in exercise and fat weight control is not the percentage of exercise energy coming from fat but the total energy cost, or how many calories are burned during the activity. The faster you walk, step or run, for example, the more calories you use per minute. However, high-intensity exercise is difficult to sustain if you are just beginning or returning to exercise, so you may not exercise very long at this level. It is safer, and more practical, to start out at a lower intensity and work your way up gradually.

The information in this chapter is © 2006 IDEA Health & Fitness Association. The individual document is cited within the text.

2. If you're not going to work out hard and often, exercise is a waste of time.

This kind of thinking keeps a lot of people from maintaining or even starting an exercise program. Research continues to show that any exercise is better than none. For example, regular walking or gardening for as little as an hour a week has been shown to reduce the risk of heart disease.

3. Yoga is a completely gentle and safe exercise.

Yoga is an excellent form of exercise, but some styles are quite rigorous and demanding both physically and mentally. As with any form of exercise, qualified, careful instruction is necessary for a safe, effective workout.

4. If you exercise long and hard enough, you will always get the results you want.

In reality, genetics plays an important role in how people respond to exercise. Studies have shown a wide variation in how different exercisers respond to the same training program. Your development of strength, speed, and endurance may be very different from that of other people you know.

5. Exercise is one sure way to lose all the weight you desire.

As with all responses to exercise, weight gain or loss is impacted by many factors, including dietary intake and genetics. All individuals will not lose the same amount of weight on the same exercise program. It is possible to be active and overweight. However, although exercise alone cannot guarantee your ideal weight, regular physical activity is one of the most important factors for successful long-term weight management.

6. If you want to lose weight, stay away from strength training because you will bulk up.

Most exercise experts believe that cardiovascular exercise and strength training are both valuable for maintaining a healthy weight. Strength training helps maintain muscle mass and decrease body fat percentage.

7. Water fitness programs are primarily for older people or exercisers with injuries.

Recent research has shown that water fitness programs can be highly challenging and effective for both improving fitness and losing weight. Even top athletes integrate water fitness workouts into their training programs.

8. The health and fitness benefits of mind-body exercise like tai chi and yoga are questionable.

In fact, research showing the benefits of these exercises continues to grow. Tai chi, for example, has been shown to help treat low-back pain and fibromyalgia. Improved flexibility, balance, coordination, posture, strength, and stress management are just some of the potential results of mind-body exercise.

9. Overweight people are unlikely to benefit much from exercise.

Studies show that obese people who participate in regular exercise programs have a lower risk of all-cause mortality than sedentary individuals, regardless of weight. Both men and women of all sizes and fitness levels can improve their health with modest increases in activity.

10. Home workouts are fine, but going to a gym is the best way to get fit.

Research has shown that some people find it easier to stick to a home-based fitness program. In spite of all the hype on trendy exercise programs and facilities, the "best" program for you is the one you will participate in consistently.

Chapter 18

Measuring Exercise Intensity

The intensity of physical activity, or how hard your body is working, is typically categorized as light, moderate, or vigorous based on the amount of energy or effort a person expends in performing the activity.

This chapter describes the following methods of estimating the relative intensity of any physical activity as it applies to your own level of health.

Talk Test

The talk test method of measuring intensity is simple. A person who is active at a light intensity level should be able to sing while doing the activity. One who is active at a moderate intensity level should be able to carry on a conversation comfortably while engaging in the activity. If a person becomes winded or too out of breath to carry on a conversation, the activity can be considered vigorous.

Target Heart Rate and Estimated Maximum Heart Rate

A second way of monitoring physical activity intensity is to determine whether a person's pulse or heart rate is within the target zone during physical activity.

Excerpted from "Physical Activity for Everyone," a publication of the Division of Nutrition and Physical Activity, National Center for Chronic Disease Prevention and Health Promotion, part of the Centers for Disease Control and Prevention (CDC), www.cdc.gov/nccdphp/dnpa, October 28, 2005.

For moderate-intensity physical activity, a person's target heart rate should be 50 to 70% of his or her maximum heart rate. This maximum rate is based on the person's age. An estimate of a person's maximum age-related heart rate can be obtained by subtracting the person's age from 220. For example, for a 50-year-old person, the estimated maximum age-related heart rate would be calculated as 220 - 50 years = 170 beats per minute (bpm). The 50% and 70% levels would be:

- 50% level: 170 x 0.50 = 85 bpm, and
- 70% level: 170 x 0.70 = 119 bpm.

Thus, moderate-intensity physical activity for a 50-year-old person will require that the heart rate remains between 85 and 119 bpm during physical activity.

For vigorous-intensity physical activity, a person's target heart rate should be 70 to 85% of his or her maximum heart rate. To calculate this range, follow the same formula as used above, except change "50 and 70%" to "70 and 85%." For example, for a 35-year-old person, the estimated maximum age-related heart rate would be calculated as 220 - 35 years = 185 beats per minute (bpm). The 70% and 85% levels would be:

- 70% level: 185 x 0.70 = 130 bpm, and
- 85% level: 185 x 0.85 = 157 bpm.

Thus, vigorous-intensity physical activity for a 35-year-old person will require that the heart rate remains between 130 and 157 bpm during physical activity.

Taking Your Heart Rate

Generally, to determine whether you are exercising within the heart rate target zone, you must stop exercising briefly to take your pulse. You can take the pulse at the neck, the wrist, or the chest. We recommend the wrist. You can feel the radial pulse on the artery of the wrist in line with the thumb. Place the tips of the index and middle fingers over the artery and press lightly. Do not use the thumb. Take a full 60-second count of the heartbeats, or take for 30 seconds and multiply by 2. Start the count on a beat, which is counted as zero. If this number falls between 85 and 119 bpm in the case of the 50-year-old person, he or she is active within the target range for moderate-intensity activity.

Perceived Exertion (Borg Rating of Perceived Exertion Scale)

A third method of determining physical activity intensity is the Borg Rating of Perceived Exertion (RPE). Perceived exertion is how hard you feel like your body is working. It is based on the physical sensations a person experiences during physical activity, including increased heart rate, increased respiration or breathing rate, increased sweating, and muscle fatigue. Although this is a subjective measure, a person's exertion rating may provide a fairly good estimate of the actual heart rate during physical activity (Borg, 1998). A high correlation exists between a person's perceived exertion rating times 10 and the actual heart rate during physical activity; so a person's exertion rating may provide a fairly good estimate of the actual heart rate during activity (Borg, 1998). For example, if a person's rating of perceived exertion (RPE) is 12, then 12 x 10 = 120; so the heart rate should be approximately 120 beats per minute. Note that this calculation is only an approximation of heart rate, and the actual heart rate can vary quite a bit depending on age and physical condition. The Borg Rating of Perceived Exertion is also the preferred method to assess intensity among those individuals who take medications that affect heart rate or pulse.

Practitioners generally agree that perceived exertion ratings between 12 to 14 on the Borg Scale suggests that physical activity is being performed at a moderate level of intensity. During activity, use the Borg Scale to assign numbers to how you feel. Self-monitoring how hard your body is working can help you adjust the intensity of the activity by speeding up or slowing down your movements.

Through experience of monitoring how your body feels, it will become easier to know when to adjust your intensity. For example, a walker who wants to engage in moderate-intensity activity would aim for a Borg Scale level of "somewhat hard" (12-14). If he describes his muscle fatigue and breathing as "very light" (9 on the Borg Scale) he would want to increase his intensity. On the other hand, if he felt his exertion was "extremely hard" (19 on the Borg Scale) he would need to slow down his movements to achieve the moderate-intensity range.

Instructions for Borg Rating of Perceived Exertion (RPE) Scale

While doing physical activity, we want you to rate your perception of exertion. This feeling should reflect how heavy and strenuous the exercise feels to you, combining all sensations and feelings of physical stress, effort, and fatigue. Do not concern yourself with any one factor such as leg pain or shortness of breath, but try to focus on your total feeling of exertion.

Look at the rating scale below while you are engaging in an activity; it ranges from 6 to 20, where 6 means "no exertion at all" and 20 means "maximal exertion." Choose the number from below that best describes your level of exertion. This will give you a good idea of the intensity level of your activity, and you can use this information to speed up or slow down your movements to reach your desired range.

Try to appraise your feeling of exertion as honestly as possible, without thinking about what the actual physical load is. Your own feeling of effort and exertion is important, not how it compares to other people's. Look at the scales and the expressions and then give a number.

- 6 = No exertion at all
- 7 = Extremely light (7.5)
- 8
- 9 = Very light
- 10
- 11 = Light
- 12
- 13 = Somewhat hard
- 14
- 15 = Hard (heavy)
- 16
- 17 = Very hard
- 18
- 19 = Extremely hard
- 20 = Maximal exertion

Nine corresponds to "very light" exercise. For a healthy person, it is like walking slowly at his or her own pace for some minutes.

Thirteen on the scale is "somewhat hard" exercise, but it still feels OK to continue.

Seventeen ("very hard") is very strenuous. A healthy person can still go on, but he or she really has to push himself or herself. It feels very heavy, and the person is very tired.

Nineteen on the scale is an extremely strenuous exercise level. For most people this is the most strenuous exercise they have ever experienced.

Metabolic Equivalent (MET) Level

A fourth way of measuring physical activity intensity is by the metabolic equivalent, or MET, level. Although the intensity of certain activities is commonly characterized as light, moderate, or vigorous, many activities can be classified in any one or all three categories simply on the basis of the level of personal effort involved in carrying out the activity (i.e., how hard one is working to do the activity). For example, one can bicycle at intensities ranging from very light to very vigorous. MET is used to estimate the amount of oxygen used by the body during physical activity (Ainsworth et al., 1993).

1 MET = the energy (oxygen) used by the body as you sit quietly, perhaps while talking on the phone or reading a book.

The harder your body works during the activity, the higher the MET.

- Any activity that burns 3 to 6 METs is considered moderate-intensity physical activity.

- Any activity that burns more than 6 METs is considered vigorous-intensity physical activity.

References

1. Ainsworth BE, Haskell WL, Leon AS, et al. Compendium of physical activities: classification of energy costs of human physical activities. *Medicine and Science in Sports and Exercise* 1993;25(1):71–80.

2. Borg G. *Perceived exertion and pain scales.* Champaign (IL): Human Kinetics, 1998.

Chapter 19

Hiring a Personal Trainer

The Importance and Benefits of Physical Activity

It has been firmly established that individuals who engage in some form of physical activity, either by lifestyle or occupation, are likely to live longer and healthier lives. Research shows that even moderate caloric expenditure from physical activity has a significant impact on longevity. A physically active person who possesses risk factors like hypertension, high cholesterol, diabetes, and even a smoking habit can derive significant gains from incorporating regular physical activity into his or her daily activities.

Regular physical activity is also likely to help modify a number of risk factors. As an adjunct to weight loss, exercise is likely to help you stay on a diet and lose weight. Additionally, regular exercise is associated with reductions in blood pressure, improved glucose regulation, promotion of better lipid profiles, and stronger, denser bones.

Benefits of a Personal Trainer

A qualified and properly trained personal trainer can help you safely start and maintain an effective exercise program. A personal trainer will understand your "fitness goals" and help you achieve them. A personal trainer can be a great source of motivation and encouragement, as well as a resource for the latest objective health and

ACSM Personal Trainer brochure, 2003. Reprinted with permission of the American College of Sports Medicine.

133

fitness information. He or she can also help you fit exercise into your busy schedule and teach you how to make the most out of your time in the gym.

But beware: The title "personal trainer" does not guarantee that a person is qualified to do the job. Currently, there is no national standard or minimum requirement for carrying this job title. Working with an underqualified trainer could actually threaten your safety. This chapter will arm you with the knowledge of what to look for when seeking a personal trainer that is educated, qualified, and most importantly, right for you.

Locating a Personal Trainer

Begin by asking about personal trainers at a health club or fitness facility. Many fitness facilities have in-house personal trainers, which you can use. Consult www.acsm.org or call the American College of Sports Medicine (ACSM) at 317-637-9200 to ask about the appropriate qualifications for personal trainers. Also at www.acsm.org, you can find ACSM's Pro Finder, an online database of ACSM-certified professionals. Personal trainers will also be listed in the phone book under such headings as: "Personal Trainers," "Health Clubs, "Exercise," and "Physical Fitness."

Choosing a Personal Trainer

Certification and Education

- Does the personal trainer hold a four-year degree (from an accredited university) in Exercise Science, Kinesiology, Exercise Physiology, Physical Education, or a related health and fitness field? A trainer with a degree in one of these areas will have a better understanding of the body and how it responds to exercise.

- Does the personal trainer have additional training and a certification by a nationally recognized organization, preferably a not-for-profit organization?

- What continuing education is required to maintain the certification?

- Is the trainer certified in first aid and CPR?

- Does the trainer have liability insurance?

All certifications should be obtained from a nationally recognized organization and based on job-related performance criteria, which has been validated by scientific research in the field. There are many certifying organizations that do not comply with industry standards. Ask about the trainer's educational background and professional certifications. Check to make sure the certification is from a credible and reputable organization.

Experience and References

- How long has he or she been a personal trainer?
- What types of clients does he or she work with?
- Can he or she provide you with an updated resume?
- Can he or she provide you with a list of references?
- The trainer should have more education and experience than just having been a "weightlifter," a "bodybuilder," or "active in fitness."

Safety and Preactivity Screening: Client Evaluation

The trainer should be able to respond to any reasonable and foreseeable emergency situation that threatens the safety of a client. The trainer should be able to provide information regarding potential risks associated with exercise.

- Every client should be offered a preactivity screening that is appropriate for the activity he or she will perform.
- Every client should be screened before training to assess whether he or she has medical conditions or risk factors that should be addressed by a physician.
- Does the trainer offer fitness assessments?
- Does the trainer ask specific questions, before the exercise program begins, about medical conditions, medications currently being taken, previous injuries, surgery as it relates to exercise, and aches and pains?

Resource Network

Does the trainer have a network of other health professionals he or she works with? The trainer should be aligned with other health professionals as sources for answering specific questions and for referrals outside his or her area of expertise.

Some of the health professionals a personal trainer can be aligned with include: physicians, physical therapists, nutrition specialists, and other professionals with expertise in fitness.

Personality and Gender

- Would you prefer a male or female trainer?

- Do you like the trainer's personality? Will he or she be a good fit for your personality and your fitness goals?

- Is the trainer friendly and open to answering questions?

- Does the trainer communicate well and explain exercises in an easy-to-understand manner?

- Will the trainer motivate you to exercise and make you want to continue your program?

- The trainer should motivate you without being intimidating or pushing you beyond reasonable fitness limits.

- Is the trainer sensitive to your needs?

- Are you comfortable with the trainer?

Personal Training for Children and Adolescents

If you are choosing a personal trainer for your son or daughter, the trainer should have a good understanding of the unique characteristics of young people.

- Does he or she relate and communicate well with young people?

- Has he or she trained young athletes before?

- Is the trainer aware of special sports medicine needs and training precautions for young athletes?

- Does the trainer understand the specific needs for the sport in which your son or daughter participates? At the same time, does the trainer advocate a well-rounded fitness program?

- If your son or daughter is not an athlete and just wants "to get into shape," does the trainer understand the guidelines for training young people?

Fees

- What does the personal trainer charge?
- How long is each session?
- What services are included in the price?
- Is there an additional "gym membership" fee?
- Are there "package" or long-term package prices?
- Does the trainer require you to sign a contract for long-term training?

The fees personal trainers charge may vary according to qualifications, experience, location, length of session, and sometimes the specialization of the work-out. Typically, a personal trainer will charge $20 to $100 an hour. Some trainers will offer reduced hourly rates for long-term packages or prepaid sessions.

Scheduling, Cancellation Policies, and Business Practices

- Is the trainer available to meet your schedule?
- What is the cancellation policy?
- Will you be charged if you do not cancel within a certain time frame?

The trainer should provide you with a written copy of all policies on contracts, billing, scheduling, and cancellations.

Hiring a personal trainer is an investment in your health, fitness, and your quality of life, as well as an investment of time and money. Make sure the trainer has a good reputation, proper education and certification(s), and is well respected by other trainers and clients.

The trainer should conform to all relevant laws, regulations, and published standards, including United States federal laws (Americans with Disabilities Act [ADA] and Occupational Safety and Health Administration [OSHA]), and local government laws and regulations.

Special Needs

The trainer may or may not be able to accommodate special needs. Ask questions to see if he or she can meet your needs regarding modification of equipment and/or programs.

Important Points to Remember

Ask a lot of questions so that you will have accurate information. Making an informed decision can help you avoid making a wrong decision, which may end up costing you money.

There are many considerations that you should investigate prior to hiring a personal trainer. These considerations do not ensure the exercise program with a personal trainer will be risk-free, or that you will be satisfied with the trainer or the program(s). But these guidelines can help you make a decision based upon industry standards.

Your exercise program should be part of your lifestyle, and the trainer you choose can play a major role in the success of your program. Selecting a professional and qualified personal trainer is a sound investment for your health.

A Complete Physical Activity Program

There are three principal components to a rounded program of physical activity: aerobic exercise, strength training exercise, and flexibility training. It is not essential that all three components be performed during the same workout session. Try to create a pattern that fits into your schedule and one to which you can adhere. Commitment to a regular physical activity program is more important than the intensity of the workouts. Therefore, choose exercises you believe you are likely to pursue and enjoy. ACSM's Position Stand "The Recommended Quantity and Quality of Exercise for Healthy Adults" ©1998 states that aerobic training should be performed three to five days per week with a minimum of 20 minutes per day. Remember, if your schedule is tight, it is better to exercise for a shorter period of time than not at all. Typical forms of aerobic exercise are walking and running (treadmills), stair climbing, bicycling (bicycle ergometers), rowing, cross-country skiing, and swimming. Many devices offer a combination of these motions. For general purposes, strength training should be done two to three times per week. Strength training is performed with free weights or weight machines. For the purposes of general training, two to three upper body and lower body exercises should be done. Additionally, abdominal exercises are an important part of strength training. Flexibility training is important and frequently neglected, resulting in increased tightness as we age and become less active. Stretching is most safely done with sustained gradual movements lasting a minimum of 15 seconds per stretch. At a minimum, strive to stretch every day.

Chapter 20

Choosing a Health and Fitness Facility

The Importance and Benefits of Physical Activity

It has been firmly established that individuals who engage in some form of physical activity, either by lifestyle or occupation, are likely to live longer and healthier lives. Research shows that even moderate caloric expenditure from physical activity has a significant impact on longevity. A physically active person who possesses risk factors like hypertension, diabetes, and even a smoking habit can derive significant gains from incorporating regular physical activity into his or her daily activities.

Regular physical activity is also likely to help modify a number of risk factors. As an adjunct to weight loss, exercise is likely to help you stay on a diet and lose weight. Additionally, regular exercise is associated with reductions in blood pressure, improved glucose regulation, promotion of better lipid profiles, and stronger, denser bones.

The First Step

Before you begin an exercise program, take a fitness test, or substantially increase your level of activity, answer the questions below. This physical activity readiness questionnaire (PAR-Q) will help determine your suitability for beginning an exercise routine or program.

ACSM Health/Fitness Facility brochure, 2003. Reprinted with permission of the American College of Sports Medicine.

- Has your doctor ever said that you have a heart condition and that you should only participate in physical activity recommended by a doctor?

- Do you feel pain in your chest during physical activity?

- In the past month, have you had chest pain when you were not doing physical activity?

- Do you lose your balance because of dizziness, or do you ever lose consciousness?

- Do you have a bone or joint problem that could be made worse by a change in your physical activity?

- Is your doctor currently prescribing drugs for your blood pressure or heart condition?

- Do you know of any reason you should not participate in physical activity?

If you answered yes to one or more questions, if you are over 40 years of age and have been inactive, or if you are concerned about your health, consult a physician before taking a fitness test or substantially increasing your physical activity. If you answered no to each question, you have reasonable assurance of your suitability for fitness testing and training.

Selecting a Facility

According to the International Health, Racquet and Sportsclub Association (IHRSA), there are more than 17,000 health clubs in the United States with a membership representing more than 33 million individuals. These facilities can offer an attractive, safe, and effective venues for exercise and health promotion. The quality of the facilities, staffing, and programs vary greatly; therefore, you will want to evaluate the facility before making your decision. It is important to understand that you could actually be putting yourself at risk of harm if you select a facility that does not provide a safe environment, adequate screening, a properly trained staff, and safe programs. This chapter was developed to help you make an informed decision.

Benefits of a Health and Fitness Facility

A quality health and fitness facility will allow you the opportunity to exercise in a safe environment under the direction of qualified personnel. It will also allow you the opportunity to use state-of-the-art exercise equipment and participate in any number of beneficial activity programs. Group exercise programs will afford you the opportunity to meet new people and exercise in a social environment.

Before Joining

It is strongly suggested that you shop around and visit several facilities prior to making your investment. Some facilities offer a trial membership for a day or a week. Before joining, take a tour and ask questions. Observe the classes and/or programs. Take notes on what you like and dislike regarding the facility. You should consider whether the facility is located in an area that is convenient for you.

Safety

The staff of the facility should be able to respond to any reasonable and foreseeable emergency situation that threatens the safety of its members. Staff should also provide you with any information regarding potential risks associated with using the facility. Check for these safety features:

- Does the facility have a posted emergency response/evacuation plan?
- Is staff qualified to execute the emergency response/evacuation plan?
- Does the facility have automated external defibrillator(s) (AEDs) on site? These devices can be used to aid someone suffering a cardiac arrest.
- Is the facility clean and well maintained?
- Is the facility free from physical or environmental hazards?
- Is the facility appropriately lit?
- Does the facility have adequate heating, cooling, and ventilation?
- Does the facility have adequate parking, especially at peak times?

Preactivity Screening

Every adult member should be offered a preactivity screening. Check to see if the facility provides for or adheres to the following:

- Does the facility offer a preactivity screening, such as the PAR-Q, to assess whether members have medical conditions or risk factors that should be addressed by a physician?

- Aside from an initial general health and wellness screening, does the facility have a health and fitness screening method appropriate for the type of exercise you will undertake?

- Does the facility offer fitness assessments?

Personnel

The facility should have a professional staff that has the appropriate education and training related to the duties they perform. Professional qualifications optimally should include a college degree in a health-related field such as exercise science, physical education, or kinesiology. Additionally, staff should hold an exercise certification from a nationally recognized, preferably non-profit organization such as the American College of Sports Medicine (ACSM). Any certification should be based upon job-related performance criteria that have been validated by scientific research in the field and analyzed for reliability and validity. Many certification programs do not comply with the industry standards, so when asking what certifications facility staff possess, remember to inquire about how the certification examination was developed and administered and what the prerequisites were for participating in the certification program. Check to make sure the credentials and education are from credible institutions for not only the personal trainers, but also the supervisors and managers of the facility.

Checklist for personnel:

- Do staff members have appropriate education, certification, and/or training that is recognized by the industry and the public as representing a high level of competence and credibility?

- Is there sufficient staff on site?

- Are staff members easy to recognize? Do they wear name tags?

- Are the staff members friendly and helpful?

- Do staff members receive ongoing professional training?

- Do staff members provide each new member with an orientation as to instruction in using the equipment and/or facility?

- Are the staff members trained in cardiopulmonary resuscitation (CPR), in the use of AEDs, and in first aid?

- Are staff knowledgeable about my health conditions?
- Can staff help me set realistic exercise goals?

Youth Services

There are important considerations for facilities that offer youth programs. Youth programs should be appropriately supervised at all times. In certain parts of the country, background screening, specific training, and/or licensure is required. Check to make sure that the facility provides for your needs regarding child care and/or youth programs.

Programs

The health/fitness facility should provide a variety of equipment and programs to meet your personal fitness goals and interests. First, establish your exercise/fitness goals, then talk to personnel to see if they provide the programs and/or equipment in which you are interested. Consider the following:

- Does the facility offer the type of exercise or program in which you are interested (i.e., personal training, aerobics, spinning, martial arts, strength training, yoga, Pilates, etc.)?
- Do qualified exercise instructors develop the programs?
- Will staff members modify the programs to meet your needs?
- Does the facility offer programs to address medical conditions (i.e., weight loss, diabetes, hypertension, or smoking cessation)?
- Does the facility offer programs for the age group in which you are interested (i.e., elderly, adolescents, children, infants)?
- Does the facility offer fitness assessments and a personalized exercise program or prescription?

Special Needs

The facility may or may not be able to accommodate your special needs. Ask questions to see if the staff of the health/fitness facility can meet your needs regarding modification of equipment, facilities, and/or programs. If you are interested in a rehabilitation program, check to see if such programs are available and check with an appropriate medical doctor for recommendations regarding programming.

The facility should conform to all relevant laws, regulations, and published standards, including United States federal laws (Americans with Disabilities Act [ADA] and Occupational Safety and Health Administration [OSHA]), local government laws and regulations (local health departments), and local building codes and ordinances.

Business Practices

Joining a health and fitness facility is an investment in your health, fitness, and quality of life. Purchasing a membership is also an investment of time and money. You want to make sure the facility has a good reputation, and is well respected by its members.

- Consider how the facility is operated before signing a contract.
- Does the staff pressure you into purchasing a membership?
- Does the membership fee fit into your budget?
- Is there a trial membership program?
- Is there a grace period in which you can cancel your membership and receive a refund?
- Are there different membership options and are all the fees for services posted?
- Does the facility provide you with a written set of rules and policies, which govern the responsibilities of members as well as the facility?
- Does the facility have a procedure to inform members of any changes in charges, services, or policies?
- Make sure you read and understand everything before signing a contract. Do not rely on verbal responses.

Important Points to Remember

Ask a lot of questions so that you will have accurate information. Making an informed decision can help you avoid choosing a facility that does not fit your needs and ends up costing you money.

There are many considerations that you should investigate prior to joining a health/fitness facility. These considerations do not ensure the health and fitness facility will be risk free or that you will be satisfied with the programs. But these guidelines can help you make a decision based upon industry standards.

Your exercise program should be part of your lifestyle, and the facility you choose can play a major role in the success of your program. Selecting a facility with professional and qualified staff, state-of-the-art equipment, and a variety of programs is a sound investment of your money and in your health.

A Complete Physical Activity Program

There are three principal components to a rounded program of physical activity: aerobic exercise, strength training exercise, and flexibility training. It is not essential that all three components be performed during the same workout session. Try to create a pattern that fits into your schedule and one to which you can adhere. Commitment to a regular physical activity program is more important than intensity of the workouts. Therefore, choose exercises you believe you are likely to pursue and enjoy. ACSM's Position Stand "The Recommended Quantity and Quality of Exercise for Healthy Adults" © 1998 states that aerobic training should be performed three to five days per week with a minimum of 20 minutes per day. Remember, if your schedule is tight, it is better to exercise for a shorter period of time than not at all. Typical forms of aerobic exercise are walking and running (treadmills), stair climbing, bicycling (bicycle ergometers), rowing, cross-country skiing, and swimming. Many devices offer a combination of these motions. For general purposes, strength training should be done two to three times per week. Strength training is performed with free weights or weight machines. For the purposes of general training, two to three upper body and lower body exercises should be done. Additionally, abdominal exercises are an important part of strength training. Flexibility training is important and frequently neglected, resulting in increased tightness as we age and become less active. Stretching is most safely done with sustained gradual movements lasting a minimum of 15 seconds per stretch. At a minimum, strive to stretch every day.

145

Chapter 21

Using Exercise Equipment at Home

Chapter Contents

Section 21.1

How to Design Your Own Home Gym

Exercising at home is a good alternative for people who are short on time, can't afford a club membership, or just can't seem to make it across town to the local gym.

Many people are interested in setting up a home gym, but are intimidated by the many available choices. Before you invest time and money in designing a gym of your own, take a minute to consider your fitness needs, available space, budget, and other factors that will determine how much time you are able to devote to home fitness.

Quality Matters

Home gym equipment is of higher quality and more space efficient than ever before. The real challenge is choosing from the many options. Before purchasing a piece of equipment, make sure you test it out yourself. Here are some factors to consider when creating a home gym.

What Is Your Budget?

You get what you pay for. Expensive equipment is usually priced that way for a reason. High-quality equipment that is reliable and will work for years to come can't be made cheaply. However, there are options for every budget.

For example, if you really want a $1,500 stair stepper, but it's not in your budget, some quality step-training tapes and a set of benches with risers for around $150 is feasible. This would be a better choice than spending $300 on a low-quality machine that will quickly wear out. You may also want to consider purchasing used commercial equipment from a reputable dealer who offers a warranty.

Consider This

Will other people in your household be using the gym? If so, keep in mind that a treadmill may need enough programming features and a long enough deck to accommodate the different body shapes and fitness goals of multiple users. Similarly, weight machines and free weights should adjust to safely accommodate a range of sizes and abilities.

A home gym represents a significant investment. Trimming the budget on cardiovascular equipment is a false economy. Any equipment in this category should suit your interests and fitness level and should be able to maintain at least 20 minutes of smooth continuous motion. The activity you choose to do should be enjoyable as well as challenging and you should be able to increase the resistance, incline, or duration.

Strength Equipment for Any Budget

Choosing strength-training tools is a matter of budget and safety. Novice exercisers may be better off with a multigym, which is safer to use unsupervised than free weights. The key with any home gym is to make sure it's easy to adjust. If a multigym isn't in your budget, a set of free weights is an affordable alternative, as is resistance tubing.

Think about the Space

Even equipment designed for home use can be a space hog, once you've put in a treadmill and multigym. Space limitations may mean you have to opt for a space-saving rack of dumbbells instead of a multigym. Also look at ceiling height, since some equipment sits high off the ground.

Consider the Design and Features

Before purchasing a piece of equipment, inspect it for safety, serviceability, design, and appropriate features. The equipment should be adjustable, easy to learn, and your body should move in a correct and safe manner. Parts should be easily removed and replaced, and moving parts should lattice well. There shouldn't be any design flaws or weaknesses that could increase the risk of injury.

Finally, be honest with yourself about how motivated you will be to exercise at home before you make the investment. It is also important that you understand how to exercise safely and that your doctor has cleared you to exercise. Once you have made the decision to design your own home gym, your next step could be on a new treadmill.

Square Footage

Use these guidelines to determine approximately how much room you'll need:

- Treadmills—30 square feet
- Single-Station Gym—35 square feet
- Free Weights—20 to 50 square feet
- Bikes—10 square feet
- Rowing Machines—20 square feet
- Stair Climbers—10 to 20 square feet
- Ski Machines—25 square feet
- Multi-Station Gym—50 to 200 square feet

Section 21.2

Using an Elliptical Trainer

ACSM Elliptical Trainer brochure, 2002. Reprinted with permission of the American College of Sports Medicine.

The Importance and Benefits of Physical Activity

It has been firmly established that individuals who engage in some form of physical activity, either by lifestyle or occupation, are likely to live longer and healthier lives. Research shows that even moderate caloric expenditure from physical activity has a significant impact on longevity. A physically active person who possesses such risk factors as hypertension, diabetes, and even a smoking habit can derive significant gains from incorporating regular physical activity into his or her daily activities.

Regular physical activity is also likely to help modify a number of risk factors. As an adjunct to weight loss, exercise is likely to help you stay on a diet and lose weight. Additionally, regular exercise is associated with reduction in blood pressure, improved glucose regulation, promotion of better lipid profiles, and stronger, denser bones.

The First Step

Before you begin an exercise program, take a fitness test, or substantially increase your level of activity, answer the questions below. This physical activity readiness questionnaire (PAR-Q) will help determine your suitability for beginning an exercise routine or program.

- Has your doctor ever said that you have a heart condition and that you should only participate in physical activity recommended by a doctor?

- Do you feel pain in your chest during physical activity?

- In the past month, have you had chest pain when you were not doing physical activity?

- Do you lose your balance because of dizziness, or do you ever lose consciousness?

- Do you have a bone or joint problem that could be made worse by a change in your physical activity?

- Is your doctor currently prescribing drugs for your blood pressure or heart condition?

- Do you know of any reason you should not participate in physical activity?

If you answered yes to one or more questions, if you are over 40 years of age and have been inactive, or if you are concerned about your health, consult a physician before taking a fitness test or substantially increasing your physical activity. If you answered no to each question, you have reasonable assurance of your suitability for fitness testing and training.

Selecting a Home Elliptical Trainer

Elliptical trainers have become one of the most popular machines for cardiovascular exercise. These trainers engage the legs in a movement pattern that combines the motion of stair stepping with cross-country skiing, providing a low-impact workout. Some elliptical devices also include poles that can be maneuvered with the arms while the legs are in motion, similar to cross-country machines. This option increases the amount of muscle mass used to perform the exercise.

Following are guidelines that should be considered when purchasing an elliptical trainer. These recommendations will help you select a trainer that suits your specific needs. Before making any purchases, always be sure to try out the machine so that you can familiarize yourself with its options.

Safety

Make sure the equipment is properly fitted to your size and movement range. If the machine is motorized, there should be a safety turn-off control.

When in use, the machine should be very sturdy and should neither move nor have the tendency to tip over. The side rails should also be sturdy and provide for adequate balance.

Check the area around the machine for adequate headroom and space for leg and arm motion.

Maintenance and Durability

- Is the machine manufacturer reputable and reliable?
- Does the trainer come with a warranty?
- What does the warranty cover and how long is the warranty period?
- Is the machine durable, easily assembled, and easily maintained?
- Elliptical machines tend to be rather large—is the space in which it is to be used large enough?
- If it is to be stored between use, is there adequate space for storage?
- Are local technicians available for service?

Power, Performance, and Operation

- Is the trainer motorized or non-motorized?
- Does your home have the proper power supply? (Motorized machines may require 120 to 220 volts)

- Does the trainer require calibration?
- How often does the trainer have to be serviced?
- Is the noise level acceptable?
- Is the trainer sturdy and stable?
- Is there a control panel/read-out? Is it easy to read? Is it accurate?
- Does the control panel offer the information that is important for your needs (time, distance, resistance level, calories expended, etc.)?
- Is the instruction manual easy to read and follow?

Other Considerations

Make certain the pedals will comfortably accommodate the size of your feet. Pedals with a textured "non-slip" surface and high curved ridges will also prevent your feet from sliding around or even off the pedal when exercising.

The stride length permitted by the trainer is also an important factor. Avoid purchasing a trainer if the stride length is too limited for your leg movement range. Some machines allow you to adjust the stride length.

Overall fit is very important. A good fit should allow you to move comfortably and smoothly, with a good upright posture and without the chance of your knees bumping into the console. The fixed hand-support rails should also allow you to maintain a comfortable upright posture versus a tendency to lean too far forward (which can be stressful to the back).

If the machine provides upper body handles or poles, make sure that the handles are sturdy, easy to reach, and that the handgrips are comfortable. Avoid trainers with upper body poles that infringe on your range of motion or cause contact with your knees.

Familiarize yourself with the options that increase the intensity of the workout. Some machines have elevating ramps under each pedal. Others increase the intensity through faster movement or by changing the resistance of the pedals with a tension control.

Using an Elliptical Trainer

Follow the manual regarding directions for proper set-up and use of the machine. Make certain the trainer operates properly and be sure

153

that adequate space is available and that the power supply is nearby. Adjust the machine to suit your size and range of movement. Get comfortable with any programming features such as exercise time, distance goal, resistance level, speed level, and caloric expenditure.

When exercising, maintain the correct posture by keeping your shoulder back, head up, chin straight, abdominals tight, and arms relaxed. Do not lean forward or grab and grip the balance bars tightly. The participant's weight should be supported by the lower body.

Important Points to Remember

Before you start exercising on the elliptical trainer, make sure that you are familiar with the controls that increase speed and/or resistance. Make sure that the emergency shut-off switch or button works.

- **Maintain a good posture:** Shoulders should be back, head up and slightly forward, chin up and abdominals tight. Look forward, not down at your feet. Do not grip the handrails too tightly. Make sure that your weight is evenly distributed and that your lower body supports the majority of your weight.

- **Stride:** Relax and maintain a good stride going through your normal range of motion.

- **Make it a habit:** An elliptical trainer is only as good for your health as the frequency with which you use it. Set a specific time of day, set a specific number of minutes and make it routine.

Start out slowly and make sure that you have checked with your doctor before beginning any exercise program.

A Complete Physical Activity Program

There are three principal components to a rounded program of physical activity: aerobic exercise, strength training exercise, and flexibility training. It is not essential that all three components be performed during the same workout session. Try to create a pattern that fits into your schedule and one to which you can adhere. Commitment to a regular physical activity program is more important than intensity of the workouts. Therefore, choose exercises you believe you are likely to pursue and enjoy. ACSM's Position Stand "The Recommended Quantity and Quality of Exercise for... Healthy Adults" ©1998 states that aerobic training should be performed three to five days per week with a minimum of 20 minutes per day. Remember, if your schedule is tight, it is better to exercise for a shorter period of time than not at all. Typical forms of aerobic exercise are walking and running (treadmills), stair climbing, bicycling (bicycle ergometers), rowing, cross-country skiing, and swimming. Many devices offer a combination of these motions. For general purposes, strength training should be done two to three times per week. Strength training is performed with free weights or weight machines. For the purposes of general training, two to three upper body and lower body exercises should be done. Additionally, abdominal exercises are an important part of strength training. Flexibility training is important and frequently neglected, resulting in increased tightness as we age and become less active. Stretching is most safely done with sustained gradual movements lasting a minimum of 15 seconds per stretch. At a minimum, strive to stretch every day.

Section 21.3

Using a Home Treadmill

ACSM Home Treadmill brochure, 2002. Reprinted with permission of the American College of Sports Medicine.

The Importance and Benefits of Physical Activity

It is now firmly established that individuals who engage in some form of physical activity, either by lifestyle or occupation, are likely to live longer and healthier lives. Research shows that even moderate caloric expenditure from physical activity has a significant impact on longevity. Importantly, a physically active person who possesses other risk factors like hypertension, diabetes, and even a smoking habit can derive significant gains from incorporating regular physical activity into his or her daily activities.

Regular physical activity is also likely to help modify a number of risk factors. As an adjunct to weight loss, exercise is likely to help you stay on a diet and lose weight. Additionally, regular exercise is associated with reductions in blood pressure, improved glucose regulation, promotion of better lipid profiles and stronger/denser bones.

The First Step

Before you begin an exercise program, take a fitness test, or substantially increase your level of activity, answer the questions below. This physical activity readiness questionnaire (PAR-Q) will help determine your suitability for testing or training.

- Has your doctor ever said that you have a heart condition and that you should only participate in physical activity recommended by a doctor?

- Do you feel pain in your chest when you participate in physical activity?

- In the past month, have you had chest pain when you were not involved in physical activity?

- Do you lose your balance because of dizziness, or do you ever lose consciousness?

- Do you have a bone or joint problem that could be made worse by a change in your physical activity?

- Is your doctor currently prescribing drugs for your blood pressure or heart condition?

- Do you know of any other reason you should not participate in physical activity?

If you answered yes to one or more questions, if you are over 40 years of age and have been inactive, or if you are concerned about your health, consult your physician before taking a fitness test or substantially increasing your physical activity.

If you answered no to all the questions, you have reasonable assurance of your suitability for fitness testing and training.

Selecting a Home Treadmill

Treadmills are a popular choice of equipment for those who want to engage in physical activity. Here are useful guidelines for you to consider before making a purchase. Be sure to try it out before you buy. Doing so will allow you to find a treadmill that meets your specific needs.

A treadmill may be either motorized or human-powered. Manual treadmills are less expensive and safer because the running belt stops moving when you do. However, manual treadmills usually have smaller running belts, making it difficult to jog or run, let alone maintain a brisk walk. Often, the difficulty in getting the belt to move smoothly on a non-motorized treadmill increases the likelihood of holding on to the handrail in an effort to generate power, causing an inconsistent pace.

This inconsistent pace may cause muscle strain or difficulty in elevating your heart rate. Additionally, the holding on may elevate blood pressure from breath holding. Exercise at home should be easy and something to look forward to. If it is difficult to get the machine to work, you are less likely to exercise. For these reasons, you may want to consider a motorized treadmill.

Safety

- Stability of platform when level and with elevation: feels solid, not wobbly.

- Doesn't have parts that hit you or cramp your movements in an unnatural fashion.

- Automatic emergency shut-off key, clip or tether.

- Side rails or safety bars for balance: They should be reachable and sturdy, but out of the way of swinging arms.

Maintenance and Durability

- Is the company reliable and reputable?

- Can the treadmill be easily assembled and maintained?

- Cost of maintenance?

- Does the treadmill come with a warranty? What does the warranty cover and for how long?

- Are local technicians available for service?

Power and Performance

- Treadmill motor: should have a minimum continuous duty rating of 1.5 h.p. [horsepower] motor (2.5 to 3.0 h.p. is preferred). To test the motor, plant your feet firmly on the belt while the machine is running at its lowest speed, checking for any hesitation, groaning, or grinding.

- Power supply: Does the treadmill require 110 or 220v? 220v will probably require circuit alterations in the room where it will be used.

- Belt size: Should be at least 18 to 20 inches wide and 48 inches long. Narrow, short running belts make it more difficult and less enjoyable because the chances of tripping or falling off of the belt increase with a narrow belt. The platform should be low to the floor and have ample space to straddle the treadmill belt.

- Speed range should be 0.1 to a minimum of 8 mph. This speed range should satisfy most walkers as well as runners. Low starting speed is an important issue. We recommend a safe starting speed of 0.1 mph with slow incremental increase in belt speed. The stop should be smooth stop (not sudden). The motor should be able to maintain speed regardless of treadmill elevation and weight of user.

- Incline should range from 0 percent to at least 10 percent. Incline mechanisms can be either electric or manual. Manual cranks are found generally on lower end treadmills to keep the price down. The treadmill should not wobble at high elevations.

Operation

- Is the control panel accessible and easy to read?
- Does the control panel have the capacity for manual use separate from software used for automated programming?
- Is the noise level acceptable?
- Is the belt heavy duty as to not stretch with extended use?

Other Considerations

- Weight of treadmill
- Space available and height of ceiling
- Aesthetics
- Storage potential
- How accurate is the calibration?

Using a Home Treadmill

Treadmills should be positioned away from walls to avoid injury due to falls. Be sure that the back of the treadmill has at least six to eight feet of clearance from a ledge, wall, or window. The power supply and wiring should be located away from walking paths or taped to prevent tripping when stepping on or off of the running belt.

Make sure the running belt is properly adjusted before use. Belts that are too loose or too tight will cause wear and tear on the treadmill, which result in expensive repair or replacement costs. The deck beneath the belt should be laminated to protect it from friction wear and tear. This deck absorbs the hundreds of pounds of force from each step.

Make sure that you follow the directions included with purchase for maintaining the belt deck connection. Increased friction and heat will cause "amp draw," which pulls power away from the electrical components of your machine. Discuss appropriate lubrication and maintenance with the sales people at the store where you purchased your treadmill.

Your treadmill should come equipped with arm grips, siderails, or safety bars. These are excellent for defining the running/walking area for your exercise bout. They allow you to catch yourself it you trip or fall.

When stepping off a treadmill while the belt is moving it is advisable to use these rails for safety. The treadmill should come equipped with an emergency shut-off key, clip, or tether. These are a safety must, especially with young children around. The tether feature is preferred, since an automatic stop button may not be in reach as you fall.

Many treadmills come with sophisticated electronic displays that allow you to design workouts to your needs. For some, this programming is basically a motivation and selling point. All you need is enough variety to keep your workouts motivating and interesting. The bare minimum display and programming features should include distance, speed, time, incline, and possibly calories expended. It is important that you be able to use the treadmill in the manual mode.

Important Points to Remember

- **Before you get on:** Before you get on the treadmill, experiment with the controls. Speed it up, slow it down, increase and decrease the incline and test the emergency off button.

- **Posture when walking or running:** Shoulders back, head up and slightly forward, chin up and abdominals tight. Look forward, not down at your feet.

- **Stride length:** Relax and maintain the normal stride you would use when walking on the ground. Don't chop your steps.

- **Where you are:** It is important to pay attention to where you are on the treadmill. Don't drift sideways or allow yourself to go to the back of the belt.

- **Make it a habit:** A treadmill is only as good for your health as the frequency with which you use it. Set a specific time of day, set a specific number of minutes, and make it routine.

A Complete Physical Activity Program

There are three principle components to a rounded program of physical activity: aerobic exercise, strength training exercise, and flexibility training. It is not essential that all three components be performed during the same workout session. Try to create a pattern that fits into your schedule and one to which you can adhere. Commitment to a regular physical activity program is more important than intensity of the workouts. Therefore, choose exercises you believe you are likely to pursue and enjoy.

ACSM's Position Stand "The Recommended Quantity and Quality of Exercise for Healthy Adults" ©1998 states that aerobic training should be performed three to five days per week with a minimum of 20 minutes per day. Remember that if your schedule is tight, it is better to exercise for a shorter period of time than not at all. Typical forms of aerobic exercise are walking and running (treadmills), stair climbing, bicycling (bicycle ergometers), rowing, cross-country skiing, and swimming. Many devices contain combinations of these motions.

For general purposes, strength training should be done two to three times per week. Strength training is performed with free weights or weight machines. For the purposes of general training, two to three upper body and lower body exercises should be done. Additionally, abdominal exercises are an important part of strength training.

Flexibility training is important and frequently neglected, resulting in increased tightness as we age and become less active. Stretching is most safely done with sustained gradual movements lasting a minimum of 15 seconds per stretch. At a minimum, strive to stretch every day.

Section 21.4

Using Free Weights

ACSM Free Weights brochure, 2003. Reprinted with permission of the American College of Sports Medicine.

The Importance and Benefits of Physical Activity

It has been firmly established that individuals who engage in some form of physical activity, either by lifestyle or occupation, are likely to live longer and healthier lives. Research shows that even moderate caloric expenditure from physical activity has a significant impact on longevity. A physically active person who possesses such risk factors as hypertension, diabetes, and even a smoking habit can derive significant gains from incorporating regular physical activity into his or her daily activities. Regular physical activity is also likely to help modify a number of risk factors. As an adjunct to weight loss, exercise is likely to help you stay on a diet and lose weight. Additionally, regular exercise is associated with reduction in blood pressure, improved glucose regulation, promotion of better lipid profiles, and stronger/denser bones.

The First Step

Before you begin an exercise program, take a fitness test, or substantially increase your level of activity, answer the questions below. This physical activity readiness questionnaire (PAR-Q) will help determine your suitability for beginning an exercise routine or program.

- Has your doctor ever said that you have a heart condition and that you should only participate in physical activity recommended by a doctor?

- Do you feel pain in your chest during physical activity?

- In the past month, have you had chest pain when you were not doing physical activity?

- Do you lose your balance because of dizziness, or do you ever lose consciousness?

- Do you have a bone or joint problem that could be made worse by a change in your physical activity?

- Is your doctor currently prescribing drugs for your blood pressure or heart condition?

- Do you know of any reason you should not participate in physical activity?

If you answered yes to one or more questions, if you are over 40 years of age and have been inactive, or if you are concerned about your health, consult a physician before taking a fitness test or substantially increasing your physical activity. If you answered no to each question, you have reasonable assurance of your suitability for fitness testing and training.

Selecting Free Weights

Using free weights as part of an exercise program can be a safe and effective means of improving strength and fitness for all ages and fitness levels, for men and women. They provide a stimulus for muscle-fitness development, which can increase the amount of calories you burn (body fat reduction), increase muscle size, enhance muscle strength, power, and endurance, and increase strength of bones. Increased muscle strength can also have a positive impact on quality of life for older adults.

It is important to realize that some instruction is necessary if you have never used free weights before, or are not that familiar with the use of free weights. Technique, safety precautions, and the exercises that can be performed with free weights are the most important considerations.

Free weights come in two basic types:

- Barbell: Long bars (4-6 ft.) with weights attached or slots to add weight plates
- Dumbbell: Smaller, single handheld weights

Free weights, and more specifically dumbbells, come in more varieties and are easier to use. Dumbbells come in chrome, unfinished metal, plastic, thin foam covering, and concrete. They can be purchased in weight increments of five pounds ranging in weight from five to 150 pounds each.

The handles on free weights are important because they provide friction for a better grip. The size of the handle in relation to your own weight is also an important consideration. The handle should feel comfortable in your hand and should not cause undue muscle fatigue when lifting the weights. It is important to practice some exercises with the weights before purchasing a set.

An important first step in the purchase process is to decide on the correct amount of weight for your strength and strength development. The salesperson or exercise professional should be able to help you.

Safety

- The term "free weight" means the equipment will not restrict movement. Thus, the use of barbells and dumbbells requires more muscular coordination than machines. Because movement is not restricted, the risk of injury is higher than with machines. Precautions must be taken when using free weights. Specifically, ensure you have a good grip, maintain a stable position sitting or standing, use good technique or form, and solicit proper instruction from an exercise professional.

- When picking weights up off the floor (or putting them down), lift with your legs, not your back.

- Most accidents occur when a weight falls on a body part. This happens when a weight plate is not secure on a bar or when a dumbbell falls out of a person's hand.

- Consider how you intend to use the weights. If you are using the weights for general fitness, you probably do not need a partner to spot for you. If you are buying free weights to increase muscle size, therefore lifting heavy weights, find a training partner to spot you.

- Do not attempt to lift too much weight.

- Consider your children and/or pets and potential safety hazards when storing or not using your free weights.

Maintenance and Durability

- **Warranty**—Ask the sales representative if the set comes with a warranty.

- **Durability**—Consider your exercise motivation for the quality and durability of the weights you are purchasing. If you plan to use the weights a lot, buy a high quality and durable product. Generally speaking, free weights are rather durable.

163

- **Assembly**—Consider the time and convenience of buying weights that are set at a specific weight, or to purchase weights that can be changed according to your strength. For a set weight of dumbbells, no assembly is required.

- **Storage**—Ensure you have adequate space to safely store the weights, depending on how many or how much weight you are going to purchase. Free weights can be stored on the floor or on specialized racks.

- **Maintenance**—Consider the maintenance requirements. Chrome weights require higher maintenance than metal, concrete, or foam-covered weights.

Power, Performance, and Operation

Performance of free weights: The performance of free weights is dependent on the amount of use they receive, the care taken when putting them down or placing them back on a rack, and maintenance. The better you care for the weights, the better performance you get from your purchase.

User-Friendliness: Free weights are perhaps the most user-friendly type of exercise equipment a person can buy. The key to being user-friendly is the confidence a person has with the knowledge of the exercises that can be performed. The more knowledgeable you are about the exercises you can perform, the more you will get out of your purchase. Consult with a certified personal trainer to learn more about techniques and exercises that are right for you.

Using Free Weights

Free weights can develop muscle-fitness depending on how you use them.

- Muscle Strength: 5-8 reps, 1-3 sets
- Muscle Endurance: 15-20 reps, 1-3 sets
- Muscle Power: 3-5 reps, 1-3 sets

Rep is short for repetition. This means how many times you lift the weight. Set means a group of repetitions. Rest approximately one to two minutes between sets of each exercise or long enough to catch your breath.

Muscle Groups to Train

Exercising the major muscle groups is important for developing fitness.

- Upper body: front and back of arms, shoulders, chest, and upper back
- Torso: abdominals, sides of torso (obliques), and lower back
- Legs: front and back of thighs, calves, and buttocks

Exercises

- Upper body: Bicep curls, tricep extension, shoulder press, bench press, and bent-over row
- Torso: Abdominal curls (hands across chest), "Bird-Dog" (on hands and knees, lift opposite arm and leg 5-10 reps, then opposite arm/leg), and side-plank
- Legs: Squats or lunges and heel raises

Technique Is Important

- Learn the proper technique for each exercise before proceeding.
- Exercise both sides of the body. Whatever you exercise on the front of the body, proceed with the corresponding exercise for the back of the body.
- Breathe. Exhale when the exercise is the hardest, and inhale when the exercise is the easiest.
- Move your joints through a full range of motion when performing each exercise.
- Move in a controlled manner. Do not let momentum move the weight.

Posture

- Maintain a straight spine when performing all exercises.
- Do not hyperextend your spine.
- When picking weights up from the floor (or putting them down), use your legs, not your back.

Using a Spotter

When lifting very heavy weights, you should use a spotter in case the weights become too much for you to handle.

A spotter can offer feedback about your technique and give you a margin of safety to avoid injury.

Important Points to Remember

- **Before you buy:** Consider the space you have in which to safely engage in a weight training program.

- **When you buy:** Consider your exercise motivation in terms of the cost of the weights. Consider the size of the handles as they fit in your hand.

- **Excellent for fitness:** Using free weights is an excellent way to improve your fitness. You can increase the rate at which you burn calories, increase your muscle strength and size, and increase the strength of your bones. Increased strength through weight training can also improve the quality of life for older adults.

- **Your abilities:** Consider your level of fitness before you purchase your weights. Be careful not to buy weights that are too heavy (or too light).

- **Make it a habit:** Since you are considering buying exercise equipment, structure your lifestyle to make time to exercise and it will eventually become a lifelong habit.

A Complete Physical Activity Program

There are three principal components to a rounded program of physical activity: aerobic exercise, strength training exercise, and flexibility training. It is not essential that all three components be performed during the same workout session. Try to create a pattern that fits into your schedule and one to which you can adhere. Commitment to a regular physical activity program is more important than intensity of the workouts. Therefore, choose exercises you believe you are likely to pursue and enjoy. ACSM's Position Stand "The Recommended Quantity and Quality of Exercise for Healthy Adults" ©1998 states that aerobic training should be performed three to five days per week with a minimum of 20 minutes per day. Remember, if your schedule is tight, it is better to exercise for a shorter period of time than not at all. Typical forms of aerobic exercise are walking and running (treadmills), stair climbing, bicycling (bicycle ergometers), rowing, cross-country skiing, and swimming. Many devices offer a combination of these motions. For general purposes, strength training should be done two to three times per week. Strength training is performed with free weights or weight machines. For the purposes of general training, two to three upper body and lower body exercises should be done. Additionally, abdominal exercises are an important part of strength training. Flexibility training is important and frequently neglected, resulting in increased tightness as we age and become less active. Stretching is most safely done with sustained gradual movements lasting a minimum of 15 seconds per stretch. At a minimum, strive to stretch every day.

Section 21.5

Using a Pedometer

From "General Guidance for Pedometer Use," by the National
Institutes of Health Division of Nutrition Research Coordination,
November 19, 2004.

A digital step-counter pedometer is a reasonably accurate and reliable device that can be used for most physical activities for which there is a stepping motion. These activities include not only walking, but exercise that involves movement of the trunk, hips, and legs, such as stair climbing, cross-country skiing, dancing, household chores, running, and ball sports. There are dozens of models of pedometers. A step-only pedometer is one of the simplest and requires no calibration or adjustment, other than daily resetting to 0.

Basic Instructions for Beginners

1. Clip the step-counter onto your belt or waistband midway between your side and the crease-line of your shorts/pants. Some authorities suggest placing the step-counter at the side, either

in the 3 o'clock or 9 o'clock position. If your pedometer has a strap or leash, attach the leash to your belt to prevent losing the pedometer if it accidentally becomes unclipped.

2. Reset the step counter to 0 steps before starting your exercise and at the end of each day or exercise session.

3. For the first 3 to 4 days, assess your total number of steps and movements during a routine day at home and work. Most relatively sedentary individuals take 1,000 to 3,000 steps per day. After establishing a baseline number of steps per day, some individuals elect to count steps per week, rather than steps per day. Both approaches are acceptable.

4. With a goal of increasing your steps every day or week, begin an organized and systematic walking program. Your level of progress will depend upon your starting fitness level and health. Most apparently healthy, but sedentary adults can safely add 2,000 steps per day, or approximately one additional mile, the first week. Continue to add steps regularly. At least 10,000 steps per day is a good goal for currently sedentary people.

5. A healthful level of activity is at least 30 minutes per day of moderate-level physical activity. To achieve a moderate level of activity, increase your walking pace to 6,000 to 8,000 steps, or 3 to 4 miles, per hour for at least 30 minutes each day.

Remember that the total on a step-counter reflects all daily physical activity that involves a stepping-motion or other movement of the trunk, hips, and legs. A step-counter can be used as an activity meter, as a testing tool for evaluating walking endurance and distance, and as an educational or motivational tool to encourage physical activity.

Chapter 22

Avoiding Exercise Scams

Chapter Contents

Section 22.1

Pump Fiction: Deciphering Advertisements for Exercise Equipment

Federal Trade Commission (www.ftc.gov), November 2003.

The benefits of exercise are well documented. Unfortunately, that's not always the case with advertising claims for exercise equipment.

Some advertisers claim—without evidence—that their exercise products offer a quick, easy way to shape up, keep fit, and lose weight. The truth is, there's no such thing as a no-work, no-sweat way to a healthy, toned body. Deriving the benefits of exercise requires doing the work.

Before you jump into the next home fitness fad, the Federal Trade Commission (FTC) offers this advice: Exercise good judgment and evaluate advertising claims for exercise products carefully.

Evaluating Claims

Read the performance claims critically. Be leery of those that say the equipment or device can:

- provide easy or effortless results or burn excessive calories. The claims may be true for athletes in top physical condition, but not for most people.

- help you burn more calories or lose weight faster than other types of equipment. In general, exercise equipment that works the whole body or major parts of it probably helps you burn more calories than devices that work one part of the body. And, the more you use the equipment, the more calories you'll burn. That's a good reason to select equipment that suits you and your lifestyle. A study might show that one type of equipment burns more calories per hour than another type. But if the exercise is uncomfortable—or the equipment hard to use—chances are it will gather dust—not help you burn calories.

- help you spot reduce; for example, help you trim your hips or lose the proverbial spare tire. Toning and losing weight in one particular area of the body require regular exercise that works the whole body. Your weight depends on the number of calories you eat and use each day; increasing your physical activity helps you burn extra calories.

Always read the fine print. The advertised results may be based on more than just the use of the machine; they also may be based on restricting calories. The fine print may explain this. Even if it doesn't, keep in mind that diet and exercise together are much more effective for achieving a healthy, toned body than either tactic is alone.

Be skeptical of testimonials or before-and-after pictures from "satisfied" customers. Their experiences may not be typical: Just because one person had success with the equipment doesn't mean you will, too. As for those popular celebrity endorsements, they, too, are no proof that the equipment will work as claimed.

Finding the Right Equipment

After you've evaluated the advertised claims—but before you make a final purchasing decision—consider these questions:

- Will the equipment help you achieve your desired goal—whether it's to build strength, increase flexibility, improve endurance, or enhance your health?

- Will you stick to the program? Keeping with an exercise program can be rough: Think of all the basements, rec rooms, and yard sales stocked with costly stationary bikes, treadmills, and rowing machines that have gone unused and now serve merely as places to hang clothes. Before you buy, prove to yourself that you're ready to act on your good intentions.

To help you choose the best equipment for your needs, check out consumer and fitness magazines that rate exercise equipment. Then test various pieces of equipment at a local gym, recreation center, or retailer to find the machine or device that feels comfortable to you.

- **Shop around.** Exercise equipment advertised on TV or in newspapers or magazines may be available at local sporting goods, department, and discount stores. That can make it easier to shop for the best price. Don't be fooled by companies that advertise "three easy payments" or "only $49.95 a month." The advertised price may not include shipping and handling fees, sales tax, and delivery and set-up fees. Ask about the costs before you close the deal.

- **Get details on warranties, guarantees, and return policies.** A "30-day money-back guarantee" may not sound as good if you're responsible for paying a hefty fee to return a bulky piece of equipment you bought.

- **Check out the company's customer and support services.** Call the advertised toll-free number to get an idea of how easy it is to reach a company representative and how helpful he or she is.

You may get a great deal on a piece of fitness equipment from a secondhand store, consignment shop, yard sale, or the classified ads. Buy wisely: Items bought secondhand usually aren't returnable and don't carry the warranties that new equipment does.

Section 22.2

Electrical Muscle Stimulators: Do They Work?

"Six-Pack Abs Electronically?" *FDA Consumer* magazine, published by the U.S. Food and Drug Administration, July-August 2002.

You've probably seen the ads on television that promise "six-pack abs" without a workout. Can you really tone your muscles using an electrical muscle stimulator while lounging around the pool like the models on TV?

In May [2002], the Federal Trade Commission (FTC) filed complaints against three manufacturers of these devices, alleging that they have made false claims in their advertising, seen in heavily aired infomercials on national cable television, shorter television commercials, and ads in the print media.

The unfounded claims cited by the FTC include the promise of "six pack" or "washboard" abs without exercise, claims that the devices will give users a trimmer waist or cause fat loss, and that use of the device is equivalent to (or better than) regular abdominal exercises, such as sit-ups or crunches. The FTC complaints also allege that the advertising claimed falsely that the stimulators are safe for all to use, and did not disclose adequately the possible health hazards for some people.

Here's more information about the devices, what they can and can't do, and how they are regulated by the Food and Drug Administration's Center for Devices and Radiological Health.

Why does the FDA regulate electrical muscle stimulators?

Electrical muscle stimulators are considered medical devices under the Federal Food, Drug, and Cosmetic Act. Under this law and the agency's regulations, the FDA is responsible for regulating the sale of all electrical muscle stimulators in the United States. Therefore, firms must comply with appropriate FDA premarket regulatory requirements before they can legally sell their stimulators. Most electrical muscle stimulators (EMS devices) that have been reviewed by the FDA are intended for use in physical therapy and rehabilitation under the direction of a health-care professional. If a company wants to sell EMS devices directly to consumers, the company needs to show the FDA that the device can be used safely and effectively in that setting.

These electrical muscle stimulators are advertised not only to tone, firm, and strengthen abdominal muscles, but also to provide weight loss, girth reduction, and rock-hard abs. Do they really work?

Although an EMS device may be able to temporarily strengthen, tone or firm a muscle, no EMS devices have been cleared at this time for weight loss, girth reduction, or for obtaining rock-hard abs.

Is the FDA concerned about the unregulated marketing of these devices?

Yes. The FDA has received reports of shocks, burns, bruising, skin irritation, and pain associated with the use of some of these devices. There have been a few recent reports of interference with implanted devices such as pacemakers and defibrillators. Some injuries required hospital treatment. It is very important that these devices be properly designed, manufactured, and labeled with clear and complete instructions for use and that all users follow the instructions carefully. The FDA is also concerned because many of these devices have cables and leads. If those cables and leads do not comply with electrical safety standards, there is the possibility that users and other household members could be electrocuted. The FDA is currently investigating firms that are illegally marketing EMS devices.

Why should I select an electrical muscle stimulator that is legally marketed according to FDA regulations?

Electrical muscle stimulators that have not met FDA requirements are illegal, and the FDA has not determined whether they are properly designed, manufactured, and labeled to provide reasonable assurance that they are safe and effective.

Does that mean that it's unsafe to use an electrical muscle stimulator that has not met FDA requirements?

Using a product that has not met FDA requirements isn't necessarily unsafe or dangerous. But it could be. The FDA has received reports of injuries and interference with other critically important medical devices associated with the use of unregulated products. Unregulated devices also may have safety problems associated with cables and leads that can lead to accidental shock and electrocution of users and other household members, including children.

If I use an electrical muscle stimulator that has met FDA regulatory requirements, will it give me the same kind of effect that lots of sit-ups, stomach crunches, and other abdominal exercises will?

Using these devices alone will not give you six-pack abs. Applying electrical current to muscles may cause them to contract. Stimulating muscles repeatedly with electricity may eventually result in muscles that are strengthened and toned to some extent but will not, based on currently available data, create a major change in your appearance without the addition of weight loss and regular exercise.

But hasn't the FDA cleared electrical muscle stimulators to treat medical conditions?

Yes. The FDA has cleared many electrical muscle stimulators for prescription use in treating medical conditions. Doctors may use electrical muscle stimulators for patients who require muscle re-education, relaxation of muscle spasms, increased range of motion, prevention of muscle atrophy, and for treating other medical conditions that usually result from a stroke, a serious injury, or major surgery. Again, the effect of using these devices is primarily to help a patient recover from impaired muscle function due to a medical condition, not to increase muscle size enough to affect appearance.

Are there any over-the-counter EMS devices that have met the FDA's regulatory requirements?

Yes. At this time, Slendertone Flex, marketed by BMR NeuroTech Inc. of Phoenix, has been cleared by the FDA for toning, strengthening, and firming abdominal muscles.

Chapter 23

Choosing an Athletic Shoe

One of the major considerations when purchasing athletic shoes is what type of activity the shoes will be worn for. A runner, for example, should seek a different type of shoe than a tennis player. According to the American Orthopaedic Foot and Ankle Society (AOFAS), if you participate in a sport at least three times a week, you need a shoe specific to that sport.

Runners should select footwear that provides cushioning and support for the straight-ahead motion of the sport. Cushioning in the heel is also important. Tennis and basketball players should select court shoes that provide support for lateral, or side-to-side, movement. Because these athletes spend much of their time on the balls of their feet, cushioning of the forefoot is important. The same is true of people who aerobicize.

Cross-training shoes try to provide the best of both worlds without doing either very well. Buying a more specialized shoe properly fitted to your foot will provide greater comfort and more protection from injury. Furthermore, extremely lightweight racing shoes are meant only for competing; they should not be worn for training because they have sacrificed support and cushioning for speed. So-called "walking" shoes generally do not provide as much support and cushioning as running shoes; running shoes are thus preferable for walkers.

"Consider Use When Selecting Athletic Shoes," August 2001. © 2001 Medical College of Wisconsin. Reprinted with permission of Medical College of Wisconsin HealthLink, www.healthlink.mcw.edu. Reviewed by David A. Cooke, M.D., on August 1, 2006.

Another consideration involves the stability of the foot in the shoe. By checking the pair of shoes they're currently using, athletes can get an idea of how their shoes wear. Some people's feet roll or lean to the inside, for example. These people may want a thicker, firmer midsole on the inside of the foot to cradle the foot and keep it from rolling. For people whose feet roll to the outside or remain upright, more cushioning is recommended to absorb shock rather than transferring it up the leg to the knee and hip.

People with a higher arch may want to buy over-the-counter arch supports or insoles and replace the sock liner that is removable in most shoes.

An experienced salesperson can be a great help. He or she can help fit shoes properly to address the individual's concerns and explain about cushioning and shoe structure. Some brands are cut wider in the forefoot or narrower in the heel. Typically, the better cushioning, the more expensive a shoe will be. Weekend or casual athletes may actually need a higher quality shoe than those individuals who train a lot and whose bodies (and feet) are accustomed to exercise.

Be sure to try on both shoes as most people have one foot larger than the other. When you stand while trying on shoes, there should be about one thumb's width space between the tip of thc longest toe and the inside of the tip of the shoe. When simultaneously holding the toe and heel and pressing them toward one another, the shoe should bend over the ball of the foot, not in the middle of the arch (except for racing shoes).

Be sure to wear the same type of sock for the fitting as you will when exercising. Try on your shoes when your feet are at their largest—at the end of the day or after a workout. The shoe should grip your heel firmly without slipping. You should be able to freely wiggle all your toes when wearing the shoe. The shoe should be comfortable immediately.

Athletic shoes should be replaced after 300-500 miles of use. Note that a new pair of athletic shoes loses 50% of its cushioning capability just sitting in a box unused over a year's time. Some manufacturers imprint the shoe's date of production on the tongue or elsewhere on the shoe so you can be sure of purchasing a "fresh" shoe.

By Chris Geiser, Physical Therapist and Athletic Trainer, Froedtert & Medical College Sports Medicine Center, and Mark W. Niedfeldt, MD, Associate Professor of Family and Community Medicine, Medical College of Wisconsin, Froedtert & Medical College Sports Medicine Center.

Chapter 24

Facts about Aerobic Exercise

Chapter Contents

179

Section 24.1

Getting Ready for Aerobic Exercise: Warm up and Cool down

"Exercise and Injury Prevention: Warmups and Cooldowns" was provided by the Better Health Channel. Material on the Better Health Channel is regularly updated. For the latest version of this information please visit: www.betterhealth.vic.gov.au.

Warming up before exercise is the best way to reduce the risk of injury. Cold joints, tendons, and muscles are more likely to get strained or sprained by sudden movement or exertion. In normal conditions, a five- to 10-minute warmup is all you'll need—add a few extra minutes in colder weather. Concentrate on warming up the specific muscle groups you will be using in your exercise and include stretches. Cooling down after exercise is also an important injury prevention strategy. Your physiotherapist can help you devise warmup and cooldown routines appropriate to your sport.

The Health Benefits of Warming up

Some of the many health benefits of warming up before exercise or sport:

- It raises the heart rate so that the body is prepared for physical exertion.
- It speeds up nerve impulses so that reflexes are enhanced.
- It reduces muscle tension.
- It sends oxygenated blood to the muscle groups.
- It reduces the risk of injury, particularly to connective tissue like tendons.
- It increases flexibility and joint mobility.

Warmups for Specific Sports

A thorough warmup routine should not only raise the heart rate, but also warm the particular muscle groups that will be used during your sport. Some examples include:

- Cycling—Begin by cycling at a slow, leisurely pace and gradually increase the speed.
- Running—Begin by walking at a brisk pace. As your heart rate and breathing increase, pick up the speed.
- Swimming—Perform arm circles. When you get in the pool, start by performing slow and easy laps.
- Tennis—Hold the tennis racquet and gently perform your strokes.

Stretching Suggestions

Stretching should be part of both your warmup and cooldown routines. Suggestions include:

- Stretch your muscles after your warmup exercises.
- Only stretch a muscle to the point of mild discomfort. If it hurts, you're pushing too hard—ease off.
- Don't bounce. Instead, hold the stretch for around 10 to 30 seconds.
- Stretch opposing muscle groups one after the other. For example, stretch your quadriceps (muscles on the front of the thigh) then stretch the hamstrings (muscles on the back of the thigh).
- Remember to keep breathing normally as you stretch.

The Health Benefits of Cooling Down

Some of the many health benefits of cooling down after exercise or sport:

- It helps to gently return heart rate, breathing, and blood pressure to normal.
- It improves flexibility.
- It reduces the risk of injury.
- It removes waste products from muscle tissue (such as lactic acid) and helps to reduce the risk of soreness.

Cooldown Suggestions

It is important to cool down after exercise to further reduce the risk of injury. Suggestions include:

- Your cooldown should last several minutes.

- Taper off your activity. For example, if you have been running, cool down by slowing down to a jog then a brisk walk for a few minutes.

- Finish your cooldown routine with 10 minutes or so of gentle stretches.

Other Injury Prevention Suggestions

Taking sufficient time to warm up and cool down significantly reduces the risk of injury during sport. Other suggestions include:

- Don't exercise or perform beyond your physical capabilities.

- Take into consideration that equipment may need to be adapted to your needs—for example, bike pedals, gym equipment, and skiing equipment. Always wear protective equipment particular to your sport—for example, helmets, elbow and knee guards, and mouth guards.

- Avoid heavy exertion in extreme heat as it can lead to heat exhaustion or heat stroke.

- Use tape or bandages to brace vulnerable joints and prevent them from slipping beyond their comfortable range of motion.

- Consider having a massage after your cooldown to promote muscle flexibility.

- Ensure you have enough rest and recovery days.

Where to Get Help

- Your doctor
- Physiotherapist

Things to Remember

- Cold joints, tendons, and muscles are more likely to get strained or sprained by sudden movement or exertion.

- Warming up before exercise is the best way to reduce the risk of injury.

- Concentrate on warming up the specific muscle groups you will be using in your exercise and include stretches.

- It is important to cool down after exercise to further reduce the risk of injury.

Section 24.2

Common Types of Aerobic Exercise

"What Is the Best Type of Aerobic Exercise?" reprinted with permission from The Cleveland Clinic Heart Center, http://www.clevelandclinic.org/heartcenter. © 2004 The Cleveland Clinic Foundation. All rights reserved.

There is no one best exercise for everyone. The benefits to your heart are similar as long as the type of exercise satisfies some basic requirements and you follow the recommended program goals, as prescribed by your doctor or exercise physiologist.

Your aerobic exercise program should have four goals:

- It is aerobic. It uses large muscle groups repetitively for a sustained amount of time.

- You perform it for 30 to 60 minutes, three to five days a week.

- It meets the cardiovascular goals your doctor or exercise physiologist has prescribed for you.

- It is something you will enjoy doing for an extended period of time.

Safety First

The type of exercise you choose is a personal decision, but you should take certain factors into consideration to reduce the risk of injury or complications and make exercise more enjoyable.

- Always speak to your doctor first before starting any new exercise program.

- Choose a type of exercise you are more likely to stay with over the long term.

- Perform your activity at a level in which you can carry on a conversation or speak clearly while exercising. This talk test provides a general rule of thumb to help you determine if a particular activity is too strenuous for you. It is especially helpful if you have not been given a heart rate (pulse) zone to stay in during exercise.

Exercise Options

Let's look at some of the common types of aerobic exercise. See which one is best suited for you.

Walking

Walking is one of the simplest and most available aerobic exercises. You can vary the intensity to match your fitness level. Other than walking shoes, it does not require any special equipment. You can walk almost anywhere: outdoors or indoors (malls, indoor tracks, or a treadmill). This makes walking easy to continue throughout the year. Walking is a good choice for those starting their first exercise program or those who find other exercises too hard on their joints.

Cycling

Cycling is another type of aerobic exercise with wide appeal and value. You can use a stationary or regular bike. Cycling may be ideal for individuals who, due to arthritis or other orthopedic problems, are unable to walk for an extended period of time without pain or difficulty. A program that combines walking and cycling may provide cardiovascular benefits without inducing the limiting pain as quickly. Cycling is also a good choice for people who are greater than 50 pounds overweight. It helps the heart without the mechanical stress on the back, hips, knees, and ankles that walking can cause. One drawback—if you cycle outdoors, exclusively, the weather may limit your activity.

Ski Machines, Stair Climbers, Steppers, and Ellipticals

These types of machines can provide a good aerobic workout and each has its own unique strengths and drawbacks. First, exercise on these machines may be too strenuous to be enjoyable. To determine if this type of machine is within your capability, give the machine of your choice a trial run at the store or fitness center.

You should be able to pass the talk test while exercising at a moderate pace. People with knee or hip problems should avoid stair climbers and steppers as these machines can put extra stress on these joints. Ski machines require above-average coordination to master. The advantage to the machines is that they are indoor activities that can be pursued regardless of the weather.

Swimming Activities

Swimming is an excellent aerobic exercise, but considerations should be made before starting a program. For exercise beginners, people with low fitness levels, or non-swimmers it might be a difficult activity to maintain at the appropriate intensity for the recommended 30 to 60 minutes. Also, because the focus of swimming is on the smaller upper body musculature and swimming is a less efficient activity than cycling or walking, one can easily exceed their target heart rate range with swimming. Therefore, those with heart conditions should address a swimming program with their physician before starting. Water aerobics and water walking are good alternatives for those with joint pain. The buoyancy provided by the water eases stress on the joints.

Jogging and Aerobic Dance

These can be safe and beneficial exercises for the highly fit person. Both can be done indoors, which makes them year-round activities. Anyone with orthopedic problems or who experiences symptoms such as chest pain or shortness of breath should not engage in these activities. Remember to check with your doctor or cardiac rehabilitation instructor before starting any exercise program.

Section 24.3

Cross Training: What It Is and How It Works

Reproduced with permission from Cross Training, in Johnson TR, (ed): *Your Orthopaedic Connection*, Rosemont, IL, American Academy of Orthopaedic Surgeons. Available at http://orthoinfo.aaos.org.

If the thought of doing the same old exercises every day keeps you from starting an exercise program, cross training may be the answer. Cross training simply means that you include a variety of activities in your fitness program. For example, you could alternate jogging and swimming during the week, and play a game of tennis on the weekend. All three are aerobic activities and use similar muscles, but in different ways.

Cross training began to build in popularity during the 1980s. Now, with increasing numbers of multi-sport events such as triathlons, it is a common training technique. Cross training is an ideal way to develop a "balanced" fitness program and has several benefits, whether you are a serious athlete or just someone interested in becoming more fit and active.

- Cross training can provide a "total body tune-up," something you won't get if you concentrate on just one type of activity.

- Including a variety of activities in your fitness program will help prevent boredom. That can help you stick to the program.

- Exercising various muscle groups may help your muscles adapt more easily to new activities.

- Because you won't be using the same muscles in the same way all the time, you may experience fewer overuse injuries.

- If you do become injured, you usually won't have to give up your entire fitness program. You may be able to modify or substitute activities, based on your physician's suggestions.

How to Cross Train

A general fitness program has three components:

1. Aerobic exercises (stair climbing, walking, skating) improve cardiovascular capabilities.

2. Strength training (weight lifting, push-ups) helps develop muscle mass.

3. Flexibility exercises (stretches, yoga) help keep muscles limber.

With cross training, you can easily incorporate all three components in your fitness routine. First, talk to your physician and make sure that it's safe for you to begin a program. Some activities are not appropriate for people with certain physical limitations.

Then consider what kinds of activities are readily available to you. Select activities that are convenient and enjoyable. You should be doing at least 30 minutes of moderate activity on most days. You can break your exercise routine into shorter periods, as long as it adds up over the course of the day. Remember that physical activity isn't limited to sports like jogging or weight lifting. Dancing, gardening, and housework count, too.

A Sample Program

A balanced weekly cross training program might look like this:

1. **Three times a week:** 30 minutes of aerobic exercises, alternating activities such as walking, swimming, and stair climbing.

2. **Twice a week (not consecutive days):** 30 minutes of strength training, working each major muscle group.

3. **Every day:** 5 to 10 minutes of stretching. It's also safe to walk every day.

Start slowly and gradually increase the duration and intensity of your exercises. Try to follow the 10% rule—increase the frequency, duration, or intensity of an activity by no more than 10% each week.

You may not see results overnight, but cross training will have a beneficial effect on your health and fitness level. Regular physical activity increases your chances for a longer, healthier, and more independent life. Keep at it!

Section 24.4

Interval Training

Lack of time is the number one reason people give for not exercising. And lack of results once they do start exercising isn't far behind. Interval training is a great solution for both of these common problems.

Interval training involves alternating short bursts of intense activity with what is called active recovery, which is typically a less-intense form of the original activity.

The Swedes came up with a term for this type of training: fartlek, which means speed play. Not only is it an efficient training method, fartlek training can help you avoid injuries that often accompany nonstop, repetitive activity, and provides the opportunity to increase your intensity without burning yourself out in a matter of minutes.

Unlike traditional interval training, fartlek training does not involve specifically or accurately measured intervals. Instead, intervals are based according to the needs and perceptions of the participant. In other words, how you feel determines the length and speed of each interval.

The Advantages of Intervals

Interval training utilizes the body's two energy-producing systems: the aerobic and the anaerobic. The aerobic system is the one that allows you to walk or run for several miles, that uses oxygen to convert carbohydrates from various sources throughout the body into energy.

The anaerobic system, on the other hand, draws energy from carbohydrates (in the form of glycogen) stored in the muscles for short bursts of activity such as sprinting, jumping, or lifting heavy objects. This system does not require oxygen, nor does it provide enough energy for more than the briefest of activities. And its byproduct, lactic acid, is responsible for that achy, burning sensation in your muscles that you feel after, say, running up several flights of stairs.

Interval Basics

Interval training allows you to enjoy the benefits of anaerobic activities without having to endure those burning muscles. In its most basic form, interval or fartlek training might involve walking for two minutes, running for two, and alternating this pattern throughout the duration of a workout.

The intensity (or lack thereof) of each interval is up to how you feel and what you are trying to achieve. The same is true for the length of each interval. For example, if it is your habit to walk two miles per day in 30 minutes, you can easily increase the intensity of your walk (as well as up its calorie-burning potential) by picking up the pace every few minutes and then returning to your usual speed.

A great trick is to tell yourself that you'll run a particular distance, from the blue car to the green house on the corner, for example, and then walk from the green house to the next telephone pole.

When you first start fartlek training, each interval can be a negotiation with yourself depending on how strong or energetic you happen to feel during that particular workout. This helps to break up the boredom and drudgery that often comes from doing the same thing day after day.

A More Advanced Approach

Despite its simplicity, it also is possible to take a very scientific approach to interval training, timing both the work and recovery intervals according to specific goals. See below for a list of the four variables to keep in mind when designing an interval training program.

An ACE-certified personal trainer can help you design an interval training program based on your particular goals.

Consider the following four variables when designing an interval training program:

- Intensity (speed) of work interval
- Duration (distance or time) of work interval
- Duration of rest or recovery interval
- Number of repetitions of each interval

Chapter 25

Common Forms
of Aerobic Exercise

Chapter Contents

Section 25.1

Walking for Fitness: A Step in the Right Direction

"Walking: A Step in the Right Direction" is a brochure produced by the Weight-control Information Network (WIN), part of the U.S. Department of Health and Human Services, NIH Publication No. 04-4155, September 2004.

Walking is one of the easiest ways to be physically active. You can do it almost anywhere and at any time. Walking is also inexpensive. All you need is a pair of shoes with sturdy heel support. Walking will:

- give you more energy;
- make you feel good;
- help you to relax;
- reduce stress;
- help you sleep better;
- tone your muscles;
- help control your appetite; and
- increase the number of calories your body uses.

For all these reasons, people have started walking programs. If you would like to start your own program, read and follow the information provided here.

Is it OK for me to walk?

Answer the following questions before you begin a walking program.

- Has your health care provider ever told you that you have heart trouble?
- When you are physically active, do you have pains in your chest or on your left side (neck, shoulder, or arm)?

- Do you often feel faint or have dizzy spells?

- Do you feel extremely breathless after you have been physically active?

- Has your health care provider told you that you have high blood pressure?

- Has your health care provider told you that you have bone or joint problems, like arthritis, that could get worse if you are physically active?

- Are you over 50 years old and not used to a lot of physical activity?

- Do you have a health problem or physical reason not mentioned here that might keep you from starting a walking program?

If you answered yes to any of these questions, please check with your health care provider before starting a walking program or other form of physical activity.

How do I start a walking program?

Leave time in your busy schedule to follow a walking program that will work for you. In planning your walking program, keep the following points in mind:

- Choose a safe place to walk. Find a partner or group of people to walk with you. Your walking partner(s) should be able to walk with you on the same schedule and at the same speed.

- Wear shoes with thick flexible soles that will cushion your feet and absorb shock.

- Wear clothes that will keep you dry and comfortable. Look for synthetic fabrics that absorb sweat and remove it from your skin.

- For extra warmth in winter, wear a knit cap. To stay cool in summer, wear a baseball cap or visor.

- Do light stretching before and after you walk.

- Think of your walk in three parts. Walk slowly for 5 minutes. Increase your speed for the next 5 minutes. Finally, to cool down, walk slowly again for 5 minutes.

- Try to walk at least three times per week. Add 2 to 3 minutes per week to the fast walk. If you walk less than three times per week, increase the fast walk more slowly.

- To avoid stiff or sore muscles or joints, start gradually. Over several weeks, begin walking faster, going further, and walking for longer periods of time.

- The more you walk, the better you will feel. You also will use more calories.

What are some safety tips?

Keep safety in mind when you plan your route and the time of your walk.

- Walk in the daytime or at night in well-lighted areas.
- Walk in a group at all times.
- Notify your local police station of your group's walking time and route.
- Do not wear jewelry.
- Do not wear headphones.
- Be aware of your surroundings.

How do I warm up?

Before you start to walk, do the stretches shown. Remember not to bounce when you stretch. Perform slow movements and stretch only as far as you feel comfortable.

How do I take the first step?

Walking right is very important.

- Walk with your chin up and your shoulders held slightly back.
- Walk so that the heel of your foot touches the ground first. Roll your weight forward.
- Walk with your toes pointed forward.
- Swing your arms as you walk.

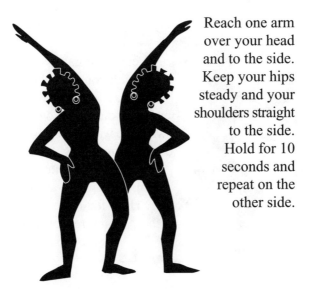

Reach one arm over your head and to the side. Keep your hips steady and your shoulders straight to the side. Hold for 10 seconds and repeat on the other side.

Figure 25.1. Side Reaches

Lean your back against a wall. Keep your head, hips, and feet in a straight line. Pull one knee to your chest, hold for 10 seconds, then repeat with the other leg.

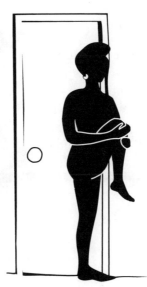

Figure 25.2. Knee Pull

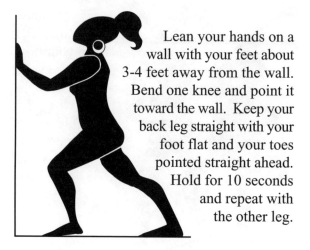

Lean your hands on a wall with your feet about 3-4 feet away from the wall. Bend one knee and point it toward the wall. Keep your back leg straight with your foot flat and your toes pointed straight ahead. Hold for 10 seconds and repeat with the other leg.

Figure 25.3. Wall Push

Pull your right foot to your buttocks with your right hand. Keep your knee pointing straight to the ground. Hold for 10 seconds and repeat with your left foot and hand.

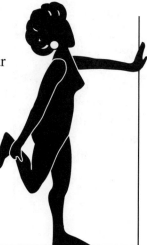

Figure 25.4. Leg Curl

	Warm Up Time	*Fast Walk Time*	*Cool Down Time*	*Total Time*
WEEK 1	Walk slowly 5 min.	Walk briskly 5 min.	Walk slowly 5 min.	15 min.
WEEK 2	Walk slowly 5 min.	Walk briskly 8 min.	Walk slowly 5 min.	18 min.
WEEK 3	Walk slowly 5 min.	Walk briskly 11 min.	Walk slowly 5 min.	21 min.
WEEK 4	Walk slowly 5 min.	Walk briskly 14 min.	Walk slowly 5 min.	24 min.
WEEK 5	Walk slowly 5 min.	Walk briskly 17 min.	Walk slowly 5 min.	27 min.
WEEK 6	Walk slowly 5 min.	Walk briskly 20 min.	Walk slowly 5 min.	30 min.
WEEK 7	Walk slowly 5 min.	Walk briskly 23 min.	Walk slowly 5 min.	33 min.
WEEK 8	Walk slowly 5 min.	Walk briskly 26 min.	Walk slowly 5 min.	36 min.
WEEK 9 & BEYOND	Walk slowly 5 min.	Walk briskly 30 min.	Walk slowly 5 min.	40 min.

Chart 25.1. *A sample walking program for exercise beginners. If you walk less than three times per week, increase the fast walk time more slowly.*

Section 25.2

The Health Benefits of Hiking

"Hiking for Fitness: Three Steps to Success,"
reprinted with permission Eat Right Montana, © 2006.

Tips for Hiking for Fitness

Look for fun and scenic hikes close to home.

The definition of a hike is "a long walk in the countryside, usually for pleasure." Now, what could be better for your mental and physical health than a long walk for pleasure—especially with family, friends, and/or a friendly pet!

Whether you live in the city or the country, the world is full of wonderful places to hike. City parks and river fronts often have easily accessible hiking paths, whereas state and national parks provide nature's fitness centers at no or minimal cost.

Get the right gear for fun and safety.

The gear for day hiking is really quite simple: sturdy shoes or boots for your feet and a cap or hat for sun protection are the most essential pieces of equipment. You'll also want an easy way to carry water and some tasty fuel, like fruit and nuts, for the trail.

Longer hikes or overnight trips require more gear and a well-fitting pack to carry it all. Get advice on buying the best equipment from an outdoor store. Try renting some equipment first (from a store, college, or club) to see what works best for you.

Plan regular hikes with family, friends, and dogs.

Making a commitment to regular activities with other people increases the likelihood that you will actually do them. Plan shorter, closer, once-a-week hikes for summer evenings. Plan longer weekend hikes when you have the time for greater distances.

A fun way to increase your fitness and feel a real sense of success is to set your sights on a taller or longer goal. You might want to climb a mountain or walk a historic route somewhere in the state. All it takes is some planning and training!

Section 25.3

Tips for Beginning Runners

"Starting a Running Program: Tips for Beginning Runners,"
by Matt Rogers, MS, CSCS, published by the U.S. Customs and Border
Protection (www.cbp.gov), 2006.

Take stock of your current health and fitness level.

If you have been sedentary, have or suspect health problems such as heart disease, diabetes, high blood pressure, high cholesterol, joint problems, etc., or are over 40, it is recommended that you have a physical with your doctor before starting a vigorous exercise program. If you know you have no major health problems, starting a light- to moderate-intensity exercise program such as brisk walking usually does not require a physical, but check with your doctor for his or her opinion in your specific case. Remember that the health risks of a sedentary lifestyle are much greater than the risks of exercise. A renowned exercise physiologist, Per Olaf Astrand, quipped that if one plans a sedentary lifestyle, one should have a physical to see if the heart can stand it.

Be safe.

Don't run/walk in high crime areas. When running after dark, be sure to wear reflective clothing, carry a small flashlight, and assume drivers don't see you. Well-lighted neighborhoods are a good choice. Women should run with a partner or a dog if possible, and consider carrying pepper spray. Runners and walkers should never use headphones outdoors, as it makes it impossible to hear traffic or an approaching attacker. Always carry ID.

Start slowly and build up gradually.

Most people should start with a brisk walking program and progress to a mix of alternating walking and jogging. Eventually you should be able to run the entire distance you desire at a comfortable pace. At that point you can increase weekly mileage about 10% every 3rd week, depending on your goals. For health and fitness there is generally no need to run more than about 15 miles per week, along with some strength and flexibility training. Those wishing to progress to competitive running should seek out experienced runners or coaches for advice. Check www.rrca.org for a running club in your area.

Using the right type of shoes helps prevent injuries.

Shin splints and runner's knee are preventable with proper conditioning **and** the right running shoe type. There are three basic types for different running mechanics:

- **Motion Control**—generally best choice for flat feet and "floppy ankles" (overpronation or rolling too far to the inside after foot touches down). Shoes should be straight lasted and often will have a full board last inside, plus a harder rubber or plastic area on the inner (arch support) side of heel to control excess movement.

- **Stability**—generally best for normal arches, these shoes will have a semi-curved last and a moderate amount of motion control.

- **Cushioned**—generally best for high arches and "clunk foot"; these feet are usually very rigid and underpronate. Underpronation means that feet do not roll to the inside far enough after foot touches down and therefore make poor shock absorbers. Shoes should have a curved or semi-curved last, extra cushioning, a full slip last (no board inside), and be very flexible.

Another choice for off road running are trail running shoes. These are made low to the ground and more stable to help prevent ankle sprains, have good traction, and help prevent foot bruises from roots and rocks.

Don't use any type running shoes for other sports, as they are not made for lateral movements, making ankle sprains more likely. They also last longer and maintain cushioning better if only used for running. Use only good quality court shoes or cross-trainers for other conditioning activities. Wrestling shoes are recommended for defensive tactics training on matted floors.

Do the "wet test" to see what type of foot you have.

Wet feet and step onto some paper on a hard surface. (Even better is to run a short distance barefoot on sand.) A "blob" footprint with little arch indicates flat feet. Two 'islands' with a lot of space between the heel and ball indicates high arches. A normal arch will look like the classic cartoon footprint.

Make sure the shoe fits.

The best shoe for you is one that fits your foot type and running mechanics and also is the right length and width. Try on running shoes with the socks you plan to run in and toward the end of the day when feet are larger. You should have about one thumb's width of room between your longest toe and the end of the shoe. Shoes should be wide enough that foot does not feel pinched on the sides, but not a sloppy fit or one that slips at the heel. Jog a bit in the store to see how the shoes feel and fit. Most running specialty stores will have the expertise and take the time to fit you properly in several models and watch you run in them before you choose. Don't count on the employees of a general sporting goods or discount footwear store to understand any of the above running shoe information.

Dress for the weather.

In cold weather wear several lightweight layers, hat, and gloves to trap body heat. You can unzip or remove layers if you get too warm. In hot weather wear as little as the law allows, and don't forget the sunscreen. Drink plenty of fluids throughout the day to avoid dehydration and plan ahead so you can get fluids during longer runs.

Run with good form.

Shoulders should be relaxed with elbows bent to about 90 degrees as arms swing smoothly forward and back with no twisting of the torso. Arms should not cross the center of body and hands should pass just above the "hip pocket" on each forward and backward motion. The upper body should be nearly upright, with a very slight forward lean. Don't run on the toes or hit hard with the heel, but rather land as softly as possible with foot nearly flat. The foot should be flexed upward slightly just before foot lands. Breathe naturally through both the nose and mouth. If you're gasping for air—slow down.

Most running injuries are avoidable.

Following the tips on proper footwear, form, and starting slowly will greatly reduce your chances of common beginners' complaints such as shin splints and knee pain. Basic strength and flexibility exercises can prevent and correct muscle imbalances responsible for most running injuries. If you do have a running injury, find the cause rather than just treating the symptoms.

Ignore the myths.

The bulk of scientific evidence shows that running, even in ultra-marathon runners, does not cause osteoarthritis in the hips or knees if these joints were healthy to begin with. In fact, weight-bearing exercise such as running probably prevents arthritis, since the incidence in long-time runners is about half that of non-runners, including swimmers.

Matt Rogers began running and working out at age 13 in order to overcome childhood obesity, and has maintained a healthy weight for nearly 3 decades. He is an exercise physiologist, NSCA Certified Strength and Conditioning Specialist, and a long-distance runner. Rogers competed in cross-country and track and field in high school and at Eastern Kentucky University. He is employed in the Department of Health Promotion and Wellness by Southeast Georgia Health System and is currently assigned to the U.S. Customs & Border Protection Academy in Glynco, Georgia.

Section 25.4

Bicycling for Health and Fitness

The documents "Bicycling for Health and Fitness" and "Getting Back on Your Bicycle" are reprinted from the Pedestrian and Bicycle Information Center, http://www.bicyclinginfo.org. Accessed June 6, 2006.

Bicycling for Health and Fitness

Remember the feeling of first learning to ride a bicycle on your own—without training wheels and without a parent's balancing hand? Remember that sudden rush of freedom?

If you have to strain to think back that far, well, maybe it's time to strap on a helmet and saddle up. Because not only is bicycling fun and freeing, it's an excellent way to get healthy exercise.

That's one of the reasons that sixty million Americans bicycle. Whether you're an avid mountain biker or simply trying to incorporate cycling into your daily routine, you too can reap the many health benefits of bicycling.

This has never been more important until now. An alarming number of Americans are becoming more sedentary and obese and consequently risking their lives, reports the Centers for Disease Control and Prevention (CDC). "Obesity is an epidemic and should be taken as seriously as any disease epidemic," warns CDC director Jeffrey Kaplan.

In recent studies the CDC found that thanks to the American lifestyle of convenience and inactivity, cycling and walking have been replaced by automobile travel for all but the shortest distances. That's why we have to make bicycling convenient again.

Even small increases in light to moderate activity will produce measurable benefits among those who are least active. Cycle for pleasure, but try to integrate bicycling wherever you can: a trip to the store, to a sporting event or party, to a concert, to a friend's house. Try cycling to work at least once a month and then once a week.

You'll shape up, and your body will thank you. Because you'll reduce your risk of coronary heart disease, stroke, and other chronic and life-threatening illnesses. You'll lower your health care costs. And while you're enhancing your physical health, you'll improve your mental outlook and overall quality of life.

Even older adults can cycle. Just visit any country outside the United States and you'll see the proof positive. Regular exercise provides a myriad of health benefits for senior adults including a stronger heart, a positive mental outlook and an increased chance of remaining indefinitely independent—a benefit that will become increasingly important as our population ages in the coming years.

Once upon a time, kids represented the largest cycling population. But thanks to a number of contributing factors—among them, unsafe neighborhoods, heavy traffic, and a de-emphasis on physical activity— American children spent 15% less time bicycling in 1998 than they did eight years ago. And kids who cycle infrequently grow up to be adults who cycle less- or not at all.

The solution? It's easy. In fact, it's just like learning to ride a bicycle all over again.

Getting Back on Your Bicycle

If it's been too long since you've ridden your bicycle last, now is the time to dust off your bicycle. Here are a few tips to save some embarrassment and to keep you safe!

Get Your Bicycle Checked Out

Take your bicycle to your local bicycle shop and get a tune-up. Your bike is a wonderfully simple and efficient machine, but needs some TLC—and you don't want to break down your first time out. Most bike dealers have spring specials to check the essentials, such as brakes, gears, and tires, and squirt oil in all the right places.

Get Yourself Checked Out

If you really haven't ridden in a long time, it might be wise to check in with your doctor and see if there's any reason you shouldn't be saddling up and going for a spin. Bicycling is such a great way to get the recommended daily dose of exercise that chances are your doctor will encourage you to go for it. Don't try to ride 50 miles right away; take it slowly and you'll enjoy the ride and still be able to walk again the next day.

Deck Yourself out with the Latest Gear

Simplicity is certainly one of the attractions of bicycling—you can just hop on your bike and start riding. But there's also a lot of equipment available to make your ride safer and more comfortable. Things have come a long way since the days of the wool cycling shorts. For example:

- A wide variety of helmets are available in different styles and price ranges. Your local bike dealer will help you get the right size and fit.

- A sturdy lock is essential if you're planning on riding your bike and leaving it somewhere for awhile.

- Front and rear lights and reflectors are required, and make good sense, if you're going to be riding at night or dusk.

- Padded shorts, gloves, and other special clothing will make longer rides more comfortable, but probably aren't necessary for riding to the video store and back.

Find a Safe Place to Practice

Again, if you really haven't ridden in a long time, it makes sense to regain your confidence on the bike and practice somewhere safe as opposed to on the main road to work. Find a quiet street, trail, playground, or empty parking lot and get back in touch with your bike handling skills. Practice looking behind you, making turns, stopping suddenly, dodging rocks or potholes, changing gears, and even getting on and off. If you are using toe clips or clipless pedals, take a few extra minutes to remind yourself how to get your feet out in a hurry.

Follow the Rules of the Road

When you're ready to hit the road or trail, remembering a few basic safety rules will help you avoid the most common mistakes that cause crashes.

- **Always ride with traffic.** Forget what you heard in the past, you are better off riding with the flow of traffic, not against it. You are much more predictable and visible to motorists, especially at intersections and driveways.

- **Don't ride on the sidewalk.** Although you might think it's a safer option, motorists are simply not looking for bicyclists on the sidewalk, especially those riding against traffic. So at every driveway and intersection, you are at much greater risk of being hit by a motorist than if you were riding on the road with traffic. Pedestrians will thank you for riding on the road as well.

- **Ride on the trail, paved shoulder, bike lane, or bike route.** But you still need to follow the rules of the road and watch out for your fellow travelers. Ride to the right, signal your turns, and obey traffic signs and signals.

- **Be predictable and visible.** Try not to be hesitant or do things that motorists and other travelers may not be expecting. Make sure everyone can see you and knows where you are and where you are going.

- **Watch for turning traffic.** Perhaps rather surprisingly, the crash data tells us that getting hit from behind is extremely unlikely. Most car/bike collisions happen at intersections and driveways when motorists or bicyclists are turning. So at every intersection and driveway, keep a careful eye out for:

  - motorists turning right in front of you—you may be going faster than they think; and

  - motorists turning left across your path—drivers are looking for gaps in traffic and may not be paying attention to anything other than other motor vehicles.

- **Watch for stuff on the road or trail that might make you fall or swerve**. Rocks, trash, wet leaves, potholes, gravel, railroad tracks and even wet pavement markings can all send you flying.

Have Fun

Bicycling is fun, healthy, safe, convenient, and by riding you are setting a great example to others. So above all have a great time riding.

Section 25.5

Aquatic Exercise

Are you considering a water fitness program? More people than ever are exploring pool activity programs, and for good reason: Water fitness can improve strength, flexibility, and cardiovascular health; decrease body fat; facilitate rehabilitation; improve functionality for daily living; and even enhance sports skills. Water fitness classes today offer more variety than ever before, but how do you find the right class for your goals, interests, and skills?

We asked water fitness experts Mary Sanders, MS, an adjunct faculty member at the University of Nevada at Reno, and Tatiana Kolovou, assistant director of fitness and wellness for the Division of Recreational Sports at Indiana University in Bloomington. They offered these recommendations for making sure your pool time is spent wisely.

1. Check out the facility.

Start with the basics, says Kolovou. Look for a clean, safe, well-maintained pool. The water temperature should be comfortable: 82 to 84 degrees Fahrenheit (28 to 29 degrees Celsius); and there should be a lifeguard on duty—your instructor shouldn't have to do it all! Check out the equipment, too. You want to see a variety—for example, buoyancy belts and dumbbells, gloves, noodles, and paddles.

2. Look for professionalism.

Ask about the water fitness staff itself. Are instructors professionally trained in fitness, not just swimming or lifeguard skills? The staff should be certified in fitness and have additional training in water fitness. Also inquire about the types of classes available and the results you can expect from each class. If the course descriptions are vague or confusing, ask for more detailed explanations.

207

3. Know your limitations.

In general, water fitness is so versatile and safe it is the ideal choice for people with a variety of conditions, including pregnancy, orthopedic problems, and arthritis. Before joining a class, however, always check with the instructor to make sure it will be appropriate for you. Don't attempt a deep-water fitness class unless you are comfortable in deep water; you can't rely on a buoyancy device to give you complete confidence.

4. Try a variety of classes, and practice basic skills.

Remember that all classes are not alike; training in the water is muscle- and function-specific. Once in the pool, ensure your comfort and safety by learning the fundamentals—for instance, how to scull for balance (making figures of eight with your hands) and how to recover to a stand, or vertical position, with correct posture.

Your instructor should encourage you to go at your own pace, and teach you how to progressively increase and decrease the intensity of each exercise. The pool is a liquid weight machine, says Sanders. The harder you press, the more intense your workout is, so you have great control of your exercise program.

5. Know your goals.

This may be the most important key to having a satisfying water fitness experience, says Sanders. She suggests you look for classes that focus on some or all of the following, depending on the results you'd like to achieve:

- **Cardiovascular health and weight management.** To provide these benefits, a class should focus primarily on working the legs, using the arms (with webbed gloves on the hands) for balance. Interval training is the ideal. You should be able to adjust your speed and effort as needed to create a progressive training program.

- **Muscular endurance.** To improve muscular endurance, a class should work isolated muscle groups along with the muscles that stabilize the joints and body. Shallow-water jumping, buoyancy devices, an aquatic step, or surface area equipment such as giant sandals (called Sloggers) may be used to add overload.

- **Functional fitness.** If your goal is functional fitness, look for exercises that target the activities of daily living. For example, aquatic step exercise can improve stair climbing, and a program that includes dynamic reaching and leaping can enhance range of motion and flexibility. Your instructor should teach proper postural alignment for each activity.

- **Sports skills.** Do you want to hone your skills on the court or field? Check for sport-specific drills that will improve your ability to run, jump, change directions, etc.

- **Physical therapy.** If you need rehabilitation, you should seek a licensed therapist for your water fitness program. Postrehabilitation can be conducted by a trained water fitness professional who is willing to work closely with your health care providers and can design progressions to help you regain function.

Chapter 26

Cardiorespiratory Exercise in Everyday Activities and Recreation

Chapter Contents

Section 26.1

How Environment and Community Affect Physical Activity

"Design," © 2006 Active Living by Design. Reprinted with permission. For additional information, visit www.activelivingbydesign.org.

Design is a key component for creating active living environments. By designing buildings, communities, and environments that reduce automobile reliance and support pedestrian and bicycle activity, physical structures can help improve public health by promoting active living, a way of life that integrates physical activity into daily routines.

Design and Public Health

The built environment by definition is planned and designed by humans and can ultimately support or inhibit physical activity. The built environment encompasses all of the buildings, spaces, and products created or modified by people. For example: buildings (housing, schools, workplaces); land use (industrial or residential); public resources (parks, museums); zoning regulations; and transportation systems. Design is defined as the intentional change to an existing environment or the creation of a new one, but is more than just urban planning or architecture. It is a process that encompasses everything from the micro (stairwells, bike racks, promotional signs), to the design of buildings and spaces between them, to the macro (how cities are laid out). Routine physical activity is necessary to prevent premature death, unnecessary illness and disability, enhance physical and mental health, and help maintain a high quality of life for everyone. A healthy environment that is designed to positively affect physical activity by providing pedestrian-friendly amenities would: encourage walking and biking; promote human interaction and social adhesion; remove barriers to activity for everyone; and make healthy levels of physical activity attainable for large numbers of people during their daily routine.

Historically, design of the built environment and public health developed close ties, especially in the past two hundred years. In colonial times, evolving urban environments fostered infectious diseases due to inadequate housing conditions (crowded, dark, unventilated housing), unpaved and littered streets, and inadequate or non-existent drinking water and sewage systems. By the beginning of the twentieth century, as the industrial era emerged, environmental pollutants, bad air quality, and related social problems such as high density have dominated health profiles of the urban environment.

Health threats of the urban environment (infectious diseases, industrial pollutants and social conditions) gained prominence, especially in the twentieth century.[1] Reactions to the environmental and social problems of the industrial revolution and their health consequences, supported by the GI Bill, cheap capital, mass automobile ownership, and emerging land development strategies, converged to legitimize a new urban planning and design paradigm. Changing zoning regulations, fostered by an anti-urban movement, also facilitated these changes.

Beginning in the post-WWII era of the 1950s, provisions developed to overcome infectious diseases and other health issues, dramatically changing the characteristics of what were originally considered healthy living environments. However, their support of auto-dependent, sedentary lifestyles has now produced the chronic diseases of the twenty-first century and "sprawl" development.

Design Affects Our Level of Physical Activity

Research is beginning to show how the built environment is designed has a direct influence on the amount of physical activity users of that environment receive. Evidence suggests that ranging from the nearby environ of one's home or work place (micro); one's neighborhood (meso); to the larger domain of our cities (macro), the built environment is an important variable in physical activity.

- Primarily, different land uses (shops, restaurants, cafes, schools, parks, beaches etc.) within an accessible distance increases physical activity by offering destinations for both leisure and utilitarian physical activity.[1,2,4]

- Similarly, increase in density corresponds to increases in physical activity levels by offering accessible nearby destinations.[1]

- Connectivity of streets is another spatial variable that affects physical activity. More connected street networks (e.g., grid-iron) offer more direct and accessible distances for different destinations and increase the route options in the environment compared to less connected street networks (e.g., cul-de-sacs)[3,4]

Established design disciplines that can have a significant impact in promoting physical activity include architecture, landscape architecture, graphic design, and urban design, all of which can have a significant impact in promoting physical activity.

Physical Activity and Urban Design

Urban design, as a field, is concerned with creating livable and healthy environments with a special focus on the design of the intermediate or "meso"-scale built environments such as neighborhoods, public spaces, and streets. Urban design principles applied to a locale have environmental as well as social outcomes. Design features of the urban landscape determine activity opportunities for different user groups, influence the probability of social encounters, and thus affect the health behavior of individuals and communities. Different dimensions of urban design, such as the design of street networks (cul-de-sac, grid-iron etc.), the location and content of public spaces and amenities (parks, plazas, recreational and commercial uses), and accessibility to and from these places, have direct influences on the physical and social activity patterns of individuals.

Research from planning, transportation, urban design, and public health literatures suggest that the presence of certain attributes of the built environment is related to a higher propensity for moderate intensity physical activity. For instance connectivity of accessible pedestrian routes, continuity of sidewalks, diversity of land uses, and streetscape design features such as set-back distances provide safer and more pleasant environments promoting physical activity in daily routines such as walking and cycling.

Physical Activity and Architecture

Architecture is concerned with creating, preserving, and adapting buildings; with supporting and shaping the social interactions that take place among people in buildings, neighborhoods, and cities; with using and inventing building technology; and with creating a physical world that is rich in diversity and expressive meaning. In these means, architects have a hands-on influence in providing physical structures that promote physical activity.

Through practice, architects use design innovations or building modifications to increase active living user behavior. Decisions affecting the location of parking, the attractiveness of pedestrian spaces between buildings, access to staircases, provision of roof gardens and interior spaces, and local government zoning and building regulations are important in promoting pedestrian activity such as walking.

Research has shown that the architectural design of buildings and nearby environments can affect physical activity by affording possible areas for social encounters and thus by increasing perceived safety levels[5] and social capital[6] in the community.

A prime example of how architecture can affect physical activity is through the provision of bicycle storage facilities. A key factor in deciding when to use bicycling as a mode of transportation is whether the destination has adequate facilities to secure bicycles. Architectural building designs should include areas for adequate bicycle storage, including bike racks, benches, adequate lighting, water fountains, and a covered shelter.

Physical Activity and Landscape Architecture

Landscape architecture works to protect the integrity of natural ecosystems during urban development by shaping the places where people live, work, and play. In this process, landscape architecture can support physical activity by serving the needs of user groups by designing outdoor spaces that express the cultural meaning of communities and by using vegetation as an aesthetic enhancement in daily life.

As landscape architects shape outdoor space, they can design opportunities for active living in all environments, including campuses, residential neighborhoods, community parks, bike and pedestrian trails, urban plazas, and commercial development. However, to encourage individuals to be active in their community, they must first feel comfortable and safe in their surrounding environment. Landscape architecture plays an important role in this goal by creating pedestrian-scale environments that are geared toward improving the street experience for pedestrians. By designing human-scale communities with buildings, signs, lighting, vegetation, and other street improvements, people can feel more comfortable interacting in and moving around their environment.

Research is mounting that the presence and continuity of sidewalks,[1] existence of trees or other shade elements in the streetscape,[7] and aesthetics of the streetscape[8] (attractiveness of the environment, adjacent facades) promote physical activity by offering safe and pleasant environments for movement.

To maximize their potential contribution to design for active living, landscape architects must take an active leadership role throughout a project's design process as well as in the preparation of general plans at the local level, including pedestrian and bicycle plans, parks, trails and greenways plans, and other green infrastructure components.

Physical Activity and Graphic Design

Graphic design is concerned with bringing meaningful visual form to all aspects of communication, including printed, environmental, and electronic presentations of information and using those works to express messages that inform, persuade, and incite action of individuals and audiences.

Graphic design has an important role to play in the active living movement by designing attractive and informative messages and to communicate them effectively to local leaders, city planners, public health officials, and the greater public in general to achieve social change toward more active lifestyles.

Physical Inactivity Affects Our Health

Physical inactivity plays a significant role in the most common chronic diseases in the United States, including coronary heart disease, stroke, high blood pressure, and diabetes; each of these is a leading cause of death.[9] Specifically:

- Physical inactivity and poor diet are responsible for an estimated 400,000 deaths annually from coronary heart disease, colon cancer, stroke, and diabetes.[10]

- Health scientists have recently declared a new epidemic of children diagnosed with adult-onset diabetes, a disease that was rarely seen in children as recently as the early 1990s.[11]

- Obesity and overweight play a significant role in death and disability and are strongly influenced by physical inactivity. Obese individuals have a 50 to 100 percent increased risk of premature death versus individuals at a healthy weight.[12]

- The proportion of young people who are overweight has increased drastically in recent years. Among children aged 6 through 19 years in 2002, 31.5 percent were overweight or at risk of overweight and 16.5 percent were overweight.[13]

- In 2002, the National Health and Nutrition Examination Survey (NHANES) found that 65.7 percent of adults are overweight or obese, and 30.6 percent of adults are obese, or approximately 30 pounds overweight.[13]

- In 2000, 26.2 percent of U.S. adults reported they received recommended levels of physical activity; 27.5 percent of white individuals, 21.9 percent of black individuals, and 21.1 percent of Hispanic individuals reported meeting recommended levels.[14] Twenty-eight percent of adults reported no leisure time physical activity (i.e., sedentary).[15]

- People who meet or exceed the recommended levels of physical activity report higher levels of perceived quality of life and health status. In 2001, individuals across all age groups meeting recommended levels of physical activity were significantly less likely to report "unhealthy days" compared to physically inactive adults.[16]

How Much Is Enough? Physical Activity Recommendations

The U.S. Surgeon General's Physical Activity Recommendations are:

- In order to reduce the risk of chronic disease, adults should accumulate 30 minutes or more of moderate intensity physical activity on five or more days per week. Moderate activities include a brisk walk, bicycling on level ground, mowing the lawn, etc.

- Alternatively, adults can participate in vigorous exercise for 20 minutes or more on three or more days per week. Vigorous activities include bicycling on hills, aerobics classes, etc.

Community Solutions

Partnerships addressing community and site design can counteract sedentary lifestyles by implementing the following activities:

Preparation

- Recruit design professionals, e.g., building engineers, architects, landscape architects, and industrial and graphic designers to participate in community active living planning projects.

- Work with local governments and developers to conduct design charettes [*Note:* A charette is a creative process used by design professionals to develop solutions to a design problem] in order to engage citizens in design and redesign processes for streets, plazas, parks, and other public spaces.

- Disseminate information among design professionals about the need for creating environments that support routine physical activity.
- Educate design students about the link between design and physical activity—include allied disciplines (health, urban planning, transportation, etc.).
- Evaluate existing community housing and open spaces for their support of active lifestyles.
- Include nontraditional partners such as public health professionals, parents and children, and active living advocates in design processes.

Promotion

- Create active living award programs to provide incentives for good design.
- Educate and engage the local media to recognize the importance of how the built environment impacts physical activity.
- Publicize new designs and environments that have been created with active living principles in mind.
- Disseminate information about design/health recommendations through professional organizations.
- Publicize community planning events, such as charettes and citizen input meetings, related to future designs in public spaces, e.g., parks, road corridors.

Programs

- Establish programs to connect communities with local designers in order to enhance their environments to support physical activity (e.g., loan-a-landscape-architect programs to support community gardens and parks initiatives).
- Develop art walk programs that bring together artists, designers, trail advocates, and the public.
- Train extension agents to work with communities and individuals to address the issue of sedentary lifestyles and promote changes in their environments.

- Work with teachers and schoolchildren to incorporate community design exercises as learning experiences.
- Establish demonstration programs at schools.

Policies

- Produce active living design guidelines and recommendations for architecture, landscape architecture, graphic design, and industrial design.
- Create overlay districts that create incentives for or require active living designs close to transit stations (e.g., bike racks, pedestrian zones with community and commercial facilities).
- Work with government officials to implement building guidelines and codes affecting public indoor spaces that promote active movement; e.g., prominent, open, and inviting staircases; showers; exercise rooms.
- Work with county and municipal governments to require site design elements that promote active living in their development ordinances; e.g., buildings oriented to the street, prominent walkways, bicycle parking/storage accommodations.
- Work with higher education institutions and local school boards to incorporate active living designs in new and existing campuses; e.g., on-site trail systems, remote parking trails, bike facilities, campus promenades, attractive staircases.

Physical Projects

- Emphasize clear sight lines and visual connections between destination points to increase safety and encourage walking.
- Design school outdoor recreation and learning areas to accommodate a diversity of uses during and after school hours.
- Design buildings with windows facing streets, plazas, and parks to create natural surveillance of public spaces, prevent crime, and increase perceptions of safety.
- Promote sidewalk upkeep by local governments and by community members(e.g., by trimming shrubbery near walkways and planting attractive perennial borders).
- Create safe play settings in parks and schools for individuals of all ages and abilities.

- Work with horticulturists and landscape architects to develop community gardens to support physical activity and healthy nutrition.

- Work with city officials to develop in-fill locations in recreation environments and places for physical activity.

- Create spaces that attract people of different ages and socioeconomic strata to the same area.

- Ensure that public space surfaces are walkable, smooth for bicycles, scooters, in-line skates, wheelchairs, etc.

- Design public places to facilitate a variety of transportation choices and physical activities.

- Add surprises, landmarks, ever-changing elements, a variety of materials, and sensory interest to create dynamic environments for pedestrians.

- Provide "point-of-decision" prompts in indoor spaces to encourage stair use over elevators.

Resources

For more information on how design affects public health and for more resources to improve design and health in your community, please see the Active Living by Design website at www.activelivingby design.org. The site is rich with data sources, funding sources, tools, publications, presentations, and links to potential partners.

Active Living by Design

Active Living by Design is a national program of The Robert Wood Johnson Foundation and is a part of the University of North Carolina School of Public Health in Chapel Hill, North Carolina. The program will establish and evaluate innovative approaches to increasing physical activity through community design, public policies and communications strategies. For more information, please visit our website (www.activelivingbydesign.org) or call 919-843-2523.

Thanks to Nilda Cosco and the North Carolina State University School of Design for their assistance.

1. Frank, L.D., Engelke, P.O., and Schmid, T.L., 2003. *Health and Community Design: The Impact of the Built Environment on Physical Activity*. Washington, DC: Island Press.

2. Cervero, R, 1996. Mixed Uses of Land and Commuting: Evidence from the American Housing Survey. Transportation and Research A. 30(5):361–377.

3. Frank, L.D., and Engelke, P., 2001. The built environment and human activity patterns: Exploring the impacts of urban form on public health. *Journal of Planning Literature*, 16(2): 202–218.

4. Owens, P.M, 1993. Neighborhood form and pedestrian life: Taking a closer look. *Landscape and Urban Planning* (26):115–135.

5. Newman, O. 1972. *Defensible Space: Crime prevention through urban design*. New York: Macmillan.

6. Leyden, K., 2003. Social capital and the built environment: The importance of walkable neighborhoods. *American Journal of Public Health*, 93 (9):1546–1551.

7. King, A.C., Stokols, D., Talen E., Brassington G.S., Killingsworth, R., 2002. Theoretical approaches to the promotion of physical activity: Forging a transdisciplinary paradigm, *American Journal of Preventive Medicine* 23(2S):15–25.

8. Ball K., Bauman A., Leslie, E., Owen, N., 2001. Perceived environmental aesthetics and convenience and company are associated with walking for exercise among Australian adults. *Preventive Medicine*, 33:434–440.

9. McKenna, M.T., Taylor, W.R., Marks, J.S., and Koplan, J.P., 1998. Current issues and challenges in chronic disease control. In: *Chronic Disease Epidemiology and Control*, (2nd ed.). Brownson, R.C., Remington, P.L., Davis, J.R. (eds.). Washington, DC: American Public Health Association.

10. Mokdad, A., Marks, J., Stroup, D., and Gerberding, J., 2004. Actual causes of death in the United States, 2000. *JAMA*, 291(10):1238–1245.

11. Kaufman, F. (2002). Type 2 diabetes mellitus in children and youth: A new epidemic. *Journal of Pediatric Endocrinology and Metabolism*, 15(Suppl 2):737–744.

12. United States Department of Health and Human Services, Public Health Services, Office of the Surgeon General. (2001). *The Surgeon General's call to action to prevent and decrease overweight and obesity, 2001*. Rockville, MD: Author.

221

13. Hedley, A.A., Ogden, C.L., Johnson, C.L., Carroll, M.D., Curtin, L.R., and Flegal, K.M., 2004. Prevalence of overweight and obesity among U.S. children, adolescents, and adults, 1999-2002. *JAMA,* 291(23):2847–2850.

14. Behavioral Risk Factor Surveillance System (BRFSS), 2000. Centers for Disease Control and Prevention. Physical Activity Statistics 1986-2000. http://www.cdc.gov/nccdphp/dnpa/physical/stats/stats.htm.

15. Behavioral Risk Factor Surveillance System (BRFSS), 2000. Centers for Disease Control and Prevention. http://apps.nccd .cdc.gov/brfss.

16. Brown, D.W., Balluz, L.S., Heath, G.W., Moriarty, D.G., Ford, E.S., Giles, W.H., and Mokdad, A.H., 2003. Associations between recommended levels of physical activity and health-related quality of life: Findings from the 2001 Behavioral Risk Factor Surveillance System (BRFSS) survey. *Preventive Medicine,* 37(5):520–528.

Section 26.2

Trails and Greenways Encourage Everyday Exercise

Physical Activity and the American Health Crisis

The evidence continues to mount that an emerging health crisis in the United States is related to physical activity.

*   The Centers for Disease Control and Prevention (CDC) published a study in 2003 reporting that the rate of obesity in American adults had reached 20.9 percent, climbing from 19.8 percent in only a one-year period.[1]

- A 2001 "call to action" by the Surgeon General highlighted an alarming trend: Overweight and obesity may soon cause as much preventable disease and death as cigarette smoking. Approximately 300,000 U.S. deaths a year currently are associated with obesity and overweight, and the total direct and indirect costs attributed to these conditions amounted to $117 billion in the year 2000.[2]

Most Americans make the connection between exercise and health, but many people still lead sedentary lives. According to the Surgeon General's "call to action," less than one third of Americans meet the federal recommendation of at least 30 minutes of moderate physical activity at least five days a week, and 40 percent of adults engage in no leisure-time physical activity at all.[3] Both the Surgeon General's "call to action" and the CDC report emphasize the connection between exercise and health.

- In addition to helping control weight, physical activity helps prevent heart disease, helps control cholesterol levels and diabetes, slows bone loss associated with advancing age, lowers the risk of certain cancers and helps reduce anxiety and depression.[4] The power of physical activity to improve mood and prevent disabilities and chronic diseases is especially pronounced for older adults.[5]

- For people who are inactive, even small increases in physical activity can bring measurable health benefits.[6] A 2000 study in Denmark found that leisure-time physical activity improves longevity across genders and age groups. Even moderate activity yielded benefits, with further positive effects derived from bicycling as transportation.[7]

What Are Trails and Greenways?

Greenways are corridors of protected open space managed for conservation and recreation purposes. Greenways often follow natural land or water features, and link nature reserves, parks, cultural features and historic sites with each other and with populated areas. Greenways can be publicly or privately owned, and some are the result of public/private partnerships. Trails are paths used for walking, bicycling, horseback riding, and other forms of recreation or transportation. Some greenways include trails, while other do not. Some appeal to people, while others exist primarily as a habitat for wildlife.

From the hills and plains of inland America to the beaches and barrier islands of the coast, greenways provide a vast network linking America's special places.

How Can Trails and Greenways Help Make a Healthier Community?

Trails and greenways create healthy recreation and transportation opportunities by providing people of all ages with attractive, safe, accessible places to bike, walk, hike, jog, skate, or ski. In doing so, they make it easier for people to engage in physical activity.

- Trails connect people with places, enabling them to walk or cycle to run errands or commute to work. A majority of the daily trips people make are short, providing an opportunity for physical activity that can be built into the daily routine.

- Trails and greenways provide natural, scenic areas that cause people to actually want to be outside and physically active. Cities, such as Chattanooga, Tennessee and Providence, Rhode Island have transformed unsightly urban decay into inviting and popular greenways and walkways that make their communities more livable and walkable. Both cities promote their riverside greenways to attract visitors, businesses, and residents.

- Trails connect neighborhoods and schools so children can cycle or walk to their friends' homes or to school, especially in communities that lack sidewalks. In Denver, the Weir Gulch Trail provides a safe neighborhood route for elementary-aged children, the trail's primary users.[8]

- In this age of expensive indoor gyms and health clubs, trails and greenways offer cost-effective places to exercise. Like gyms and health clubs, they also serve as a place where people can see and interact with other people exercising. Researchers have found that a lack of this type of social support is often a barrier to participation in exercise.[9]

- A North Carolina State University study conducted to gauge potential use of a trail in Cary, North Carolina, found that 72 percent of respondents indicated it was likely the trails would provide a place for them to exercise, and 57 percent said they likely would exercise more if the trail were created.[10] Even if only half those respondents actually end up increasing their exercise because of the trail, the impact on public health is substantial.

Creating Healthy Habits by Building Healthy Communities

Individuals must choose to exercise, but communities can make that choice easier. Lack of time or access to convenient outlets for healthy transportation and recreation opportunities are reasons commonly cited by all demographic groups as barriers to regular exercise. Communities can use trails and greenways as the tools to help make exercise more convenient and neighborhoods more exercise-friendly. By doing so, they can help change bad habits into healthy ones. Some of the steps communities can take to encourage physical activity and health are:

- Use trails and greenways as tools to provide alternative transportation options. Connect neighborhoods and business districts so that people can walk or cycle to work and school, to complete errands, or to visit friends and neighbors. This may help efforts to reduce road congestion and mitigate its polluting effects.

- Build trails and greenways through neighborhoods and along rivers and other natural landscapes to create attractive and accessible places to exercise.

- Connect parks and playgrounds with trails and greenways to create a network of recreational areas.

- Supplement public health promotion with concrete efforts to make more facilities like trails available and accessible. After completing a study of environmental and policy factors associated with physical activity, Dr. Ross Brownson of St. Louis University concluded, "There certainly is no shortage of health messages reminding people to be physically active. But this study suggests that changing communities by making them safer and offering people access to community parks, public recreation facilities, and walking and biking trails may help reduce the prevalence of overweight by promoting physical activity and healthy lifestyles."[11]

With such evidence in hand, as well as poll numbers indicating strong support for the use of government funds to provide areas to engage in physical activity,[12] many communities are beginning dedicated programs to encourage physical activity, including advocating and creating trails and greenways. In addition, the federal government has made physical activity a research and promotion priority.

225

- In *Healthy People 2010*, the U.S. Department of Health and Human Services set specific goals and objectives for increasing physical activity. These objectives call for substantial increases in the percentages of both adults and adolescents who get at least 30 minutes of moderate physical activity five days a week or more. They also call for walking to be the mode of choice for more than 25 percent of adult trips under one mile and 50 percent of trips to school under one mile. Among several other prescribed actions, the report recommends providing more facilities like trials to provide a space for activity to help reach these goals.[13]

- The White House HealthierUS Initiative, launched in 2002, identifies four keys for a healthier America. The first of these is to "be physically active every day." Toward this goal, the HealthierUS Initiative also highlights the Rivers, Trails and Conservation Assistance Program of the National Park Service, which works with community groups and local and state governments to develop trails and greenways.[14]

- The Missouri Department of Health and Senior Services recently announced the creation of the Missouri Council on the Prevention and Management of Overweight and Obesity. The council aims to fill the need for a coordinated approach, including a focus on strategies and policies to improve environmental factors that determine physical activity, like the presence of trails.[15]

- The Rhode Island Prevention Coalition and the American Heart Association made Rhode Island the first state to start a Path to Health program. The program's purpose is to encourage walking for health and enjoyment by establishing safe walking routes, which are marked with signs every half-mile and at every turn. The Coalition provides informational brochures about all existing paths, and hopes to install a Path to Health in each of the 39 communities in Rhode Island.[16]

Trails and Greenways Making a Difference

With more health-focused initiatives in progress and more trails on the ground than ever before, the evidence is beginning to accumulate showing the extent of the positive impact trails and greenways have had on public health.

- In southeastern Missouri, 55 percent of trail users (who responded to the Bootheel and Ozark Health Projects survey) are exercising more now than before they had access to a trail.[17]

- Japanese researchers found that simply living in areas with walkable green spaces positively influenced the longevity of older citizens in large cities, independent of their age, gender, marital status, baseline functional status and socioeconomic status. Their report concludes that such public spaces should be further emphasized in planning for densely populated areas.[18]

- The Indiana Trails Study, which surveyed trail users on six different trails in Indiana, found that in all six locations, over 70 percent of trail users reported that they were getting more exercise as a direct result of the trail.[19]

References

1. Centers for Disease Control and Prevention, National Center for Chronic Disease Prevention and Health Promotion, Press Release, January 1, 2003.

2. U.S. Department of Health and Human Services, *Surgeon General's Call to Action to Prevent and Decrease Overweight and Obesity,* 2001.

3. *Surgeon General's Call to Action.*

4. *Surgeon General's Call to Action.*

5. Partnership for Prevention, "Creating Communities for Active Aging: A Guide to Developing a Strategic Plan to Increase Walking and Biking by Older Adults in Your Community," 2001.

6. Centers for Disease Control and Prevention and the President's Council on Physical Fitness and Sports, *Healthy People 2010, Conference Edition* (2000), Section 22—Physical Activity and Fitness.

7. Lars Bo Andersen, Peter Schnohr, Marianne Schroll and Hans Ole Hein, *Arch Intern Med.,* Vol. 160, pg. 1621–1628, 2000.

8. The Conservation Fund and Colorado State Parks State Trails Program, *The Effect of Greenways on Property Values and Public Safety,* March 1995.

9. Ross C. Brownson, Elizabeth A. Baker, Robyn A. Housemann, Laura K. Brennan and Stephen J. Bacak, "Environmental and Policy Determinants of Physical Activity in the United States," *American Journal of Public Health,* Vol. 91 No. 12, pg. 1995-2003, 2001.

10. Mark I. Ivy and Roger L. Moore, "2000 Cary Greenway Neighbor Study: Assessing Landowner Attitudes Towards Proposed Greenway Trail Development," North Carolina State University, Department of Parks, Recreation and Cultural Resources, April 2, 2001.

11. Saint Louis University, School of Public Health, "New Study Finds Overweight Linked to Poor Community Environment," Press Release, March 5, 2003.

12. See Ross et al. (9).

13. *Healthy People 2010.*

14. "HealthierUS: The President's Recommendations for Improving Physical Fitness," Chapter Three, www.whitehouse.gov/infocus/fitness/chapt3.html, accessed March 11, 2003.

15. See Saint Louis University (11).

16. "Path to Health: History" and "Path to Health Routes in Rhode Island," www.pathtohealth.org/history.htm and www.pathtohealth.org/rimap.htm, accessed March 11, 2003.

17. Ross C. Brownson, "Promoting and Evaluating Walking Trails in Rural Missouri," Saint Louis University School of Public Health, 1999.

18. T. Takano, K. Nakamura, and N. Watanabe, "Urban Residential Environments and Senior Citizens' Longevity in Megacity Areas: The Importance of Walkable Green Spaces," *Journal of Epidemiology and Community Health,* Vol. 56, pg. 913–918, 2002.

19. Eppley Institute for Parks and Public Lands, School of Health, Physical Education and Recreation, Indiana University, *Indiana Trails Study: Summary Report,* November 30, 2001.

Section 26.3

Housework and Daily Activities Count in Health and Fitness

"Daily Activities Count in Health and Fitness," by Dixie L. Thompson, Ph.D., FACSM, and David R. Bassett, Jr., Ph.D., FACSM, from the ACSM Fit Society® Page, Spring 2002, p. 3. Reprinted with permission of the American College of Sports Medicine.

Few people would argue that regular exercise provides health benefits. Numerous studies have documented the role that regular aerobic exercise plays in reducing disease risk, such as coronary artery disease and type 2 diabetes, lowering cardiovascular disease risk factors, such as blood pressure and blood lipids, and increasing longevity. Traditional exercise prescriptions recommend that vigorous, sustained exercise be performed at least three days a week in order to increase fitness and promote health. However, national studies have shown that only a small percentage of Americans perform regular, vigorous exercise. It is possible that many Americans dislike hard exercise, or lack the necessary fitness to participate in it.

In the past several years, researchers and policy makers have begun to recognize that routine daily activity, as well as planned exercise, can promote health. In fact, many public health recommendations now focus on accumulation of moderate intensity activities throughout the day. Although debate continues about the optimal amount and intensity of exercise for promoting health, it is clear that individuals who are active tend to be healthier than those who are sedentary. Unfortunately, the Healthy People 2010 report indicates that approximately 40 percent of American adults get no leisure-time physical activity. This suggests that there is a huge need to find ways to promote exercise among the general population.

The U.S. Surgeon General, the U.S. Centers for Disease Control and Prevention, as well as the American College of Sports Medicine have suggested that adults accumulate at least 30 minutes of moderate intensity activity on most, preferably all, days of the week. But what is moderate exercise, and what types of activities fit this recommendation?

Although these seem like simple questions, quantifying and classifying activity is complex. For example, running at 6.0 mph is a very slow jog for a trained runner, but this same pace can exceed the maximal capacity of an untrained person. Researchers often use a percentage of maximal capacity to classify exercise intensity. Exercise that requires an effort equivalent to 40-60 percent of the individual's maximal oxygen uptake (VO_{2max}) is often considered moderate exercise. The difficulty with using this type of system is that it requires knowledge of VO_{2max} and monitoring of some physiological variable, such as heart rate. This can get cumbersome. Imagine the aggravation of trying to monitor your heart rate while you are gardening. As an alternative, researchers sometimes classify activities in terms of how much energy the task requires in comparison with resting energy consumption (referred to as a MET). In this system, one MET is equal to the energy needed to sustain the body at rest, two METs is twice as much energy as resting metabolic rate, and so forth. When using METs, moderate intensity activities are usually classified as those ranging from three to six METs.

Recently, a number of investigators documented the energy cost of various activities using portable oxygen uptake equipment. These researchers also examined the use of various devices (e.g., pedometers, accelerometers) to monitor activity. One result of that work was a clearer understanding of what activities fit the moderate intensity category.

A wide range of activities requires three to six METs. Examples of sports that are typically moderate intensity include golf while walking and carrying clubs (4.5 METs), bowling (3.0 METs), and doubles tennis (5.0 METs). Many types of lawn work are moderate intensity, including raking the lawn (4.3 METs), chopping wood (6.0 METs), and planting seedlings (4.5 METs). It should be noted that these are typical MET values for these activities, and the actual MET value could be higher or lower depending on the vigor with which one pursues the activity. Below are other types of activities that are typically performed at a moderate intensity.

Home Repair

- Cleaning gutters   5.0 METs
- Auto repair   3.0 METs
- Laying carpet   4.5 METs
- House painting   5.0 METs

Exercises

- Walking 4 mph   5.0 METs
- Leisure biking   4.0 METs
- Water aerobics   4.0 METs
- Tai chi   4.0 METs

Home Activities

- Vacuuming   3.5 METs
- Scrubbing floor   3.8 METs
- Moving furniture   6.0 METs
- Washing windows   3.0 METs

As you can see from these examples, there are numerous ways that individuals can accumulate the suggested 30 minutes per day of moderate intensity activity, some of which are more enjoyable than others! Although evidence continues to accumulate that will shape future exercise recommendations, the important take-home message is that regular, moderate activity provides many health benefits. Finding activities that fit your lifestyle and interests are keys to maintaining regular activity over a lifetime.

Section 26.4

Gardening for Fitness

"Tips on Gardening for Fitness" is reprinted with permission from Kansas State University Agricultural Experiment Station and Cooperative Extension Service. Written by Kathleen Ward, April 26, 2004.

Gardening is exercise that leads to things of value, ranging from homegrown tomatoes to curb appeal.

"No matter how beneficial it would be, I just can't get motivated to ride a bike that's going nowhere. Besides, gardening at any level is a lot better exercise than most of us realize," said Chip Miller, horticulturist with Kansas State University Research and Extension.

With any form of exercise, there is risk of injury, Miller added. Gardening is no exception.

Even so, research has found gardening can strengthen limbs, help the cardiovascular system, and develop both flexibility and hand-eye coordination, he said. It's adaptable to a range of physical disabilities. It even relieves tension while providing sunshine and fresh air. Miller offered these tips to help gardeners benefit from the exercise, but reduce the risk:

- Learn to recognize your tolerance for exertion, and don't exceed your limits. Vary activities, pace yourself and/or take rest times.

- If you get muscle aches and pains, rest and apply a cold pack at intervals through the day. Save any heat treatments for a few days later and combine it with stretching exercises.

- Don't ever get so involved that you forget heat-related illness can kill. The younger or older you are, the more vulnerable you are. For everyone, however, the risk goes up in tandem with the air temperature and dew point. So, monitor the resulting heat index—the perceived heat your body will be reacting to. (Air temperatures of 82 degrees Fahrenheit, combined with a dew point of 82, equals a heat index of 95 degrees Fahrenheit.)

- Drink water or juice, but not beer or caffeinated beverages. Alcohol and caffeine dehydrate.

- Don't depend on thirst to tell you when to drink. Research shows that it won't. Drink a pint of water before going outside and another 8 ounces after each 30 minutes of gardening.

- Use sunscreen to prevent burns and to head off the potential for skin cancer.

- Wear a brimmed hat and sunglasses." Studies at Kansas State have found wearing that kind of head gear greatly reduces your risk for developing macular degeneration of the eyes," Miller said.

- Learn to lift properly. Keep your back straight and knees partially bent. Use leg and buttocks (**not** arm and back) muscles to provide the strength.

- Make use of such labor-saving devices as garden carts and wheelbarrows to move heavy objects. "Humans aren't designed to carry half-grown balled-and-burlapped trees," the horticulturist said.

- As you buy tools, select ones that are sized to fit you. A too-long or too-short handle, for example, can quickly cause muscle strain and fatigue. "A too-large power tool can actually be exhausting to use. Then it can become a dangerous weapon when exhaustion makes you lose control," Miller warned.

- Keep power tools away from those too young or too unskilled to handle them safely.

- If tools come with an owner's manual, read it first. Then follow its directions for operating the equipment. Also follow its recommendations for wearing such safety equipment as goggles, ear plugs, leather shoes, and/or chemical-proof gloves.

- Make glove protection an absolute necessity when gardening. Cotton gloves can help reduce the number of scratches you get, plus prevent the blisters that often result from repetitive work. Leather gauntlets provide even greater protection if you're working with thorny plants. Any gloves cut the odds for cuts, abrasions, torn fingernails, and infections.

- Learn to recognize and avoid poison ivy. Do the same with stinging insects—many of which will be benefitting your garden.

- Never handle wildlife—alive or dead. If wild animals feel cornered, most will fight as hard as they can. Most also are a haven for microorganisms, ticks, lice, and a host of other critters. If you ever have to remove dead wildlife from your yard, use a shovel.

233

- Make it a practice to wash your hands, arms, and face thoroughly when you return indoors. Use lots and lots of soap and cool water if you suspect you may have been in contact with poison ivy. During tick season, also take a shower within hours of coming indoors, so you can wash ticks away before they have time to get imbedded.

"Then take time occasionally just to walk through your garden and enjoy the fruits—the value—of your labors. Some people say they feel an almost spiritual renewal from being outdoors in beautiful surroundings," Miller said. "Gardening is definitely not a form of exercise that goes nowhere."

Section 26.5

Gearing up for Golf

Golf is rapidly becoming the sport of choice for many Americans.

While some view the sport as slow paced, golf actually requires a great deal of strength and stamina, not to mention skill. While you may not have to be in the best cardiovascular shape to play golf, your muscles, particularly those of the legs and upper torso, must be both strong and flexible to keep your handicap below an embarrassing level.

The Key Components

To be successful in golf there are three components of fitness that you should focus on: strength/power, flexibility, and cardiovascular endurance. These also are the three most important components of any well-rounded fitness program.

Strength and Power

Developing muscular strength and power is essential for generating club head speed, a determining factor in how far you can hit the ball.

The list below describes specific exercises that will help you generate more power in your upper body as well as stabilizing strength in your lower body.

One or more sets of eight to 12 repetitions of each exercise should be performed three days per week.

Exercises to Improve Your Golf Swing

- abdominal curl
- biceps curl
- chest cross
- chest press
- lateral raise
- leg curl
- leg extension
- leg press
- low back extension
- neck extension
- neck flexion
- front lat pull
- triceps extension
- weight-assisted chin-up

A recent study found this regimen to be extremely effective. As similar studies have shown, strength training brings about significant improvements in lean body weight, reduced body fat, increased leg strength and joint flexibility, and a reduction in systolic blood pressure.

But more important, at least to the golfers in this study, was the significant improvement in club head speed. The 17 exercisers increased the speed of their swing by an average of 5 mph. The control group experienced no such improvements.

Flexibility

Flexibility is another important key to developing a full, fluid golf swing. Simply swinging the club is not enough, but you can increase the range of motion in your shoulders, trunk, low back, and hamstrings with just a few minutes of daily stretching.

But don't save your stretching until five minutes before you tee off. Flexibility exercises must be done every day. And always warm up your muscles before you stretch them to increase your range of motion and prevent injury.

Cardiovascular Conditioning

Finally, cardiovascular conditioning is essential to help you keep your energy up during a long round of golf. That conditioning can help you deal with the stress of making a crucial putt or of getting out of a sand trap.

Try to fit in at least 20 minutes of walking, cycling, or whatever aerobic activity you prefer, three times per week.

Improving your golf game requires a bit more than simply playing a lot of golf, but it doesn't mean you have to spend hours in the gym. Try the exercises outlined here and you'll not only come closer to par, but you'll also reap numerous health benefits, such as increased lean body weight, reduced body fat, lower blood pressure, and increased strength and flexibility.

While it may be difficult to motivate some people to stretch or begin strength training, telling them they might lower their handicap may be just the ticket to get them to head to the gym. Or work out at home. Whichever is most convenient.

The point is to do it, regardless of whether it's for health or for a better golf score.

Section 26.6

Social Dancing Offers an Entertaining Way to Exercise

Want to get a leg up on your health? Then give dancing a whirl.

"Most of us don't exercise enough," said Michele Wood, women's health manager at St. Francis Hospital & Health Centers [Indianapolis, Indiana]. "Dance is a great way to be more active and have fun at the same time."

Health Benefits of Dance

Not only is dance enjoyable, but it also can:

- lower blood pressure;
- burn about the same amount of calories as tennis (about 327 calories per hour for a 121-pound woman);
- tone muscles;
- increase energy
- boost flexibility;
- keep bones strong; and
- reduce the risk of falling in older women.

Dance Improves Your Mind, Body, and Spirit

Besides being good for the body, shaking and shimmying also may boost mental health. "Dance, like other kinds of exercise, can have a positive effect on mood," Wood said.

Dance may help people become more aware of their bodies. Wood said, "In this age of technology, we lose touch with our bodies. But through dance, people can regain that awareness, as well as a sense of playfulness."

237

There's also the spiritual side of dance. "Dance is about physical grace, and in some cases, even spiritual grace," Wood said. Take tai chi, for example. This traditional Chinese exercise combines graceful movements into a slow, choreographed dance. It is based on the Taoist belief that such movements can balance life force, or chi.

Dance can offer many social benefits, according to Wood. "Through dance, we can improve relationships or reach out and make new friends."

Chapter 27

All about Strength Training

Chapter Contents

Section 27.1

The Benefits of Strength Training

Excerpted from the brochure "Growing Stronger: Strength Training for Older Adults," by the Division of Nutrition and Physical Activity, National Center for Chronic Disease Prevention and Health Promotion, part of the Centers for Disease Control and Prevention (www.cdc.gov/nccdphp/dnpa), February 8, 2006.

Research has shown that strengthening exercises are both safe and effective for women and men of all ages, including those who are not in perfect health. In fact, people with health concerns—including heart disease or arthritis—often benefit the most from an exercise program that includes lifting weights a few times each week.

Strength training, particularly in conjunction with regular aerobic exercise, can also have a profound impact on a person's mental and emotional health.

Benefits of Strength Training

There are numerous benefits to strength training regularly, particularly as you grow older. It can be very powerful in reducing the signs and symptoms of numerous diseases and chronic conditions, among them:

- arthritis;
- diabetes;
- osteoporosis;
- obesity;
- back pain; and
- depression.

Arthritis Relief

Tufts University recently completed a strength-training program with older men and women with moderate to severe knee osteoarthritis. The results of this 16-week program showed that strength training decreased pain by 43%, increased muscle strength and general physical performance, improved the clinical signs and symptoms of the disease, and decreased disability. The effectiveness of strength training to ease the pain of osteoarthritis was just as potent, if not more potent, as medications. Similar effects of strength training have been seen in patients with rheumatoid arthritis.

Restoration of Balance and Reduction of Falls

As people age, poor balance and flexibility contribute to falls and broken bones. These fractures can result in significant disability and, in some cases, fatal complications. Strengthening exercises, when done properly and through the full range of motion, increase a person's flexibility and balance, which decrease the likelihood and severity of falls. One study in New Zealand in women 80 years of age and older showed a 40% reduction in falls with simple strength and balance training.

Strengthening of Bone

Post-menopausal women can lose 1% to 2% of their bone mass annually. Results from a study conducted at Tufts University, which were published in the *Journal of the American Medical Association* in 1994, showed that strength training increases bone density and reduces the risk for fractures among women aged 50 to 70.

Proper Weight Maintenance

Strength training is crucial to weight control, because individuals who have more muscle mass have a higher metabolic rate. Muscle is active tissue that consumes calories while stored fat uses very little energy. Strength training can provide up to a 15% increase in metabolic rate, which is enormously helpful for weight loss and long-term weight control.

Improved Glucose Control

More than 14 million Americans have type 2 diabetes—a staggering 300% increase over the past 40 years—and the numbers are steadily climbing. In addition to being at greater risk for heart and renal disease, diabetes is also the leading cause of blindness in older adults. Fortunately, studies now show that lifestyle changes such as strength training have a profound impact on helping older adults manage their diabetes. In a recent study of Hispanic men and women, 16 weeks of strength training produced dramatic improvements in glucose control that are comparable to taking diabetes medication. Additionally, the study volunteers were stronger, gained muscle, lost body fat, had less depression, and felt much more self-confident.

Healthy State of Mind

Strength training provides similar improvements in depression as antidepressant medications. Currently, it is not known if this is because people feel better when they are stronger or if strength training produces a helpful biochemical change in the brain. It is most likely a combination of the two. When older adults participate in strength training programs, their self-confidence and self-esteem improve, which has a strong impact on their overall quality of life.

Sleep Improvement

People who exercise regularly enjoy improved sleep quality. They fall asleep more quickly, sleep more deeply, awaken less often, and sleep longer. As with depression, the sleep benefits obtained as a result of strength training are comparable to treatment with medication but without the side effects or the expense.

Healthy Heart Tissue

Strength training is important for cardiac health because heart disease risk is lower when the body is leaner. One study found that cardiac patients gained not only strength and flexibility but also aerobic capacity when they did strength training three times a week as part of their rehabilitation program. This and other studies have prompted the American Heart Association to recommend strength training as a way to reduce risk of heart disease and as a therapy for patients in cardiac rehabilitation programs.

Research and Background about Strength Training

Scientific research has shown that exercise can slow the physiological aging clock. While aerobic exercise, such as walking, jogging, or swimming, has many excellent health benefits—it maintains the heart and lungs and increases cardiovascular fitness and endurance—it does not make your muscles strong. Strength training does. Studies have shown that lifting weights two or three times a week increases strength by building muscle mass and bone density.

One 12-month study conducted on postmenopausal women at Tufts University demonstrated 1% gains in hip and spine bone density, 75% increases in strength and 13% increases in dynamic balance with just two days per week of progressive strength training. The control group had losses in bone, strength, and balance. Strength training programs can also have a profound effect on reducing risk for falls, which translates to fewer fractures.

Section 27.2

How Women Build Muscle

There are more myths and misconceptions about strength training than any other area of fitness. While research continues to uncover more and more reasons why working out with weights is good for you, many women continue to avoid resistance training for fear of developing muscles of Herculean proportions.

Other women have tried it and been less than thrilled with the results. Don't worry, people say. Women can't build muscle like men. They don't have enough testosterone. This is, in fact, only partly true.

Many women, believing they wouldn't build muscle, hit the gym with a vengeance and then wondered why, after several weeks of resistance training, their clothes didn't fit and they had gained muscle weight.

The truth is, not everyone responds to training in quite the same way. While testosterone plays a role in muscle development, the answer to why some men and women increase in muscle size and others don't lies within our DNA [deoxyribonucleic acid].

We are predisposed to respond to exercise in a particular way, in large part, because of our genetics. Our genetic makeup determines what types of muscle fibers we have and where they are distributed. It determines our ratio of testosterone to estrogen and where we store body fat. And it also determines our body type.

243

A Question of Body Type

All women fall under one of three body classifications, or are a combination of types. Mesomorphs tend to be muscular, endomorphs are more rounded and voluptuous, and ectomorphs are slim or linear in shape. Mesomorphs respond to strength training by building muscle mass much faster than their ectomorphic counterparts, even though they may be following identical training regimens.

Endomorphs generally need to lose body fat in order to see a change in size or shape as a result of strength training. Ectomorphs are less likely to build muscle mass but will become stronger as a result of resistance training.

Building Just Your Heart Muscle

One of the fundamental principles of strength training is that if you overload the muscle, you will increase its size. With aerobic training, the overload is typically your body weight. Activities such as step/bench training or stair stepping result in changes in the size and shape of the muscles of the lower body. Increasing the height of the step or adding power movements increases the overload.

For those concerned about building muscle, it would be better to reduce the step height or lower the impact of the movements. While this may reduce the aerobic value of the workout, it also will decrease the amount of overload on the muscles, making it less likely that you will build more muscle.

Training by the Rules

When it comes to strength training, the old rule still applies: to get stronger, work with heavier weights and perform fewer repetitions. To promote endurance, use lighter weights and complete more repetitions.

It's encouraging to note that just like men, most women will experience a 20 percent to 40 percent increase in muscular strength after several months of resistance training.

Understanding your body type and how you might respond to exercise can help you set realistic goals and expectations. Avoid comparisons to others you see, at the gym or elsewhere, and remember that no two people are alike.

Focus on how good exercise makes you feel rather than how you would like to look. Accepting our bodies for what they are is a great way to get rid of the guilt or pressure we often feel to look a certain way.

Section 27.3

Beginning a Strength Training Program

Excerpted from "Growing Stronger: Strength Training for Older Adults," a publication of the Division of Nutrition and Physical Activity, National Center for Chronic Disease Prevention and Health Promotion, part of the Centers for Disease Control and Prevention (CDC), www.cdc.gov/nccdphp/dnpa, February 8, 2006.

Equipment Needs

Strength training requires little special equipment, but there are a few basic necessities:

A Sturdy Chair and Exercise Space

Find a strong, stable chair without arms that does not rock or sway when you sit in it or move when you stand up from it. When you're seated in the chair, your knees should be at a 90-degree angle and your feet should be flat on the ground. If the chair is too high, find one with shorter legs; if it's too low, try putting a pillow or a folded blanket on the seat to give you a slight boost.

For your exercise space, choose an open area, preferably carpeted, with at least enough space for your chair and ample room to walk around it. Carpeting will prevent the chair from sliding. On bare floor, put your chair against the wall. If you think you might like to exercise to music or while watching television, plan your space accordingly.

Good Shoes

Good shoes are essential for any exercise. For strength training, try athletic shoes with good support, such as walking, running, or cross-training sneakers. The sole should be rubber, but not too thick, as fat soles may cause you to trip. If you don't already have shoes that fit this description, you can find them at sporting goods, discount, and department stores.

Comfortable Clothing

Wear loose, cool, comfortable clothing that breathes well during exercise—for example, a cotton T-shirt and cotton shorts or pants. If you want to purchase new workout clothes, look for materials that readily absorb moisture and breathe well.

Dumbbells (Handheld Weights) and Ankle Weights

You can complete the first part of the exercise program without weights, but as you get stronger and add new exercises, you will need dumbbells and ankle weights. It's a good idea to buy these before you begin strength training, or as soon as possible after you start, so that you'll have them on hand when you're ready to add them to your program. Your minimum purchase should include a set of two dumbbells in each of the following weights:

Women

- Two pounds
- Three pounds
- Five pounds

Men

- Three pounds
- Five pounds
- Eight pounds

The best ankle weights for this program are the adjustable type. These allow you to add weight gradually in increments of a half-pound or full pound, until you reach as much as 10 or 20 pounds per leg.

Some stores and mail-order companies offer specials that include a set of one-pound, three-pound, and five-pound weights at substantial

Table 27.1. Choices for Purchasing Strength Training Equipment

Options	Benefits	Drawbacks
Newspaper, want ads	Inexpensive	Used; can't return
Sporting goods store	Can test product	Slightly more expensive
Mail order	Convenient	Shipping costly

savings. This is a good starter kit; later you can buy heavier dumb-bell sets.

Storage Container

For safety reasons, consider storing your weights in a floor-level cupboard or in a container such as a wooden box or canvas bag—preferably on a cart with wheels for easy relocation to your exercise spot. Storage containers and wheeled carts are usually available at local department and discount stores. If you choose not to use a cart, try to keep your weights in the area where you exercise to minimize transporting the weights from one area to another. Also, be mindful to store weights out of the reach of children and in a place where people will not trip over them.

Safety

At times, you will not feel like exercising. This is true for everyone. If you're just feeling a little tired or low on energy, go ahead and try to complete your routine. The workout will likely boost your energy level and your mood. However, if you're not feeling well—if you think you might be getting sick, coming down with a cold or the flu; or if you have any kind of pain or swelling—take a break from exercising and, if necessary, contact your doctor. Your health and safety are top priority.

The reasons listed below are good cause to take a day off from strength training. Be cautious. If you're not sure whether you're well enough to exercise, take a break and see how you feel the next day.

Refrain from exercising or check with your doctor first if you:

- have a cold, flu, or infection accompanied by fever;
- have significantly more fatigue than usual;
- have a swollen or painful muscle or joint;
- have any new or undiagnosed symptom;
- have chest pain, or irregular, rapid, or fluttery heartbeat;
- have shortness of breath;
- have a hernia, with symptoms; and
- have been advised by your doctor not to exert yourself for a given period of time due to illness, surgery, etc.

Listen to your body. As you get used to your exercise program, you will know when you're well enough to handle a workout and when you need to take a day off or see your doctor.

Scheduling Exercise

Look at your schedule to see where strength training may best fit in—perhaps on weekday mornings before work or during your favorite evening television program. There are no rules about the best time to exercise. But keep in mind that you should schedule your sessions on three non-consecutive days of week (say, Monday, Wednesday, and Friday; or Tuesday, Thursday, Saturday) in order to give your muscles proper rest. Alternatively, you can try doing lower body exercises one day and then upper body exercises the next; this way, you will avoid overworking the same muscle groups.

Put your scheduled strength-training appointments on your calendar and keep them faithfully, just as you would a doctor's appointment. You might also try to find an exercise partner who can join you for your scheduled sessions; working with a friend will help you adhere to your regimen and keep you motivated.

Here are some tips on scheduling exercise:

- Consider what days best suit your schedule, given your other commitments.

- Pick a time of day at which you find exercise enjoyable: Some people like to exercise first thing in the morning; others are more motivated in the evening or afternoon.

- Write your first exercise appointments on your calendar.

- After completing your first two or three sessions, evaluate whether your selected days and times work well for you. If they don't, reexamine your schedule and try to find better times.

Progression

How to Progress

After the first week or so of strength training, you should start doing each exercise with weights that you can lift at least ten times with only moderate difficulty. (If a given exercise seems too difficult— if you cannot do at least eight repetitions—then the weight you are using is too heavy and you need to scale back.)

After two weeks of strength training, you should reassess the difficulty of each exercise with your current level of weights. You may start doing the overhead press with one-pound dumbbells, for example. By the end of the second week, the exercise may feel too easy—that is, you can easily lift the one-pound dumbbell through the full range of motion and in proper form more than twelve times. You should now step up your weights to two- or three-pound dumbbells and see how the exercise feels at the new weight level.

Why Progression Is Important

To take full advantage of the many benefits of strength training, it's important to progress, or consistently advance the intensity of your workout by challenging your muscles with heavier weights. This continuous challenge allows your muscles to grow strong and stay strong. Progressing will boost your feelings of independence and will help ensure that you live well into old age without the fear of falling. It will also give you a tremendous sense of pride and accomplishment.

Staying on Track

It's important to stick to your strength-training program as much as you can. You may find that you make a few false starts before you succeed at making this program a regular part of your life. There may be times when interruptions such as vacation, illness, family, or work demands prevent you from doing your exercises for a week or two—or even longer. Try not to feel guilty or disappointed in yourself. Just restart your routine as quickly as you can. You may not be able to pick up exactly where you left off—you may need to decrease your weights a bit. But stay with it, and you will regain lost ground.

If you have trouble getting back into the swing of things, start back into the program slowly. Remember why you started strength training in the first place and why you chose your goals. It may help to reassess your goals and make new ones because your motivations may change as time passes. Most important, remember how your past successes made you feel: healthy, strong, independent, and empowered.

Exercises

Warmup: 5-Minute Walk

To get your muscles warm and loose for strength training, walk for five to ten minutes outside if weather permits, or inside around the house or on a treadmill if you have one. Walking will help direct needed blood flow to your muscles and prepare your body for exercise. Warming up is important for preventing injury as well as gaining maximal benefit from the exercise, because loose, warm muscles will respond better to the challenge of lifting weights.

If you have another piece of aerobic exercise equipment available to you, such as a bike, rowing machine, or stair stepper, this will serve as an adequate warm up as well.

Stage 1

The following exercises comprise Stage 1. When you've been doing the exercises of this stage for at least two weeks, or if you are fairly fit right now, you can add the exercises in Stage 2. Remember to always do the warmup and cooldown as part of each exercise session.

Squats

A great exercise for strengthening hips, thighs, and buttocks.

1. In front of a sturdy, armless chair, stand with feet slightly more than shoulder-width apart. Cross your arms over your chest and lean forward a little at the hips.

2. Making sure that your knees **never** come forward past your toes, lower yourself in a slow, controlled motion, to a count of four, until you reach a near-sitting position.

3. Pause. Then, to a count of two, slowly rise back up to a standing position. Keep your knees over your ankles and your back straight.

4. Repeat 10 times for one set. Rest for one to two minutes. Then complete a second set of 10 repetitions.

Note 1: If this exercise is too difficult, start off by using your hands for assistance. If you are unable to go all the way down, place a couple of pillows on the chair or only squat down four to six inches.

Note 2: Placing your weight more on your heels than on the balls or toes of your feet can help keep your knees from moving forward past your toes. It will also help to use the muscles of your hips more during the rise to a standing position.

Make sure you:

- Don't sit down too quickly.
- Don't lean your weight too far forward or onto your toes when standing up.

Wall Pushups

This exercise is a modified version of the push-up you may have done in physical education classes. It is less challenging than a classic push-up and won't require you to get down on the floor—but it will help to strengthen your arms, shoulders, and chest.

1. Find a wall that is clear of any objects—wall hangings, windows, etc. Stand a little farther than arm's length from the wall.

2. Facing the wall, lean your body forward and place your palms flat against the wall at about shoulder height and shoulder-width apart.

3. To a count of four, bend your elbows as you lower your upper body toward the wall in a slow, controlled motion, keeping your feet planted.

4. Pause. Then, to a count of two, slowly push yourself back until your arms are straight—but don't lock your elbows.

5. Repeat 10 times for one set. Rest for one to two minutes. Then complete a second set of 10 repetitions.

Make sure you don't round or arch your back.

Toe Stands

This exercise is a good way to strengthen your calves and ankles and restore stability and balance.

1. Near a counter or sturdy chair, stand with feet shoulder-width apart. Use the chair or counter for balance.

2. To a count of four, slowly push up as far as you can, onto the balls of your feet and hold for two to four seconds.

3. Then, to a count of four, slowly lower your heels back to the floor.

4. Repeat 10 times for one set. Rest for one to two minutes. Then complete a second set of 10 repetitions.

Make sure you:

- Don't lean on the counter or chair—use them for balance only.
- Breathe regularly throughout the exercise.

Finger Marching

In this exercise you'll let your fingers, hands, and arms do the walking. This will help strengthen your upper body and your grip, and increase the flexibility of your arms, back, and shoulders.

1. Stand or sit forward in an armless chair with feet on the floor, shoulder-width apart.

2. Movement 1: Imagine there is a wall directly in front of you. Slowly walk your fingers up the wall until your arms are above your head. Hold them overhead while wiggling your fingers for about 10 seconds and then slowly walk them back down.

3. Movement 2: Next, try to touch your two hands behind your back. If you can, reach for the opposite elbow with each hand— or get as close as you can. Hold the position for about 10 seconds, feeling a stretch in the back, arms, and chest.

4. Movement 3: Release your arms and finger-weave your hands in front of your body. Raise your arms so that they're parallel to the ground, with your palms facing the imaginary wall. Sit or stand up straight, but curl your shoulders forward. You should feel the stretch in your wrist and upper back. Hold the position for about 10 seconds.

5. Repeat this three-part exercise three times.

Stage 2

When you've been doing the exercises from Stage 1 for at least two weeks, or if you are fairly fit right now, you can add these Stage 2 exercises. When you've been doing the exercises from Stages 1 and 2 for at least six weeks, you can add the exercises in Stage 3. Remember to always do the warmup and cooldown as part of each exercise session.

Biceps Curl

Does a gallon of milk feel a lot heavier than it used to? After a few weeks of doing the biceps curl, lifting that eight-pound jug will be a cinch!

1. With a dumbbell in each hand, stand or sit in an armless chair, with feet shoulder-width apart, arms at your sides, and palms facing your thighs.

2. To a count of two, slowly lift up the weights so that your forearms rotate and palms face in toward your shoulders, while keeping your upper arms and elbows close to your side—as if you had a newspaper tucked beneath your arm. Keep your wrists straight and dumbbells parallel to the floor.

3. Pause. Then, to a count of four, slowly lower the dumbbells back toward your thighs, rotating your forearms so that your arms are again at your sides, with palms facing your thighs.

4. Repeat 10 times for one set. Rest for one to two minutes. Then complete a second set of 10 repetitions.

Make sure you:

- Don't let your elbows move away from the sides of your body.
- Keep your wrists straight.

Step-Ups

This is a great strengthening exercise that requires only a set of stairs. But don't let its simplicity fool you. Step-ups will improve your balance and build strength in your legs, hips, and buttocks.

1. Stand alongside the handrail at the bottom of a staircase. With your feet flat and toes facing forward, put your right foot on the first step.

2. Holding the handrail for balance, to a count of two, straighten your right leg to lift up your left leg slowly until it reaches the first step. As you're lifting yourself up, make sure that your right knee stays straight and does not move forward past your ankle. Let your left foot tap the first step near your right foot.

3. Pause. Then, using your right leg to support your weight, to a count of four, slowly lower your left foot back to the floor.

4. Repeat 10 times with the right leg and 10 times with the left leg for one set. Rest for one to two minutes. Then complete a second set of 10 repetitions with each leg.

Make sure you:

- Don't let your back leg do the work.
- Don't let momentum do the work.
- Press your weight through the heel rather than ball or toes of your front leg as you lift.

Overhead Press

This useful exercise targets several muscles in the arms, upper back, and shoulders. It can also help firm the back of your upper arms and make reaching for objects in high cupboards easier.

1. Stand or sit in an armless chair with feet shoulder-width apart. With a dumbbell in each hand, raise your hands, palms facing forward, until the dumbbells are level with your shoulders and parallel to the floor.

2. To a count of two, slowly push the dumbbells up over your head until your arms are fully extended—but don't lock your elbows.

3. Pause. Then, to a count of four, slowly lower the dumbbells back to shoulder level, bringing your elbows down close to your sides.

4. Repeat 10 times for one set. Rest for one to two minutes. Then complete a second set of 10 repetitions.

Make sure you:

- Keep your wrists straight.
- Don't lock your elbows.
- Don't let the dumbbells move too far in front of your body or behind it.
- Breathe throughout the exercise.

Hip Abduction

By targeting the muscles of the hips, thighs, and buttocks, this exercise makes your lower body shapelier and strengthens your hipbones, which may be especially vulnerable to fracture as you age.

1. Stand behind a sturdy chair, with feet slightly apart and toes facing forward. Keep your legs straight, but do not lock your knees.

2. To a count of two, slowly lift your right leg out to the side. Keep your left leg straight—but again, do not lock your knee.

3. Pause. Then, to a count of four, slowly lower your right foot back to the ground.

4. Repeat 10 times with the right leg and 10 times with the left leg for one set. Rest for one to two minutes. Then complete a second set of 10 repetitions with each leg.

Make sure you:

- Don't lock your knee on the supporting leg.

- Keep your toes facing forward throughout the move.

- Don't lean to the side when you lift your leg.

- To increase the difficulty of this exercise, you may add ankle weights.

Stage 3

When you've been doing the exercises from Stages 1 and 2 for at least six weeks, you can add these Stage 3 exercises. Remember to always do the warmup and cooldown as part of each exercise session.

Knee Extension

By targeting the quadriceps muscles in the front of the thigh (which play a primary role in bending and straightening the leg), this exercise strengthens weak knees and reduces the symptoms of arthritis of the knee. It is important to do this exercise in conjunction with the knee curl, as the muscles targeted in these two exercises—the front thigh muscles and the hamstrings—work together when you walk, stand, and climb.

1. Put on your ankle weights.

2. In a sturdy, armless chair, sit all the way back, so that your feet barely touch the ground; this will allow for easier movement throughout the exercise. If your chair is too low, add a rolled-up towel under your knees. Your feet should be shoulder-width apart, and your arms should rest at your sides or on your thighs.

3. With your toes pointing forward and your foot flexed, to a count of two slowly lift your right leg, extending your leg until your knee is straight.

4. Pause. Then, to a count of four, slowly lower your foot back to the ground.

5. Repeat 10 times with the right leg and 10 times with the left leg for one set. Rest for a minute or two. Then complete a second set of 10 repetitions with each leg.

Make sure you keep your ankle flexed throughout the move.

Knee Curl

This is an excellent exercise for strengthening the muscles of the back of the upper leg, known as the hamstrings. When done in conjunction with the knee extension, it makes walking and climbing easier.

1. Put on your ankle weights.

2. Stand behind a sturdy chair, with feet shoulder-width apart and facing forward.

3. Keeping your foot flexed, to a count of two slowly bend your right leg, bringing your heel up toward your buttocks.

4. Pause. Then, to a count of four, slowly lower your foot back to the ground.

5. Repeat 10 times with your right leg and 10 times with your left leg for one set. Rest for a minute or two. Then complete a second set of 10 repetitions with each leg.

Make sure you:

• Keep the thigh of the bending leg in line with the supporting leg at all times.

• Keep the foot on the bending leg flexed throughout the move.

Pelvic Tilt

This exercise improves posture and tightens the muscles in your abdomen and buttocks. Do this exercise in conjunction with the floor back extension to strengthen your midsection. (You should not have the ankle weights on during this exercise.)

1. On the floor or on a firm mattress, lie flat on your back with your knees bent, feet flat, and arms at your sides, palms facing the ground.

2. To a count of two, slowly roll your pelvis so that your hips and lower back are off the floor, while your upper back and shoulders remain in place.

3. Pause. Then, to a count of four, slowly lower your pelvis all the way down.

4. Repeat 10 times for one set. Rest for a minute or two. Then complete a second set of 10 repetitions.

Make sure you:

- Breathe throughout the exercise.
- Don't lift your upper back or shoulders off the ground.

Floor Back Extension

If you suffer from lower back pain, weak abdominal muscles may be to blame. The floor back extension, done in conjunction with the pelvic tilt, will strengthen these muscles and ease back pain.

1. Lie on the floor face down, with two pillows under your hips. Extend your arms straight overhead on the floor.

2. To a count of two, slowly lift your right arm and left leg off the floor, keeping them at the same level.

3. Pause. Then, to a count of four, slowly lower your arm and leg back to the floor.

4. Repeat 10 times for one set, and then switch to left arm with right leg for another 10 repetitions.

5. Rest for a minute or two. Then complete a second set of 10 repetitions.

Make sure you keep your head, neck, and back in a straight line.

Gaining Grip Strength

If you have arthritis, you may have trouble picking up things with your hands or keeping a grip on them. Some of the exercises in this program will help strengthen your hand muscles. If you're concerned about grip strength, you may also want to add a grip exercise to increase strength and decrease stiffness in your hands. The exercise is simple; it can be done easily while reading or watching TV, and most people already have the equipment at home.

To do the exercise, grasp a racquetball, tennis ball, or stress ball in one hand while sitting or standing. Slowly squeeze it as hard as you and hold the squeeze for three to five seconds. Slowly release the squeeze. Take a short rest, then repeat the exercise 10 times. Switch hands, and do two sets of 10 squeezes with the other hand.

You may do this exercise every day or every other day, depending on how your hands feel. If they feel stiff or painful, you may want to skip a day.

Section 27.4

Making Continued Progress in Your Strength Training Program

Excerpted from "Progression and Resistance Training," by William J. Kraemer, Ph.D., and Nicholas A. Ratamess, Ph.D., from the September 2005 issue (Series 6, No. 3) of *Research Digest*, a publication of the President's Council on Physical Fitness and Sports. For a complete listing of references, see http://www.fitness.gov.

Introduction

The popularity of resistance training has increased in recent times. Not only is resistance training used to increase muscular strength, power, endurance, and hypertrophy in athletes, but the adaptations to resistance training have been shown to benefit the general population as well as clinical (i.e., those individuals with cardiovascular ailments, neuromuscular disease, etc.) populations. Both scientific and anecdotal evidence points to the concept that progression is needed in order to create a more effective stimulus to promote higher levels of fitness. In fact, a threshold of activity/effort is necessary beyond the initial few months (which is characterized by enhanced motor coordination and technique) in order for the body to produce further substantial improvements in fitness. This threshold continually changes as one's conditioning level improves and is specific to the targeted goals of the exercise program. It is also bounded by each individual's genetic ceiling for improvement. Resistance training at or beyond this threshold level leads to progression.

The 1998 American College of Sports Medicine position stand has been shown to be effective for progression during the first few months of training, but then benefits tended to plateau during subsequent months when variation in the program design was minimal. However, the question then arose, "what type of programs would be recommended for those individuals who desire a higher level of fitness?" Because it is important to make exercise a lifetime commitment, recommendations based on scientific research were needed to provide specific directives for those who desire to make further goal-specific improvements via resistance training. In response to this need, the American College of Sports Medicine later published a position stand providing basic recommendations for progression during resistance training. In this document, recommendations were given to novice, intermediate, and advanced individuals who sought to improve muscle strength, power, endurance, hypertrophy, and motor performance. The general conclusion was that there were numerous ways to progress as long as one adhered to basic tenets regarding the proper manipulation of the acute program variables. How much one can progress depends on the individual's genetic makeup, program design and implementation, and training status or level of fitness (i.e., slower rates of improvement are observed as one advances). In this chapter, we will discuss the critical elements to progression during resistance training and the current recommendations for manipulating the acute program variables. It is important to note that the amount of progression sought is individual-specific, as moderate improvements have been shown to elicit significant health benefits. Once the desired fitness level is achieved, programs can be used to maintain that current level of fitness.

Basic Components of Resistance Training Programs

Maximal benefits of resistance training may be gained via adherence to three basic principles: 1) progressive overload, 2) specificity, and 3) variation.

Progressive overload necessitates a gradual increase in the stress placed on the body during training. Without these additional demands,

259

the human body has no reason to adapt any further than the current level of fitness.

Specificity refers to the body's adaptations to training. The physiological adaptations to resistance training are specific to the muscle actions involved, velocity of movement, exercise range of motion, muscle groups trained, energy systems involved, and the intensity and volume of training. The most effective resistance training programs are designed individually to bring about specific adaptations.

Variation is the systematic alteration of the resistance training program over time to allow for the training stimulus to remain optimal. It has been shown that systematic program variation is very effective for long-term progression.

Progression and Resistance Training Program Design

The resistance training program is a composite of acute variables. These variables include: 1) muscle actions used, 2) resistance used, 3) volume (total number of sets and repetitions), 4) exercises selected and workout structure (e.g., the number of muscle groups trained), 5) the sequence of exercise performance, 6) rest intervals between sets, 7) repetition velocity, and 8) training frequency. Altering one or several of these variables will affect the training stimuli, thus creating a favorable condition by which numerous ways exist to vary resistance training programs and maintain/increase participant motivation. Therefore, proper resistance exercise prescription involves manipulation of the variables to the specificity of the targeted goals.

Muscle Actions

The selection of muscle actions revolve around concentric (CON), eccentric (ECC), and isometric (ISOM) muscle actions. Most resistance training programs include mostly dynamic repetitions with both CON and ECC muscle actions, whereas ISOM muscle actions play a secondary role. Eccentric muscle actions result in larger forces generated and less motor unit activation per tension level, require less energy per tension level, are very conducive to muscle hypertrophy, and elicit greater muscle damage compared to CON actions. Muscular strength is enhanced to a greater extent when ECC actions are included. It is recommended that both CON and ECC muscle actions be included in novice, intermediate, and advanced resistance training programs. The use of ISOM actions is beneficial but adaptations to ISOM are mostly specific to joint angles trained so ISOM actions need to be performed throughout the range of joint motion.

Resistance

The amount of weight lifted is highly dependent on other variables such as exercise order, volume, frequency, muscle action, repetition speed, and rest interval length, and has a significant effect of both the acute response and chronic adaptation to resistance training. Individual training status and goals are primary considerations when considering the level of resistance. Light loads of approximately 45–50% of one repetition maximum (1 RM) or less can increase muscular strength in novices who are mostly improving motor coordination at that level. As one becomes progressively stronger, greater loading is needed to increase maximal strength (i.e., 80–85% of 1 RM for advanced training). These findings have also been recently supported by a meta-analysis, which demonstrated that 85% of 1 RM yielded the highest effect size for strength gains in athletes. It is important to note, however, that there are few data examining consistent resistance training with heavier loading. There appears to be specific motor unit recruitment patterns during the lifting of very heavy or maximal loads which may not be reproducible with light to moderate loading. In addition, muscle hypertrophy reduces the motor unit activity necessary to lift a desired load. In order to continually recruit these higher threshold motor units, progressively heavier loads are needed to advance at a faster rate.

There is an inverse relationship between the amount of weight lifted and the number of repetitions performed. Several studies have indicated that training with loads corresponding to 1–6 RM (i.e., the maximal amount of weight that can be lifted 1 to 6 times) were most conducive to increasing maximal dynamic strength. This loading range appears most specific to increasing dynamic 1 RM strength. Although significant strength increases have been reported using loads corresponding to 7–12 RM, it is believed that this range may not be as specific to increasing maximal strength in advanced resistance-trained individuals compared to 1–6 RM (although it is very effective for strength training in novice and intermediate trainees). The 7–12 RM loading zone is commonly used in programs targeting muscular hypertrophy at all levels of training. Although heavy loading (1–6 RM) is effective for increasing muscle hypertrophy, it has been suggested that the 7–12 RM range may provide the best combination of load and volume in direct comparison. Loads lighter than this (13–15 RM and lighter) have only had small effects on maximal strength and hypertrophy, but have been very effective for enhancing local muscular endurance. Each "training zone" on this continuum has its advantages and, in order to avoid encountering training plateaus or overtraining, one should not devote 100% of the training time to one general RM zone. It appears that optimal strength, hypertrophy, and endurance training requires the systematic use of various loading strategies. Therefore, the American College of Sports Medicine recommends 60–70% of 1 RM loading for novice, 70–80% of 1 RM for intermediate, and 70–100% of 1 RM (periodized) for advanced strength training.

Training Volume

Training volume consists of the total number of sets and repetitions performed during a training session. Altering training volume can be accomplished by changing the number of exercises performed per session, the number of repetitions performed per set, or the number of sets per exercise. Volume and intensity are inversely related such that use of heavy loads results in lower volumes whereas use of light to moderate loads results in higher training volumes. Typically, high volume programs are synonymous with training for muscle hypertrophy and local muscular endurance whereas low volume programs are synonymous with strength and power training.

The vast majority of studies that examined volume and resistance training have investigated the number of sets performed per exercise. Most comparisons have been made between single- and multiple-set programs. In novice individuals, similar results have been reported from single- and multiple-set (mostly 3 sets) programs, whereas some studies have shown multiple sets superior. Thus, either may be used effectively during the initial phase of resistance training. However, periodized (i.e., varied), multiple-set programs have been shown to be superior as one progresses to intermediate and advanced stages of long-term training in all but one study. Interestingly, a recent study (using a randomized, cross-over design) in trained postmenopausal women showed that multiple-set training resulted in a 3.5 to 5.5% range of strength increase whereas single-set training resulted in a 1.1 to 2.0% reduction in strength. Within multiple-set training programs, two, three, four-five, and six or more sets per exercise have all produced significant increases in muscular strength in both trained and untrained individuals. Only a few studies have made direct comparisons and they reported similar strength gains in novice individuals between two and three sets, and two and four sets, whereas three sets have been reported as superior to one and two. Therefore, it appears that similar improvements, at least in novice-trained individuals, may be gained within various multiple-set protocols. Less is known with intermediate and advanced training. Typically, 3–6 sets per exercise are common during resistance training, although more and less have been used successfully. It is important to note that each set will have a specific purpose and that each exercise may be performed with a different number of total sets. Performing each set to near or actual muscular exhaustion (as well as the impact of rest interval length) may affect the total number of sets per exercise. We have recently shown that when 2–3 min rest intervals are used during 10-repetition sets of multiple-joint exercises (i.e., squats, bench press) with 70–75% of 1 RM, acute lifting performance tends to decrease beyond the third set (when 5 or 6 sets are performed). Based on the aforementioned data, the American College of Sports Medicine has made the following strength training recommendations: 1) Novice—1–3 sets per exercise x 8–12 repetitions per set; 2) Intermediate—multiple sets of 6–12 repetitions per set; and 3) Advanced—multiple sets of 1–12 repetitions per set (periodized).

The number of sets performed per workout has not been extensively studied. In a recent meta-analysis examining 37 studies, researchers reported that 8 sets per workout (per muscles trained) yielded the largest effect size for strength development in athletes. However, few data directly compare resistance training programs of varying total sets, thus leaving numerous possibilities for the strength and conditioning professional when designing programs.

Exercise Selection

Two general types of free weight or machine exercises may be selected in resistance training: single- and multiple-joint. Single-joint exercises stress one joint or major muscle group whereas multiple-joint exercises stress more than one joint or major muscle group. Although both are effective for increasing muscular strength, multiple-joint exercises (e.g. bench press, squat) have generally been regarded as most effective for increasing muscular strength because they enable a greater magnitude of resistance to be used. Exercises stressing multiple or large muscle groups have shown the greatest acute metabolic and anabolic (e.g., testosterone, growth hormone family) hormonal responses which may play a role in muscle size and strength increases. The American College of Sports Medicine recommends that novice, intermediate, and advanced resistance training programs incorporate single- and multiple-joint exercises with emphasis on multiple-joint exercises for advanced training.

Exercise Order and Structure

The sequencing of exercises significantly affects the acute expression of muscular strength. In addition, sequencing depends on program structure. There are three basic workout structures: 1) total body workouts (e.g., performance of multiple exercises stressing all major muscle groups per session), 2) upper/lower body split workouts (e.g., performance of upper body exercises only during one workout and lower body exercises only during the next workout), and 3) muscle group split routines (e.g., performance of exercises for specific muscle groups during a workout). All three structures are effective for improving muscular strength and it appears that individual goals, time/frequency, and personal preferences will determine which one(s) will be used. One study has shown similar improvements in previously untrained women between total body and upper/lower body split workouts. Once the structure has been developed, the sequencing of exercise will ensue. For strength training, minimizing fatigue and maximizing energy are critical for optimal acute performance—especially for the multiple-joint exercises. Studies have shown that placing an exercise early vs. later in the workout will affect acute lifting performance.

Table 27.2. General Sequencing Strategies for Strength Training

Total Body Workout

1.   Large before small muscle group exercises
2.   Multiple-joint before single-joint exercises
3.   Rotation of upper and lower body exercises or opposing (agonist-antagonist relationship) exercises

Upper and Lower Body Split Workout

1.   Large before small muscle group exercises
2.   Multiple-joint before single-joint exercises
3.   Rotation of opposing exercises (agonist-antagonist relationship)

Muscle Group Split Routines

1.   Multiple-joint before single-joint exercises
2.   Higher intensity before lower intensity exercises

Rest Intervals

Rest interval length depends on training intensity, goals, fitness level, and targeted energy system, and affects acute performance and training adaptations. Acute force production may be compromised with short (i.e., 1 min) rest periods. Research showed that all participants completed 3 sets of 10 repetitions with 10 RM loads when 3-min rest periods were used. However only 10, 8, and 7 repetitions were completed, respectively, with 1-min rest intervals in the study. We have recently developed a continuum for rest interval length for the bench press in which 3–5 min rest intervals were most effective for maintaining acute lifting performance, but 30 sec to 2 min of rest produced significant reductions in set performance. Longitudinal studies have shown greater strength increases with long vs. short rest periods between sets. These studies show the importance of recovery for optimal strength training. Rest intervals will vary based on the goals of that particular exercise, i.e., not every exercise will use the same rest interval. Muscle strength may be increased using short rest periods but at a slower rate, thus demonstrating the need to establish goals (i.e., the magnitude of strength improvement sought) prior to selecting a rest interval. The American College of Sports Medicine recommends 1–2 min rest intervals for novice training, 2–3 min rest intervals for core exercise and 1–2 min rest intervals for others for intermediate training, and at least 3 min rest intervals for core exercises and 1–2 min rest intervals for others for advanced strength training.

Repetition Velocity

The velocity at which dynamic repetitions are performed affects the responses to resistance exercise. When discussing repetition velocity, it is important to note that velocity applies mostly to submaximal loading. Heavy loading requires maximal effort in order to lift weight. For dynamic constant external resistance (also called isotonic) training, significant reductions in force production are observed when the intent is to lift the weight slowly. There are two types of slow-velocity contractions, unintentional and intentional. Unintentional slow velocities are used during high-intensity repetitions in which either the loading and/or fatigue facilitate the velocity of movement (i.e., the resultant velocity is slow despite maximal effort). Intentional slow-velocity repetitions are used with submaximal loads where the individual has greater control of the velocity. Concentric force production is significantly lower for an intentionally slow lifting velocity (5-sec

CON: 5-sec ECC) compared to a traditional (moderate) velocity with a corresponding lower neural activation. These data demonstrate that motor unit activity may be limited when the individual intentionally slows contraction velocity. Lighter loads (e.g. ~30% reduction) are required for intentionally slow velocities (i.e., > 5-sec CON, > 5-sec ECC) of training (when a targeted number of repetitions are desired) and may not provide an optimal stimulus for 1 RM strength enhancement in resistance-trained individuals. Compared to slow velocities, moderate (1–2-sec CON, 1–2-sec ECC) and fast (< 1-sec CON, 1-sec ECC) velocities have been shown to be more effective for enhanced muscular performance, e.g., number of repetitions performed, work and power output, volume, and for increasing the rate of strength gains. The American College of Sports Medicine (2002) recommends slow to moderate velocities for novice training (i.e., with light loads while correct technique is learned), moderate velocities for intermediate training, and unintentionally slow (with heavy weights) and moderate to fast (with moderate to moderately heavy weights) for optimal strength training.

Frequency

Frequency refers to the number of training sessions performed during a specific period of time (e.g., 1 week) and/or the number of times certain exercises or muscle groups are trained per week. It is dependent upon several factors such as volume and intensity, exercise selection, level of conditioning and/or training status, recovery ability, nutritional intake, and training goals. Numerous studies have successfully used frequencies of 2–3 alternating days per week in novices. For increasing strength, a) 3 days per week was superior to 1 day per week and 2 days per week; b) 4 days per week was superior to 3 days per week; c) 2 days were superior to 1 day; d) 3–5 days per week was superior to 1 and 2 days; and e) 2 and 3 days per week were similar. Progression does not necessitate a change in frequency for training each muscle group, but may be more dependent upon alterations in other acute variables such as exercise selection, volume, and intensity. Advanced training frequency varies considerably. It has been shown that football players training 4–5 days/week achieved better results than those who trained either 3 or 6 days/week. Other advanced athletes have used frequencies higher than this (i.e., 8–12 workouts per week or more). It is important to note that not all muscle groups are trained specifically per workout using a high frequency. Rather, each major muscle group may be trained 2–3 times per week despite the large number of workouts. The American College of Sports Medicine recommends 2–3 days per week for novice training, 2–4 days per week for intermediate training, and 4–6 days per week for advanced strength training.

Summary

Resistance training poses numerous health and fitness benefits to all individuals, providing that a threshold of activity/effort is reached. Progressive overload, specificity, and variation are critical elements to resistance training programs targeting progression. These elements may be attained by proper manipulation of the acute program variables in order to obtain specific, individualized goals.

Section 27.5

Periodized Training: What Is It?

"Periodized Training—and Why It's Important,"
reprinted with permission from the American Council on Exercise,
www.acefitness.org. © 2005. All rights reserved.

You have the best intentions regarding your workout, but find that your motivation has been sapped.

Lately, no matter how hard or how often you work out; you just can't seem to progress any further. You're stuck on a plateau.

It turns out that the exercise you've been doing has worked so well that your body has adapted to it. You need to "shock" or "surprise" your body a bit. You need to give it a new challenge periodically if you're going to continue to make gains.

That goes for both strength and cardiovascular training. "Periodizing" your training is the key. Instead of doing the same routine month after month, you change your training program at regular intervals or "periods" to keep your body working harder, while still giving it adequate rest.

For example, you can alter your strength-training program by adjusting the following variables:

- The number of repetitions per set, or number of sets of each exercise
- The amount of resistance used
- The rest period between sets, exercises, or training sessions
- The order of the exercises, or the type of exercises
- The speed at which you complete each exercise

There are many different types of periodized strength-training programs, and many are geared to the strength, power, and demands of specific sports. The most commonly used program is one that will move you from low resistance and a high number of repetitions to high resistance and a lower number of repetitions.

Such a program will allow your muscles to strengthen gradually and is appropriate for anyone interested in general fitness.

Research Shows Better Results

Research from the Human Performance Laboratory at Ball State University has shown that a periodized strength-training program can produce better results than a non-periodized program. The purpose of the study, published in the journal *Medicine & Science in Sports & Exercise* in 2001, was to determine the long-term training adaptations associated with low-volume, circuit-type training vs. periodized, high-volume resistance training in women (volume = total amount of weight lifted during each session).

The 34 women in the study were divided into those two groups, as well as a nonexercising control group. Group 1 performed one set of eight to 12 repetitions to muscle failure three days per week for 12 weeks. Group 2 performed two to four sets of three to 15 repetitions,

Table 27.3. Progress in Training Using Periodized and Non-Periodized Programs

Marker	Periodized	Non-Periodized
Lean muscle	+ 4.6 lb (2.1 kg)	+ 2.2 lb (1 kg)
Body fat%	-4%	-1.8%
Leg press	+ 44 lb (20 kg)	+18 lb (8 kg)
Bench press	+11.21 lb (5.1 kg)	+6 lb (2.7 kg)

with periodized volume and intensity, four days per week during the 12-week period.

As Table 27.3 shows, the periodized group showed more substantial gains in lean muscle, greater reductions in body fat, and more substantial strength gains than the non-periodized group after 12 weeks.

Periodizing Your Cardiovascular Workout

You should also periodize your cardiovascular training for the same reasons—to further challenge your body, while still allowing for adequate recovery time.

If, for example, you're a recreational runner, running for fitness, fun, and the occasional short race, you'll want to allow for flat, easy runs, as well as some that incorporate hills and others that focus on speed and strength.

What you don't want to do is complete the same run every time. If you run too easily, and don't push yourself, you won't progress. And chances are you'll get bored.

Conversely, too much speed or high-intensity training will lead to injury or burnout, and most likely, disappointing race results.

If you are serious about improving your time in a 10K, in completing a half marathon, or even a full marathon, you'll need a periodized program geared to each type of race. Many such programs are available from local running clubs, in running books and magazines, from some health clubs, as well as on running websites.

Specially designed periodized training programs are also available for cycling and many other sports.

Periodized training will ensure that you continue to make measurable progress, which will keep you energized and interested in reaching your goals.

Source: Marx, J.O. et al. (2001). Low-volume circuit versus high-volume periodized resistance training in women. *Medicine & Science in Sports & Exercise,* 33:635–643.

Section 27.6

Strengthen Your Abdominals with Stability Balls

One of today's most versatile pieces of exercise equipment looks more like an overgrown beach ball than a useful fitness tool.

The stability ball—an extra-large, inflatable orb designed to improve balance while targeting specific muscle groups—has grown in popularity since its mainstream introduction in the late 1980s and early 1990s.

The stability ball can be adapted for many uses, including developing core strength, improving posture and facilitating stretching, among others. Its application is particularly widespread in the physical therapy industry, where it was first put to use nearly 30 years ago.

Thanks to fitness professionals' interest in the stability ball and its numerous benefits, there have been several exercise programs developed over the past few years for just about every need, desire, and body part.

The Stability Ball and Your Core

So much of the exercise we do, such as running and cycling, focuses on the lower body. Not much attention is paid to the trunk, or core, of the body. It is the muscles of the core—the abdomen, chest, and back—that stabilize the rest of the body.

Think of your core as a strong column that links the upper and lower body together. Having a solid core creates a foundation for all activities, and is especially important when you add a heavy load, such as weights to your workout.

It is important when you are strengthening the core that you create balance between the muscles of the abdominal and the back. Many people will naturally have an imbalance between the strength of their abdominal muscles and the lower back muscles. Exercising with stability balls helps to develop and strengthen those muscles.

Infomercials and magazine advertisements seem to be targeting the individual who wants to strengthen their abdominal muscles. Although end results such as "toning" and "shrinking" aren't totally accurate, a handful of the techniques the equipment supports are valid.

However, you don't need an ab rocker or a special track with handles to concentrate on this area. The stability ball is well equipped to help you concentrate on your core.

Here are three exercises that can be performed with a standard stability ball and target all three sections of the abdominal muscles.

Supine Trunk Curl

Start with the top of the ball beneath the center of the back. Press the lower back into the ball and tighten the abdominals as you curl the rib cage toward the pelvis. Slowly return to the starting position.

Supine Oblique Curl

Start with the top of the ball beneath the center of the back, then stagger feet and rotate hips to one side. Anchor the lower hip to the ball and move the rib cage at a diagonal direction toward the legs (for example, right elbow to left inner thigh). Make sure your neck and pelvis are stable.

Forward Transverse Roll

Kneel on the floor and place your forearms on the ball, making sure your hips and arms form a 90-degree angle. From this starting position, roll the ball forward as you extend your arms and legs simultaneously. Contract your abdominals to help support your lower back, which should not be strained.

Roll as far forward as possible without compressing the spine, drooping shoulders, or rounding the torso. Return to starting position.

The Benefits of Balls

Besides providing balance training, stability balls work the trunk in almost every exercise that is performed. By concentrating on the abdominal section, your posture will improve and you will find that you are generally more balanced and aware of your body movements.

Your core will be more prepared to support the rest of your body in whatever activity you choose to do.

How to Choose a Ball

It is important to buy the right size ball and maintain the proper air pressure. The firmer the ball, the more difficult the exercise will be. The softer the ball, the less difficult the exercise will be.

If you are just beginning, overweight, an older adult, or you are generally deconditioned, you may want to consider using a larger, softer ball. When sitting on the ball, your knees and hips should align at a 90-degree angle.

Following are general guidelines for buying the right size stability ball:

- Under 4 feet 6 inches (137 cm): 30 cm ball (12 inches)

- 4 feet 6 inches to 5 feet (137–152 cm): 45 cm ball (18 inches)

- 5 feet 1 inches to 5 feet 7 inches (155–170 cm): 55 cm ball (22 inches)

- 5 feet 8 inches to 6 feet 2 inches (173–188 cm): 65 cm ball (26 inches)

- Over 6 feet 2 inches (188 cm): 75 cm ball (30 inches)

Chapter 28

Flexibility and Balance Exercises

Chapter Contents

Section 28.1

Techniques for Stretching

Excerpted from Chapter 4 of the book *Exercise: A Guide from the National Institute on Aging*, published by the National Institute on Aging (www.nia.nih.gov), part of the National Institutes of Health, April 2004.

How to Improve Your Flexibility

Stretching exercises give you more freedom of movement to do the things you need to do and the things you like to do. Stretching exercises alone can improve your flexibility, but they will not improve your endurance or strength.

How Much, How Often?

- Stretch after you do your regularly scheduled strength and endurance exercises.

- If you can't do endurance or strength exercises for some reason, and stretching exercises are the only kind you are able to do, do them at least 3 times a week, for at least 20 minutes each session.

- Do each stretching exercise 3 to 5 times at each session.

- Slowly stretch into the desired position, as far as possible without pain, and hold the stretch for 10 to 30 seconds. Relax, then repeat, trying to stretch farther.

Safety

- If you have had a hip replacement, check with your surgeon before doing lower body exercises.

- If you have had a hip replacement, don't cross your legs or bend your hips past a 90-degree angle.

- Always warm up before stretching exercises (do them after endurance or strength exercises, for example; or, if you are doing only stretching exercises on a particular day, do a little bit of easy walking and arm-pumping first). Stretching your muscles before they are warmed up may result in injury.

- Stretching should never cause pain, especially joint pain. If it does, you are stretching too far, and you need to reduce the stretch so that it doesn't hurt.

- Mild discomfort or a mild pulling sensation is normal.

- Never "bounce" into a stretch; make slow, steady movements instead. Jerking into position can cause muscles to tighten, possibly resulting in injury.

- Avoid "locking" your joints into place when you straighten them during stretches. Your arms and legs should be straight when you stretch them, but don't lock them in a tightly straight position. You should always have a very small amount of bending in your joints while stretching.

Progressing

You can progress in your stretching exercises; the way to know how to limit yourself is that stretching should never hurt. It may feel slightly uncomfortable, but not painful. Push yourself to stretch farther, but not so far that it hurts.

About Floor Exercises

Most of the exercises are done on the floor and stretch some very important muscle groups. If you are afraid to lie on the floor to exercise because you think you won't be able to get back up, consider using the buddy system to do these. Find a buddy who will be able to help you.

Knowing the right way to get into a lying position on the floor and to get back up also may be helpful. If you have had a hip replacement, check with your surgeon before using the following method. If you have osteoporosis, check with your doctor first.

To get into a lying position:

1. Stand next to a very sturdy chair that won't tip over (put chair against wall for support if you need to).

2. Put your hands on the seat of the chair.

3. Lower yourself down on one knee.

4. Bring the other knee down.

5. Put your left hand on the floor and lean on it as you bring your left hip to the floor.

6. Your weight is now on your left hip.

7. Straighten your legs out.

8. Lie on your left side.

9. Roll onto your back.

Note: You don't have to use your left side. You can use your right side, if you prefer.

To get up from a lying position:

1. Roll onto your left side.

2. Use your right hand, placed on the floor at about the level of your ribs, to push your shoulders off the floor.

3. Your weight is on your left hip.

4. Roll forward, onto your knees, leaning on your hands for support.

5. Lean your hands on the seat of the chair you used to lie down.

6. Lift one of your knees so that one leg is bent, foot flat on the floor.

7. Leaning your hands on the seat of the chair for support, rise from this position.

Note: You don't have to use your left side; you can reverse positions, if you prefer.

Hamstrings

Stretches muscles in the back of the thigh.

1. Sit sideways on bench or other hard surface (such as two chairs placed side by side).

2. Keep one leg stretched out on bench, straight, toes pointing up.

3. Keep other leg off of bench, with foot flat on floor.

4. Straighten back.

5. If you feel a stretch at this point, hold the position for 10 to 30 seconds.

6. If you don't feel a stretch, lean forward from hips (not waist) until you feel stretching in leg on bench, keeping back and shoulders straight. Omit this step if you have had a hip replacement, unless surgeon/therapist approves.

7. Hold position for 10 to 30 seconds.

8. Repeat with other leg.

9. Repeat 3 to 5 times on each side.

Alternative Hamstring Stretch

Stretches muscles in the back of the thigh.

1. Stand behind chair, holding the back of it with both hands.

2. Bend forward from the hips (not waist), keeping back and shoulders straight at all times.

3. When upper body is parallel to floor, hold position for 10 to 30 seconds. You should feel a stretch in the backs of your thighs.

4. Repeat 3 to 5 times.

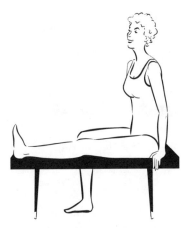

Figure 28.1. Performing the hamstrings stretch.

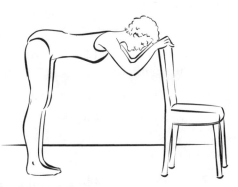

Figure 28.2. Performing the alternative hamstrings stretch.

Calves

Stretches lower leg muscles in two ways: with knee straight and knee bent.

1. Stand with hands against wall, arms outstretched and elbows straight.

2. Keeping your left knee slightly bent, toes of right foot slightly turned inward, step back 1 to 2 feet with right leg, heel, and foot flat on floor. You should feel a stretch in your calf muscle, but you shouldn't feel uncomfortable. If you don't feel a stretch, move your foot farther back until you do.

3. Hold position for 10 to 30 seconds.

4. Bend knee of right leg, keep heel and foot flat on floor.

5. Hold position for another 10 to 30 seconds.

6. Repeat with left leg.

7. Repeat 3 to 5 times for each leg.

Ankles

Stretches front ankle muscles.

1. Remove your shoes. Sit toward the front edge of a chair and lean back, using pillows to support your back.

2. Stretch legs out in front of you.

3. With your heels still on the floor, bend ankles to point feet toward you.

4. Bend ankles to point feet away from you.

5. If you don't feel the stretch, repeat with your feet slightly off the floor.

6. Hold the position for 1 second.

7. Repeat 3 to 5 times.

Triceps Stretch

Stretches muscles in back of upper arm.

1. Hold one end of a towel in right hand.

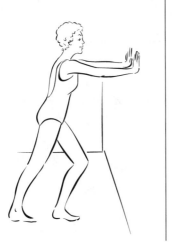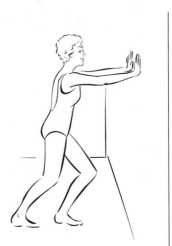

Figure 28.3. Stretching the calves.

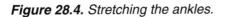

Figure 28.4. Stretching the ankles.

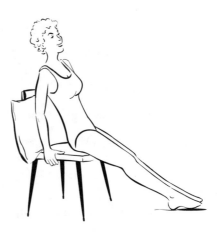

Figure 28.5. Stretching the triceps.

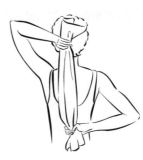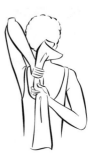

2. Raise and bend right arm to drape towel down back. Keep your right arm in this position, and continue holding onto the towel.

3. Reach behind your lower back and grasp bottom end of towel with left hand.

4. Climb left hand progressively higher up towel, which also pulls your right arm down. Continue until your hands touch, or as close to that as you can comfortably go.

5. Reverse positions.

6. Repeat each position 3 to 5 times.

Wrist Stretch

Stretches wrist muscles.

1. Place hands together, in praying position.

2. Slowly raise elbows so arms are parallel to floor, keeping hands flat against each other.

3. Hold position for 10 to 30 seconds.

4. Repeat 3 to 5 times.

Quadriceps

Stretches muscles in front of thighs.

1. Lie on side on the floor. Your hips should be lined up so that one is directly above the other one.

2. Rest head on pillow or hand.

3. Bend knee that is on top.

4. Reach back and grab heel of that leg. If you can't reach your heal with your hand, loop a belt over your foot and hold belt ends.

5. Gently pull that leg until front of thigh stretches.

6. Hold position for 10 to 30 seconds.

7. Reverse position and repeat.

8. Repeat 3 to 5 times on each side. If the back of your thigh cramps during this exercise, stretch your leg and try again, more slowly.

Double Hip Rotation

Stretches outer muscles of hips and thighs. Don't do this exercise if you have had a hip replacement, unless your surgeon approves.

1. Lie on floor on your back, knees bent and feet flat on the floor.

2. Keep shoulders on floor at all times.

3. Keeping knees bent and together, gently lower legs to one side as far as possible without forcing them.

4. Hold position for 10 to 30 seconds.

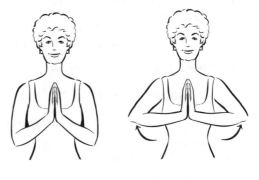

Figure 28.6. Stretching the wrists.

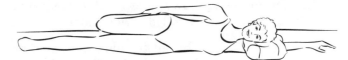

Figure 28.7. Stretching the quadriceps.

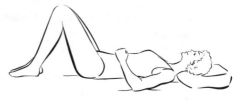

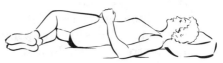

Figure 28.8. Performing the double hip rotation stretch.

5. Return legs to upright position.

6. Repeat toward other side.

7. Repeat 3 to 5 times on each side.

Single Hip Rotation

Stretches muscles of pelvis and inner thigh. Don't do this exercise if you have had a hip replacement, unless your surgeon approves.

1. Lie on your back on floor, knees bent and feet flat on the floor.

2. Keep shoulders on floor throughout exercise.

3. Lower one knee slowly to side, keeping the other leg and your pelvis in place.

4. Hold position for 10 to 30 seconds.

5. Bring knee back up slowly.

6. Repeat with other knee.

7. Repeat 3 to 5 times on each side.

Shoulder Rotation

Stretches shoulder muscles.

1. Lie flat on floor, pillow under head, legs straight. If your back bothers you, place a rolled towel under your knees.

2. Stretch arms straight out to side. Your shoulders and upper arms will remain flat on the floor throughout this exercise.

3. Bend elbows so that your hands are pointing toward the ceiling.

4. Let your arms slowly roll backward from the elbow. Stop when you feel a stretch or slight discomfort, and stop immediately if you feel a pinching sensation or a sharp pain.

5. Hold position for 10 to 30 seconds.

6. Slowly raise your arms, still bent at the elbow, to point toward the ceiling again. Then let your arms slowly roll forward, remaining bent at the elbow, to point toward your hips. Stop when you feel a stretch or slight discomfort.

7. Hold position for 10 to 30 seconds.

8. Alternate pointing above head, then toward ceiling, then toward hips. Begin and end with pointing-above-head position.

9. Repeat 3 to 5 times.

Neck Rotation

Stretches neck muscles.

1. Lie on the floor with a phone book or other thick book under your head.

2. Slowly turn head from side to side, holding position each time for 10 to 30 seconds on each side. Your head should not be tipped

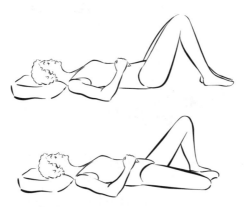

Figure 28.9. *Performing the single hip rotation stretch.*

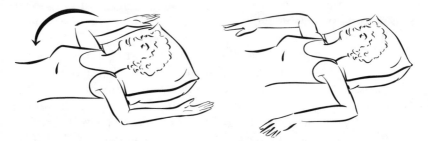

Figure 28.10. *Performing the shoulder rotation stretch.*

forward or backward, but should be in a comfortable position. You can keep your knees bent to keep your back comfortable during this exercise.

3. Repeat 3 to 5 times.

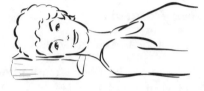
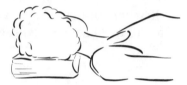

Figure 28.11. *Performing the neck rotation stretch.*

Section 28.2

Tips for Improving Your Flexibility

"Tips for Flexibility Training" is reproduced with permission of IDEA Health & Fitness Association, (800) 999-IDEA, www.IDEAfit.com. © 2006 IDEA Health & Fitness Association.

When it comes to the Big Three of exercise—cardiovascular, strength, and flexibility training—it's pretty clear which one can get overlooked. After all, while we prize cardiovascular and strength training for their role in helping us lose weight, build muscle, and get fit, the benefits of flexibility training are less immediately alluring.

However, as the population ages, more of us are learning to appreciate the rewards of stretching. Staying limber can offset age-related stiffness, improve athletic performance, and optimize functional movement in daily life. Research shows that flexibility training can develop and maintain range of motion and may help prevent and treat injury. In fact, the American College of Sports Medicine has added flexibility training to its general exercise recommendations, advising that stretching exercises for the major muscle groups be performed two to three days per week.

How can you include an effective flexibility workout in your fitness program? Here are some guidelines:

1. Think in terms of serious flexibility training, not just brief stretching.

Squeezing in one or two quick stretches before or after a workout is better than nothing, but this approach will yield limited results. What's more, generic stretches may not be effective for your particular body. The more time and attention you give to your flexibility training, the more benefits you'll experience. A qualified personal trainer, physical therapist, or health professional can design a functional flexibility program specifically for you.

2. Consider your activities.

Are you a golfer? Do you ski, run, or play tennis? Do your daily home or work routines include bending, lifting, or sitting for long periods? Functional flexibility improves "the stability and mobility of the whole person in his or her specific environment," says physical therapist Deborah Ellison. She recommends an individualized stretching program to improve both stability (the ability to maintain ideal body alignment during all activities) and mobility (the ability to use full, normal range of motion).

3. Pay special attention to tight areas.

Often the shoulders, chest, hamstrings, and hips are particularly tight, but you may hold tension in other areas, depending on your history of injuries and the existing imbalances in your muscle groups. Unless you tailor your flexibility training to your strengths and weaknesses, you may stretch already overstretched muscles and miss areas that need training.

4. Listen to your body.

Stretching is an individual thing. Pay attention to your body's signals and don't push too far. Avoid ballistic stretching, which uses bouncing or jerking movements to gain momentum; this approach can be dangerous. Instead, slowly stretch your muscles to the end point of movement and hold the stretch for about 10 to 30 seconds. Older adults, pregnant women, and people with injuries may need to take special precautions.

5. Get creative.

Varying your flexibility training can help you stick with it. You can use towels, resistance balls, and other accessories to add diversity and effectiveness to your stretching.

6. Warm up first.

If you're stretching on your own, don't forget to warm up your muscles before you begin. Walking briskly for 10 or 15 minutes is a simple way to do this.

7. Find a flexibility class that works for you.

Classes that include stretching are becoming more popular and more diverse. Some combine cardiovascular and strength components with the flexibility training; others focus exclusively on stretching.

8. Stretch yourself—mind and body.

Did you know that your emotional state may affect your flexibility? If your body is relaxed, says Ellison, it will be more responsive to flexibility training. Listening to music and focusing on your breath can help you relax as you stretch. You may also want to explore yoga or exercise inspired by the work of Joseph Pilates. In addition to stretching, classes in these disciplines may include relaxation, visualization, and other mind-body techniques designed to reduce stress and increase mindfulness.

9. It's not just for wimps.

Forget the idea that stretching is just for elderly, injured, or unconditioned people. Many Olympic and professional athletes rely on flexibility training for peak performance.

10. Do it consistently.

It doesn't help to stretch for a few weeks and then forget about it. Integrate regular stretching into your permanent fitness program. For inspiration, look to cats and dogs—they're dedicated practitioners of regular stretching!

Section 28.3

Flexibility Exercises to Try at Home

Reproduced with permission from Flexibility Exercises, in Johnson TR, (ed): *Your Orthopaedic Connection*, Rosemont, IL, American Academy of Orthopaedic Surgeons. Available at http://orthoinfo.aaos.org.

Preparing the body for exercise is important for persons at any age and fitness level. The key to preventing injuries before exercising is to warm up. One of the best ways to warm up is to do flexibility or stretching exercises.

The key to proper stretching lies in the way you perform the exercise. When you are stretching certain parts of your body, you should not feel pain. Staying relaxed is very important to stretching properly. Make sure your body is not tight. Your shoulders, hands and feet should be kept relaxed as you stretch. Breathe slowly.

Here are some exercises developed by the American Academy of Orthopaedic Surgeons. The exercises will help warm up various parts of your body.

Lower Back

- **Exercise 1:** Tighten your hip muscles and at the same time, tighten your abdominal muscles to flatten your lower back. Hold for 5 to 8 seconds, then relax. Repeat two or three times.

- **Exercise 2:** Pull your right leg toward your chest. If possible, keep the back of your head on the floor. Try to keep your lower back flat. Hold for 30 seconds. Repeat with your left leg.

Hip and Groin

- **Exercise 1:** With arms supplying slight resistance on inside of legs, slowly push down your knees. Hold for 5 to 8 seconds.

- **Exercise 2:** Place one leg forward, while your knee of the other leg is resting on the floor. Without changing the position of the knee on the floor or the forward leg, lower the front of your hip downward. Hold for 30 seconds.

Knee and Calf

- **Exercise 1:** Hold the top of your left foot with right hand and gently pull heel toward buttocks. Hold for 30 seconds. Repeat with other leg.

- **Exercise 2:** Stand close to a solid support, and lean on it with your forearms, head resting on hands. Bend one leg and place your foot on the ground in front of you, with the other leg straight behind. Slowly move your hips forward, keeping your lower back flat. Hold for 15 to 30 seconds. Do not bounce.

Shoulder

- **Exercise 1:** In a standing or sitting position, interlace your fingers. With your palms facing upward, push your arms slightly back and up. Hold for 15 seconds.

- **Exercise 2:** With your arms overhead, hold the elbow of one arm with the hand of your other arm. Gently pull the elbow behind your arm. Do slowly. Hold for 15 seconds. Stretch both arms.

- **Exercise 3:** Gently pull your elbow across your chest toward your opposite shoulder. Hold for 10 seconds. Repeat with other elbow.

Hamstring

- Sit down and straighten your left leg. The sole of your right foot should rest next to the inside of your straightened leg. Lean slightly forward and touch your foot with your fingers. Keep your left foot upright with the ankle and toes relaxed. Hold for 30 seconds. Repeat with right leg.

Section 28.4

Research Indicates Stretching Alone Does Not Prevent Injuries

"A Variety of Preparticipation Activities, Not Just Stretching, Recommended to Prevent Injuries in Sports," News release, March 3, 2004. Reprinted with permission of the American College of Sports Medicine.

Preparation for sports or exercise should involve a variety of activities and should not be limited to stretching alone, according to a report published in the March 2004 issue of *Medicine & Science in Sports & Exercise*, the official scientific journal of the American College of Sports Medicine (ACSM). Researchers examined decades of scientific evidence and caution that stretching alone may not be enough to prevent injuries.

"The use of stretching primarily as a way to prevent sports injury has been based on intuition and observation rather than scientific evidence," said lead researcher Stephen B. Thacker, M.D. "The best advice is to include a combination of warmup, strength training, plyometrics, and balance exercises to lessen injury risks."

The research team reviewed more than 350 scientific studies and articles that examined the relationship between stretching and injuries over the past four decades. While the evidence does show that stretching is important in increasing muscle and joint flexibility, in most cases researchers found little-to-no relationship between stretching and injuries or postexercise pain.

"Most injuries occur during muscle contractions within the normal range of joint motion anyway," said Thacker, "so it's unclear how increasing the range of motion through stretching would decrease injury risk." In addition, Thacker and his team point to some evidence that stretching just prior to an athletic event may actually compromise performance in elite athletes.

"We are not suggesting that athletes discontinue flexibility training and stretching altogether," Thacker continued, "but that athletes, coaches, trainers, and others look critically at preparticipation and training routines to ensure they include all the activities which, when combined, can enhance safety and performance. This might include activities such as proper warmup or strength, plyometric, and balance training."

The research team concludes that, while there is currently insufficient evidence to endorse or discontinue routine stretching to prevent injury, future research should be performed to examine the role of stretching in injury prevention for both recreational and competitive athletes. Studies are needed to determine the optimal timing (pre- or postexercise) and any optimal levels of flexibility of specific muscle groups for each sport or activity.

The American College of Sports Medicine is the largest sports medicine and exercise science organization in the world. More than 20,000 International, National, and Regional members are dedicated to advancing and integrating scientific research to provide educational and practical applications of exercise science and sports medicine.

Section 28.5

Tips for Bettering Your Balance

When we're young, we generally take our balancing skills for granted. As we get older, however, we find that our balance (the ability to sense where our bodies are positioned and adjust muscle tension to maintain alignment) isn't what it used to be. The consequences of losing our ability to balance are significant. Falls are the leading cause of injury for older adults. Every year, 30 to 50 percent of people over age 65 sustain a fall; many never recover completely. Even less serious falls can result in physical adaptations (i.e., becoming less active, moving more slowly) that negatively impact the quality of life.

While some effects of aging—such as impaired vision, reduced reflex speed, and decreased sensitivity of skin receptors—can impair balance and coordination, poor balance is not inevitable. Many physically fit older adults practice the same balance recovery strategies as younger adults and, as a result, are generally better at controlling their balance than their inactive peers.

How can you maintain good balancing skills? San Diego physical therapist Deborah Ellison, PT, an expert in functional exercise design, offers these tips:

1. Improve your cardiovascular fitness.

Improvements in this area will contribute to better gait, cardiovascular health, weight control, motor control, self-confidence, and other factors that impact balance.

2. Practice single-leg standing or yoga balancing postures.

Start by standing on a solid floor and then progress to working on a thick carpet or soft foam surface. Also do side-to-side movements, such as side-to-side step touches or small squats, moving to the right or left. To add more challenge, use a wobble board (a device used by physical therapists that consists of a circular board on an unstable base), curbs, stairs, or inclines.

3. Try tai chi, qi gong (chi kung), or Hatha yoga classes.

These offer gradual and consistent balance training.

4. Practice shifting your weight from side to side.

If you stand on two digital scales, one under each foot, you will be able to tell how much weight is on each side. As you progress in this exercise, change the base of support by moving the scales closer together or placing them on a diagonal. With your feet still on the scales, you can also try sitting, standing, or lifting an object from the floor.

5. Practice walking faster and stepping over objects in your path.

This will help improve speed and decrease hesitancy.

6. Improve your flexibility.

Take stretching classes and learn how to do a stretching routine at home. Stretching exercises help increase your range of motion, particularly at the shoulder, torso, hip, and ankle. Using a fitness ball will contribute to better pelvic mobility.

7. *Improve overall strength.*

Lower-leg strength is particularly important for walking, maintaining dynamic balance, and preventing falls. With the aid of a fitness professional, develop a complete strength program that will help you both reduce falls and recover from them.

8. *Build your self-confidence.*

Fitness programs increase your confidence and decrease your fear and apprehension about falling, thereby reducing your overall muscle tension. Develop your skills and your confidence by doing drills in which you negotiate curbs and stairs, and walk along a taped line while carrying cups of water.

9. *Consult your physician.*

In some cases, custom-made orthotics (devices worn inside shoes) can help with balance. Also, your doctor will know if any medication you are taking may be affecting your balance.

10. *Look for professionals and programs that specifically address balance.*

As the population ages, balance training is becoming a more common component of fitness programs and services offered by personal trainers and physical therapists. Find a program that works for you.

Staying grounded.

Keep safety in mind as you practice balance training. Make sure walls, chairs, or other objects are nearby to use for support, and do not practice exercises that are too challenging for you without the help of a professional.

No single factor is responsible for balance loss, Ellison notes, so it is important to participate in an integrated physical activity program that includes cardiovascular fitness, strength training, flexibility exercises, and balance and coordination work. In general, doing cross training and trying new activities—even simple ones, such as biking—will help you maintain your physical abilities as you age.

Chapter 29

Pilates for Improved Strength and Flexibility

Pilates improves your mental and physical well-being, increases flexibility, and strengthens muscles. Pilates uses controlled movements in the form of mat exercises or equipment to tone and strengthen the body. For decades, it's been the exercise of choice for dancers and gymnasts (and now Hollywood actors), but it was originally used to rehabilitate bedridden or immobile patients during World War I.

What Is Pilates?

Pilates is a body conditioning routine that seeks to build flexibility, strength, endurance, and coordination without adding muscle bulk. In addition, Pilates increases circulation and helps to sculpt the body and strengthen the body's "core" or "powerhouse" (torso). People who do Pilates regularly feel they have better posture, are less prone to injury, and experience better overall health.

Joseph H. Pilates, the founder of the Pilates exercise method, was born in Germany. As a child he was frail, living with asthma in addition to other childhood conditions. To build his body and grow stronger, he took up several different sports, eventually becoming an

"Pilates" was provided by TeensHealth, one of the largest resources online for medically reviewed health information written for parents, kids, and teens. For more articles like this one, visit www.TeensHealth.org, or www.KidsHealth .org. © 2004 The Nemours Foundation. This article was reviewed by Steven Dowshen, M.D., June 2004.

accomplished athlete. As a nurse in Great Britain during World War I, he designed exercise methods and equipment for immobilized patients and soldiers. In addition to his equipment, Pilates developed a series of mat exercises that focus on the torso. He based these on various exercise methods from around the world, among them the mind-body formats of yoga and Chinese martial arts.

Joseph Pilates believed that our physical and mental health are intertwined. He designed his exercise program around principles that support this philosophy, including concentration, precision, control, breathing, and flowing movements.

There are two ways to exercise in Pilates. Today, most people focus on the mat exercises, which require only a floor mat and training. These exercises are designed so that your body uses its own weight as resistance. The other method of Pilates uses a variety of machines to tone and strengthen the body, again using the principle of resistance.

Getting Started

The great thing about Pilates is that just about everyone—from couch potatoes to fitness buffs—can do it. Because Pilates has gained lots of attention recently, there are lots of classes available. You'll probably find that many fitness centers and YMCAs offer Pilates classes, mostly in mat work. Some Pilates instructors also offer private classes that can be purchased class by class or in blocks of classes; these may combine mat work with machine work. If your health club makes Pilates machines available to members, make sure there's a qualified Pilates instructor on duty to teach and supervise you during the exercises.

The fact that Pilates is hot and classes are springing up everywhere does have a downside, though: inadequate instruction. As with any form of exercise, it is possible to injure yourself if you have a health condition or don't know exactly how to do the moves. Some gyms send their personal trainers to weekend-long courses and then claim they're qualified to teach Pilates (they're not!), and this can lead to injury. So look for an instructor who is certified by a group that has a rigorous training program. These instructors have completed several hundred hours of training just in Pilates and know the different ways to modify the exercises so new students don't get hurt.

The Pilates mat program follows a set sequence, with exercises following on from one another in a natural progression, just as Joseph Pilates designed them. Beginners start with basic exercises and build up to include additional exercises and more advanced positioning.

Keep these tips in mind so that you can get the most out of your Pilates workout.

- **Stay focused.** Pilates is designed to combine your breathing rhythm with your body movements. Qualified instructors teach ways to keep your breathing working in conjunction with the exercises. You will also be taught to concentrate on your muscles and what you are doing. The goal of Pilates is to unite your mind and body, which relieves stress and anxiety.

- **Be comfortable.** Wear comfortable clothes (as you would for yoga—shorts or tights and a T-shirt or tank top are good choices), and keep in mind that Pilates is usually done without shoes. If you start feeling uncomfortable, strained, or experience pain, you should stop.

- **Let it flow.** When you perform your exercises, avoid quick, jerky movements. Every movement should be slow, but still strong and flexible. Joseph Pilates worked with dancers and designed his movements to flow like a dance.

- **Don't leave out the heart.** The nice thing about Pilates is you don't have to break a sweat if you don't want to—but you can also work the exercises quickly (bearing in mind fluidity, of course!) to get your heart rate going. Or, because Pilates is primarily about strength and flexibility, pair your Pilates workout with a form of aerobic exercise like swimming or brisk walking.

Most fans of Pilates say they stick with the program because it's diverse and interesting. Joseph Pilates designed his program for variety—people do fewer repetitions of a number of exercises rather than lots of repetitions of only a few. He also intended his exercises to be something people could do on their own once they've had proper instruction, cutting down the need to remain dependent on a trainer.

Before you begin any type of exercise program, it's a good idea to talk to your doctor, especially if you have a health problem.

Chapter 30

Yoga and Meditation Provide Health Benefits

Lisa, a 37-year-old mother of two, was racing through life, trying to juggle responsibilities at home, at work, and at her church, where she volunteered each week. One day, at her annual doctor's appointment, her doctor told her she had high blood pressure. Her busy schedule had slowly eroded her good eating habits and put an end to her regular fitness walks with friends. Now Lisa was 40 pounds overweight and facing the added dangers that accompany a high blood pressure diagnosis. She was intrigued when her doctor suggested yoga and meditation as part of her treatment.

Lisa is not alone. Thousands of women are learning that the ancient Indian practices of yoga and meditation can provide real health benefits. Medical studies show that yoga and meditation may be helpful for those with a variety of conditions, including heart disease, asthma, epilepsy, multiple sclerosis, premenstrual syndrome (PMS), anxiety, and stress. By stretching the body and relaxing the mind, experts say that the benefits of yoga and meditation are enormous.

"Yoga and meditation focus people," says Rachel Donnell, Community Health Nurse at Red Lake Comprehensive Health Services, which is a Red Lake Indian Reservation in Red Lake, Minnesota. "Women get so caught up in the everyday world; they have to take time to regenerate and rejuvenate." Donnell, who regularly practices yoga herself, adds, "It gives you the power to do what you want to do."

"Yoga and Meditation: An Ancient Answer to Modern Day Stress" is part of the National Women's Health Information Center's (www.4woman.gov) *Pick Your Path to Health* public health education campaign, 2004.

What Is Yoga?

Yoga is a system built on three main structures: exercise, breathing, and meditation. When yoga is practiced regularly, these systems are designed to work in unison and produce a clear mind and a strong body.

There are four types or "paths" of yoga: Jnana, the path of knowledge; Bhakti, the path of devotion; Karma, the path of action; and Raja, the path of self-control. For each path, there are a number of different styles of yoga practiced. Hatha yoga (which is actually part of Raja yoga) is the form most popular in the West and focuses on postures and breathing.

All forms of yoga should be thought of as a process rather than a type of exercise. In most fitness programs, for example, someone who has not been physically active may begin exercising with a goal of touching her fingers to her toes. A more avid athlete will train for months or even years to achieve her goal of completing a marathon. With yoga, by contrast, the focus is on what you are doing—specific postures (asana) and exercises (pranayama)—and how you feel while you are doing them.

What Is Meditation?

Meditation is a part of most yoga practices. It involves concentrating on something simple—the breath, for example—to take attention away from the random thought activity that occupies the mind. Meditation allows people to slow the high speed movies that run through their heads and put them in touch with the quiet that is so often craved. A simple meditation may involve the following technique:

- Sit in a comfortable position, either in a chair or on the floor, with your back and head straight.

- Warm up with a couple of deep, cleansing breaths.

- Close your eyes and breathe through your nose.

- Focus on your breath—slowly breathing in and out. If your mind wanders (which will likely happen), just bring your attention back to the breath.

- Start with a 5- to 10-minute meditation and work up to 15 to 20 minutes or more.

Studies show that regular meditation is great therapy for those recovering from surgery or an emotional trauma. Meditation has also been shown to relax the tension of the gross and subtle muscles and the autonomic nervous system and provide freedom from mental stress. There is no one "right" way to meditate; however, here are some guidelines to help you achieve the greatest benefit:

- Meditate every day, ideally at the same time each day (most people agree morning is best).

- Designate a special place for meditation and use it only for meditation.

- While meditating, sit straight and vertical.

- Meditate before a meal (not right after one).

Hundreds of individuals and groups teach yoga and meditation. Many different techniques are taught, some more spiritual in nature and others are mainly concerned with stress-reduction and gaining a little peace of mind. You may want to go to a couple of different classes before choosing a style that is right for you. For more information and a listing of yoga instructors by state, check out the "Yoga Site" at www.yogasite.com.

Chapter 31

Kegel Exercises: Developing Your Pelvic Muscles

Why Exercise Pelvic Muscles?

Life's events can weaken pelvic muscles. Pregnancy, childbirth, and being overweight can do it. Luckily, when these muscles get weak, you can help make them strong again.

Pelvic floor muscles are just like other muscles. Exercise can make them stronger. Women with bladder control problems can regain control through pelvic muscle exercises, also called Kegel exercises.

Pelvic Fitness in Minutes a Day

Exercising your pelvic floor muscles for just 5 minutes, three times a day can make a big difference to your bladder control. Exercise strengthens muscles that hold the bladder and many other organs in place.

The part of your body including your hip bones is the pelvic area. At the bottom of the pelvis, several layers of muscle stretch between your legs. The muscles attach to the front, back, and sides of the pelvis bone.

Excerpted from "Exercising Your Pelvic Muscles," a publication by the National Kidney and Urologic Diseases Information Clearinghouse, a service of the National Institute of Diabetes and Digestive and Kidney Diseases (NIDDK) of the National Institutes of Health. NIH Publication No. 02-4188, April 2002.

Two pelvic muscles do most of the work. The biggest one stretches like a hammock. The other is shaped like a triangle. These muscles prevent leaking of urine and stool.

How Do You Exercise Your Pelvic Muscles?

Find the right muscles. This is very important. Your doctor, nurse, or physical therapist will help make sure you are doing the exercises the right way.

You should tighten the two major muscles that stretch across your pelvic floor. They are the "hammock" muscle and the "triangle" muscle. Here are three methods to check for the correct muscles.

1. Try to stop the flow of urine when you are sitting on the toilet. If you can do it, you are using the right muscles.

2. Imagine that you are trying to stop passing gas. Squeeze the muscles you would use. If you sense a "pulling" feeling, those are the right muscles for pelvic exercises.

3. Lie down and put your finger inside your vagina. Squeeze as if you were trying to stop urine from coming out. If you feel tightness on your finger, you are squeezing the right pelvic muscle.

Don't squeeze other muscles at the same time. Be careful not to tighten your stomach, legs, or other muscles. Squeezing the wrong muscles can put more pressure on your bladder control muscles. Just squeeze the pelvic muscle. Don't hold your breath.

Repeat, but don't overdo it. At first, find a quiet spot to practice—your bathroom or bedroom—so you can concentrate. Lie on the floor. Pull in the pelvic muscles and hold for a count of 3. Then relax for a count of 3. Work up to 10 to 15 repeats each time you exercise.

Do your pelvic exercises at least three times a day. Every day, use three positions: lying down, sitting, and standing. You can exercise while lying on the floor, sitting at a desk, or standing in the kitchen. Using all three positions makes the muscles strongest.

Be patient. Don't give up. It's just 5 minutes, three times a day. You may not feel your bladder control improve until after 3 to 6 weeks. Still, most women do notice an improvement after a few weeks.

Exercise aids. You can also exercise by using special weights or biofeedback. Ask your health care team about these exercise aids.

Hold the Squeeze until after the Sneeze

You can protect your pelvic muscles from more damage by bracing yourself.

Think ahead, just before sneezing, lifting, or jumping. Sudden pressure from such actions can hurt those pelvic muscles. Squeeze your pelvic muscles tightly and hold on until after you sneeze, lift, or jump.

After you train yourself to tighten the pelvic muscles for these moments, you will have fewer accidents.

Chapter 32

Exercising away from Home

Chapter Contents

Section 32.1

Energize Your Workday with Office Exercises

"Tips for Working Out at the Office," 2006, is reprinted
with permission from the Wisconsin Governor's Challenge,
http://www.wisconsinchallenge.org.

If you think that long hours at work means no time for exercise, think again. Even at the office, there are simple ways to fit physical activity into your day.

Always remember to use discretion by knowing what's appropriate for your work environment. Always warm up, or begin your exercise gradually, and consult your health care provider before starting an exercise program.

The following are some tips to get you started.

1. Park a little further away—whether you're taking a car or bus during your daily commute, that extra walk will do you a world of good. Also think about this when you are heading to appointments, the bank, or the post office.

2. Try to plan a meeting on the run. Discuss business during an afternoon walk or jog. And use the stairs instead of the elevator as much as you can. Keep a pair of walking shoes in your briefcase.

3. Take a break every hour or so to stand, stretch, and walk around. Get up and walk down the hall to deliver your message instead of using e-mail or the phone. Not only will you get more exercise, you'll also enjoy the added personal interaction.

4. If your office is near an exercise facility, join and try to maintain scheduled visits at whatever time makes the most sense for you. Always keep a change of clothes and towel with you.

5. Just because you're on the road doesn't mean you can't fit in a workout. Invest in a small pair of speakers for your personal stereo and pack a jump rope for a lively stationary aerobic workout in your hotel room.

Some strength-training exercises for the workplace:

- **Try some squats.** Stand in front of your office chair with your feet shoulder-width apart. Bend your knees as though you're sitting on the chair, keeping your weight on your heels. When your legs are parallel with the seat of the chair, slowly rise to your original standing position.

- **Hold up the wall with wall sits.** With your back touching the wall, move your feet away from the wall so that the wall is supporting the weight of your back. Bend your knees so that your legs form a 90-degree angle. Hold as long as you can.

- **During a coffee break, try calf raises.** Holding onto your desk or a file cabinet for balance, raise your heels off the floor, then lower.

- **Peek into your neighbor's cubicle while you do toe raises.** Sitting in your chair or standing, lift and lower your toes while keeping your heels on the ground, or walk around on the heels of your feet.

- **Release tension with shoulder raises.** Raise your shoulders up to your ears, hold, then relax.

Section 32.2

Exercise at Work Benefits People with Type 2 Diabetes

Moderate physical activity can reduce cardiovascular disease deaths in people with type 2 diabetes, even if that activity comes on the job or while getting to and from work, researchers report in the July 27, 2004 issue of *Circulation: Journal of the American Heart Association.*

The protective effects of exercise are not limited to leisure-time activities, said senior author Jaakko Tuomilehto, M.D., Ph.D., professor, Diabetes and Genetic Epidemiology Unit in the National Public Health Institute in Helsinki, Finland.

"Regular physical activity should be part of standard treatment for diabetic patients. People with diabetes need to look for ways to build activity into their work, their commuting to and from work, and also their leisure time," Tuomilehto said. "Physical activity during commuting is one of the easiest, least-time consuming ways to promote health."

Diabetes increases the risk of heart disease and stroke. It's a disease in which the body doesn't make or properly respond to the hormone insulin and cannot properly control blood sugar levels. Type 2 diabetes, the most common form, usually appears in adults, often in middle age, although it's becoming an increasing problem in children and adolescents.

"We know that type 2 diabetes can be prevented or at least postponed by physical activity and a healthy diet, but too often people think only of leisure-time physical training or other aerobic activities," Tuomilehto said.

The number of people with diabetes in the world is expected to at least double in the next 25 years, and heart and blood vessel disease accounts for up to 75 percent of total deaths among patients with type 2 diabetes, researchers said.

Although occupational, commuting, and leisure-time physical activity has been associated with reductions in cardiovascular disease (CVD) deaths in the general population, this is the first large, long-term prospective study among people with type 2 diabetes, said lead researcher Gang Hu, M.D., Ph.D., M.P.H.

Researchers reviewed data on 3,316 people ages 25 to 74 who had type 2 diabetes and participated in national surveys of randomly selected samples in the Finnish population between 1972 and 1997. The data included results from questionnaires on heart disease risk factors such as smoking, medical history, and the level of physical activity on the job, on the way to and from work, and during leisure time.

Work activity was divided into three exercise levels: light (easy physical work and sitting, e.g., office work); moderate (walking and lifting light objects, e.g., store clerk), and active (walking and lifting, e.g., heavy manual labor).

Light commuting was defined as using motorized transportation; moderate was walking or bicycling up to 29 minutes daily; and active commuting was walking or cycling 30 minutes or more per day. Light leisure activity was almost completely inactive, such as reading or watching TV. Moderate was more than four hours each week of walking, cycling, or light gardening and active was more than three hours of vigorous activity per week such as swimming, running, or jogging.

During an average follow-up of 18.4 years, 1,410 of the subjects had died, including 903 (64 percent) from cardiovascular disease. After adjusting for age, gender, body mass index, systolic blood pressure, total cholesterol, and smoking, the researchers found that moderately active work was associated with a 9 percent reduction in cardiovascular death and active work was associated with a 40 percent reduction in CVD death.

An analysis of leisure-time activity found that high leisure-time physical activity was associated with a 33 percent drop in CVD death and moderate activity was linked to a 17 percent drop in CVD death compared to the most sedentary group.

"If this finding represents a causal relation, increasing exercise could be highly important to the improvement of health and the lengthening of life among working-aged patients," Hu said.

"Since the increase in computerization and mechanization has resulted in ever-increasing numbers of people being sedentary for most of their working time, adding short time exercise during working breaks, or adding walking activity during work time are recommended. We believe that it would be cost-efficient for employers."

Regular physical activity may reduce CVD and death among patients with diabetes several ways. For instance, regular exercise is associated with improvements in insulin sensitivity, blood sugar control, and other heart disease risk factors.

Commuting to work is a major source of physical activity in some populations and it can be implemented at little expense, the researchers said. More than 90 percent of workers walk or cycle to and from work each day in urban China, as did more than 40 percent of those in this study.

Co-authors include: Johan Eriksson, M.D.; Noël C. Barengo, M.D.; Timo A. Lakka, M.D.; Timo Valle, M.D.; Aulikki Nissinen, M.D.; and Pekka Jousilahti, M.D.

Section 32.3

Staying Active While You Fly

When you have little room to move and stretch on the plane, physical therapists advise doing some simple, seated exercises to keep the blood flowing, the joints mobile, and the muscles relaxed while en route.

- **Heel Raises**—Sit with feet flat on the floor, about hip-width apart. Lift heels so that only toes and the balls of the feet are on the floor. Hold for 5 to 10 seconds and lower feet back to the ground. Repeat 10 times.

- **Toe Lifts**—Sit with feet flat on the floor, about hip-width apart. Lift toes and balls of the feet so that only the heels are on the floor. Hold for 5 to 10 seconds and lower feet back to the ground. Repeat 10 times.

- **Ankle Circles**—While sitting, lift right leg slightly off the ground and rotate the foot clockwise, making a circle in the air. Do this 15 times clockwise, then 15 times counterclockwise. Repeat with left leg and foot. Alternatively, trace the letters of the alphabet in the air with the right, and then the left, foot.

- **Overhead Stretches**—Stand and reach arms straight up and stretch. Slowly lean to the left, then right, bending at the waist. Repeat this action five times to each side, holding each for 5 to 10 seconds. If you are unable to stand and stretch, then reach arms straight up while seated. If you have room, slowly stretch to each side as well.

- **Back Twists**—While sitting, reach the right arm across the body and grab the left armrest. Slowly turn the torso and head as far to the left as is comfortable. Hold for 5 to 10 seconds, repeat five times, and then switch sides.

- **Curl Downs**—While sitting, pull stomach and chin in and gently curl trunk down very slowly, reaching hands to the floor. Hold for 5 to 10 seconds then uncurl slowly back up. Repeat five times.

- **Toe-Heel Walk**—When walking down the aisle of the plane, walk on your toes one way and then return to your seat by walking on your heels.

Part Four

Fitness throughout Life

Chapter 33

Exercise Is Essential for Kids

When most adults think about exercise, they imagine working out in the gym on a treadmill or lifting weights. But for children, exercise means playing and being physically active. Kids exercise when they have gym class at school, soccer practice, or dance class. They're also exercising when they're at recess, riding bikes, or playing tag.

The Many Benefits of Exercise

Everyone can benefit from regular exercise. A child who is active will:

- have stronger muscles and bones;
- have a leaner body because exercise helps control body fat;
- be less likely to become overweight;
- decrease the risk of developing type 2 diabetes;
- possibly lower blood pressure and blood cholesterol levels; and
- have a better outlook on life.

In addition to the health benefits of regular exercise, kids who are physically fit sleep better and are better able to handle the physical

"Kids and Exercise" was provided by KidsHealth, one of the largest resources online for medically reviewed health information written for parents, kids, and teens. For more articles like this one, visit www.KidsHealth.org, or www.TeensHealth.org. © 2005 The Nemours Foundation. This article was reviewed by Mary L. Gavin, M.D., May 2005.

and emotional challenges that a typical day presents—be that running to catch a bus, bending down to tie a shoe, or studying for a test.

The Three Elements of Fitness

If you've ever watched children on a playground, you've seen the three elements of fitness in action. The child:

- runs away from the kid that's "it" (endurance);
- crosses the monkey bars (strength); and
- bends down to tie his or her shoes (flexibility).

Parents should encourage their kids to do a variety of activities so that they can work on all three elements.

Endurance is developed when someone regularly engages in aerobic activity (aerobic means "with air"). During aerobic exercise, the heart beats faster and a person breathes harder. When done regularly and for continuous periods of time, aerobic activity strengthens the heart and improves the body's ability to deliver oxygen to all its cells.

Aerobic exercise can be fun for both adults and children. Some examples of aerobic activities include:

- basketball;
- bicycling;
- ice-skating;
- in-line skating;
- soccer;
- swimming;
- tennis;
- walking;
- jogging; and
- running.

Improving strength doesn't have to mean lifting weights. Although some children benefit from lifting weights, it should be done under the supervision of an experienced adult who works with children. But most kids don't need a formal weight-training program to be strong. Push-ups, stomach crunches, pull-ups, and other exercises help tone and strengthen muscles. Children also incorporate strength activities in their play when they climb, do a handstand, or wrestle.

Stretching exercises help improve flexibility, allowing muscles and joints to bend and move easily through their full range of motion. Kids look for opportunities every day to stretch when they try to get a toy just out of reach, practice a split, or flip over the couch.

How Much Exercise Is Enough?

The percentage of children who are overweight has more than doubled over the past 30 years. Although many factors are contributing to this epidemic, kids are becoming more sedentary. In other words, they're sitting around a lot more than they used to.

According to the American Academy of Pediatrics (AAP), the average child is watching about 3 hours of television a day. And the average kid spends 5½ hours on all media combined, according to the Kaiser Family Foundation.

Parents need to ensure that their children are getting enough exercise. So, how much is enough? According to the 2005 dietary guidelines from the U.S. Department of Agriculture (USDA) and the Department of Health and Human Services (HHS), all children 2 years and older should get 60 minutes of moderate to vigorous exercise on most, preferably all, days of the week. In addition to providing more practical advice on how to give your child a healthy, balanced diet, the new dietary guidelines also suggest that kids eat more fruits, vegetables, and whole grains than in the past.

You can find out what guidelines are appropriate for your child by logging on to the USDA's interactive website for the revised food guide pyramid. The site allows you to enter your child's age, gender, and activity level to get one of 12 pyramids that make recommendations for total calories and amounts from each food, as well as some recommendations for specific foods, such as whole grains, beans, and orange veggies.

Also, here are (see Table 33.1) the current activity recommendations for children, according to the National Association for Sport and Physical Education (NASPE).

It's also important to remember that young children should not be inactive for prolonged periods of time—no more than 1 hour unless they're sleeping. And school-age children should not be inactive for periods longer than 2 hours.

One of the best ways to get children to be more active is to limit the amount of time spent in sedentary activities, especially watching TV or playing video games. The AAP recommends that children under the age of 2 years watch no TV at all and that screen time should be limited to no more than 1 to 2 hours of quality programming a day for children 2 years and older.

Table 33.1. Current Activity Recommendations for Children

Age	Minimum Daily Activity	Comments
Infant	No specific requirements	Physical activity should encourage motor development
Toddler	1½ hours	30 minutes planned physical activity AND 60 minutes unstructured physical activity (free play)
Preschooler	2 hours	60 minutes planned physical activity AND 60 minutes unstructured physical activity (free play)
School age	1 hour or more	Break up into bouts of 15 minutes or more

Raising a Fit Kid

Combining regular physical activity with a healthy diet is the key to a healthy lifestyle. By understanding the importance of being physically active, you can instill fun and healthy habits that will last a lifetime.

Here are some tips for raising a fit kid:

- Help your child participate in a variety of activities that are right for his or her age.

- Establish a regular schedule for physical activity.

- Incorporate activity into daily routines, such as taking the stairs instead of the elevator.

- Embrace a healthier lifestyle yourself, so you'll be a positive role model for your family.

- Keep it fun, so you can count on your child to come back for more.

Chapter 34

Parents Can Play Vital Role in Encouraging Children's Active, Healthy Lifestyles

Today's children may fantasize about growing up to be svelte celebrities, athletes, or models. The irony, however, is that children are, in large measure, inactive, unfit, and increasingly overstressed.

But parents that they can play a major role in encouraging their children to become more active.

"Children are more likely to continue physical activity if they enjoy it," says Dr. Jim Marks, M.D., M.P.H., director of the National Center for Chronic Disease Prevention and Health Promotion at the Centers for Disease Control and Prevention (CDC).

Encouraging a physically active lifestyle for children may be easier than parents think. Parents can start by suggesting several options that are available through local park districts, schools, and community programs.

"Children not only need to burn energy for healthy development, but also need to interact with peers, parents, and other role models in a safe, supportive environment to learn life skills, such as setting and achieving goals, competing fairly and resolving disputes peaceably," says Dr. Marks.

Assessing Youths' Needs

Experts recommend that children participate in at least 60 minutes of moderate-to-vigorous physical activity each day, such as walking

Excerpted from a press release by the Centers for Disease Control and Prevention (CDC), www.cdc.gov, 2004.

or playing hopscotch. Other ways to be active include swimming, in-line skating, Double Dutch jump roping, and dancing.

Parents also can support their children's participation in physical activity by being physically active role models, says Mike Greenwell, director of communications for CDC's chronic disease center. Family events and vacations can involve physical activities such as roller skating parties and swimming trips. For children who love to explore and search in new territories, hiking and biking are perfect ways to incorporate physical activity.

"Parents who encourage and endorse physical activities in their own lives are more likely to pass on these good habits to their children," says Dr. Marks. "By contrast, parents with little physical involvement typically have less active children."

More good news is that children who lead active lifestyles are likely to remain active as adults and pass on their healthy lifestyle habits to their own children. Consider the following benefits of regular physical activity for growing children:

- helps build and maintain healthy bones and muscles
- helps control weight, build lean muscle and reduce fat
- reduces feelings of depression, stress, and anxiety
- promotes psychological well-being, including higher levels of self-esteem and self-concept
- increases flexibility and aerobic endurance[1]

Combat Inactivity—The Number One Problem

Youth inactivity has increased continually in recent years. About 14 percent of young people report no recent physical activity. Inactivity is more common among females (14%) than males (7%) and among black females (21%) than white females (12%). Furthermore, studies have proven that as children get older, participation in all types of physical activity declines strikingly as age or grade in school increases.[2]

Physical inactivity among today's youth can be traced to several factors. Demographics and individual factors, such as confidence and lack of time, influence the level of physical activity. Family and peer support, or the lack thereof, affect children's willingness and likelihood to participate in physical activity. Parental support for physical activity is correlated with active lifestyles among children. Adequate play spaces, equipment, and transportation all affect the activity levels as well.

What Can Parents or Guardians Do to Promote Childrens' Physical Activity?

The U.S. Department of Health and Human Services' Centers for Disease Control and Prevention (CDC) stresses the importance of parents' role in encouraging healthy lifestyles and displacing risky behaviors. Following are a few suggestions to help parents promote physical activity.

- Set a good example by being physically active.
- Encourage children to be physically active.
- Play and be physically active with children.
- Inform children about sports and recreation programs in their community.
- Teach children safety rules and make sure they have the clothing and equipment needed to participate safely in physical activities.
- Be an advocate for convenient, safe, and adequate places for children to play and take part in physical activity programs.
- Encourage school administrators and community leaders to support daily physical education and other programs that promote lifelong physical activity, not just competitive sports.
- Ensure children are engaged in school and community organizations.
- Encourage children to volunteer in the community.

References

1. U.S. Department of Health and Human Services' Centers for Disease Control and Prevention. Physical Activity and Health: A Report of the Surgeon General.

2. U.S. Department of Health and Human Services' Centers for Disease Control and Prevention National Center for Chronic Disease Prevention and Health Promotion. The President's Council on Physical Fitness and Sports.

Chapter 35

Fitness for Children from Birth to Age Five

For young children, physical activity is natural. Little ones are delighted to have your company and your undivided attention. Playing actively with them will give pleasure to both of you. You do not need to be an expert on movement to promote a child's daily physical activity, and no special equipment is necessary to make meaningful activity part of children's lives.

Being active from an early age will help children become physically fit later in life. Health-related fitness involves cardiovascular endurance, muscular strength and endurance, flexibility, and body composition. The information here incorporates these elements into activities for children in three age groups: infants (birth to 18 months), toddlers (18 to 36 months), and preschoolers (3 to 5 years).

Small children need several hours of unstructured movement every day. They should never be inactive for more than 60 minutes. Toddlers need at least 30 minutes of structured activities, such as those presented here, and preschoolers need at least 60 minutes of structured activities. You can break all activity periods into smaller units of 10 or 15 minutes.

To help your child reach individual activity goals, choose several of the activities each day. Play at each one for 10 or 15 minutes. Ideally, you would have at least two or three activity sessions a day. When

Excerpted from the booklet "Kids in Action: Fitness for Children Birth to Age 5" by the President's Council on Physical Fitness and Sports (www.fitness .gov), 2003.

playing with your child, choose only activities for which he is developmentally ready. For example, don't play Creepy/Crawly until your baby is able to crawl and creep successfully. For activities that call for your infant to be seated before she can sit up unassisted, prop her up against a stable object such as the front of a sofa, or surround her with firm pillows. Most babies can sit assisted by 4 months of age and unassisted by age 9 months.

Remember that the most important thing you can do to promote an active lifestyle is to be a role model. So have fun, and let the suggestions here inspire your own creative movement ideas.

Remember, in addition to structured movements such as those described here, young children should also participate in at least 60 minutes a day of unstructured physical activity. The more the better! So be sure they have the time, space, and opportunity to crawl, walk, run, jump, climb and play actively.

Infants

Kick It!

Let your baby find out what her legs can do while she learns about cause and effect.

- Lay the baby on her back.
- Place a small pillow or a stuffed animal by the baby's feet.
- Encourage her to kick it!

Also:

- If the baby doesn't kick the object on her own, hold it just close enough to let her feel it with the bottom of her feet.
- Make sure she gets to kick with both right and left feet.
- Use language to encourage her and describe what she's doing. For example: "You're kicking the pillow!"

Crossing the Midline

Have playtime activities that help your baby's right arm or leg cross over to the left and the left arm or leg cross over to the right. This crossing over is an important step in helping your baby learn.

- Place the baby in a comfortably seated position.

- Sit or kneel in front of him and hide a favorite toy behind your back.
- Make a game of handing him the toy so he has to reach across his body to get it.

Let It Pour

This outdoor summer activity promotes both eye-hand coordination and coordination in general.

- Place a plastic sheet or old tablecloth on the porch, patio, or grass, and seat the baby on it, along with two large plastic cups—one empty and one filled with water or sand.
- Demonstrate pouring the water or sand from one cup to the other.
- Encourage the baby to try it.

Creepy/Crawly

Crawling and creeping not only help your baby get around but also use the right and left sides of the body at the same time. This helps later with reading and writing skills.

- Lay the baby on her tummy on a carpet or smooth, clean surface.
- Place a favorite toy in front of her, just out of her reach.
- Encourage her to go get it.

Toddlers

Heads, Bellies, Toes

This game helps with identifying body parts, flexibility, and understanding the concepts of up, down, low, and high.

- Stand facing your child.
- Beginning slowly, call out the names of the three body parts that are in the title, asking your child to touch each part as he hears its name.
- Once your child is successful at this, reverse—and mix up—the order of body parts.

Let's Tiptoe

Walking on tiptoe uses the child's own body weight to develop strength. It also helps with balance.

- Show your child how to tiptoe.
- Ask her to do it with you.
- Tiptoe as long as your toddler stays interested.

Row, Row, Row Your Boat

This game works on strength and flexibility, while also teaching about cause and effect.

- Sit facing your child with your legs apart and your child's legs straight out, between yours.
- Holding your child's hands, lean forward, and encourage him to lean back as far as he can.
- Pull him gently back up to a sitting position. Repeat.

Let's Gallop

Show your child how to gallop. If you do this activity for long periods of time, it helps build up your child's heart health.

- Show your child galloping (leading with one foot while the other plays catch up).
- Ask her to do it, too.
- Make a game of Follow the Leader out of it.

More Ideas for Toddlers

- **Follow the Leader:** Play this fun game using all of the traveling skills your child has learned (walking, running, tiptoeing, jumping, etc.). Stop once in a while to do a stationary (in place) skill, like stretching, bending, or twisting.

- **Tiny Steps/Giant Steps:** Move around the room with your toddler, sometimes taking tiny steps and sometimes giant steps. You can also ask her to try it on her own, giving her a signal (like two hand claps) that means it's time to switch from one kind of step to the other.

326

- **Pop Goes the Weasel:** Hum or sing this age-old favorite, asking your child to move around the room in any way he wants until the "pop," when he should jump into the air. Later, you can ask him to jump and change directions when he hears the pop.

- **Rabbits and 'Roos:** Invite your toddler to jump as though she were a rabbit. Then ask her to show you how a kangaroo would look jumping. Alternate between the two.

Preschoolers

Heel Raises

Lifting and lowering the heels is a strength-training exercise even the youngest children can do. It also helps with balance.

- Stand facing your child.
- Hold hands.
- Slowly lift and lower your heels, encouraging your child to do the same thing at the same time.

Beanbag Balance

When it comes to balancing activities, this is an all-time favorite for children.

- Place a beanbag or a small, soft toy on your child's head.
- Invite her to walk from one point in the room to another without dropping the beanbag.
- If she has to, she can hold on to it at first.

Jump the River

Jumping uses the child's own weight to build strength. If you do this for long periods of time, it can be good for the heart.

- Lay a jump rope in a straight line on the floor—or draw a line on the ground with chalk.
- Ask your child to pretend the line is a river.
- Challenge him to jump from one side of the river to the other.

Mirror Game

This cooperative game is great for social/emotional development. And it means children have to do with their bodies what their eyes are seeing. This will help later with writing, among other things.

- Talk to your child about looking in the mirror.

- Stand facing your child, explaining that you want her to do exactly as you do—just like she were your reflection in the mirror.

- Begin making slow movements that you can do in place, like raising and lowering an arm, nodding your head, or clapping hands. Take turns being leader.

More Ideas for Preschoolers

- **Bridges and Tunnels:** Forming different kinds of bridges and tunnels with the body or body parts can help with both flexibility and muscle strength.

- **The Track Meet:** Invite your child to pretend she's in a track meet at the Olympics. Can she pretend to jump hurdles, in addition to running the track?

- **Simon Says:** Play this excellent body-parts identification game without any elimination! To include fitness factors, have "Simon" issue challenges to jog or tiptoe in place, bend and stretch, or bend and straighten knees.

- **Statues:** To get your child moving, put on a piece of up-tempo music and invite him to move while the music is playing and to freeze into a statue when you pause it.

Chapter 36

Physical Activity at School

Chapter Contents

Section 36.1

The Need for Physical Education and Physical Activity in Our Schools

This information is adapted from Action for Healthy Kids' Fact Sheet, "Building the Argument: The Need for Physical Education and Physical Activity in Our Schools." Please visit www.actionforhealthykids.org for more information and resources to improve the health environment of schools nationwide.

Study after study proves what educators have long believed to be true: when children's exercise and fitness needs are met, they have the cognitive energy to learn and achieve. Given the growing epidemic of obesity and the link between physical activity and academic performance, we must work together to make quality daily physical education a priority in our schools and to give our children more opportunities to be physically active throughout the school day.

Our children are getting fatter and are developing "adult" diseases.

- Poor diet and inadequate physical activity are the second leading cause of death in the United States and together account for at least 300,000 deaths annually. Obesity and overweight have "reached epidemic proportions in the United States."[1]

- The epidemic has hit our children particularly hard: "today there are nearly twice as many overweight children and almost three times as many overweight adolescents as there were in 1980."[1] In 2000, 15% of children aged 6 to 11 were overweight and nearly 16% of adolescents were overweight.[2]

- The Centers for Disease Control and Prevention (CDC) warns that one in three U.S. children born in 2000 will become diabetic unless many more people start eating less and exercising more.[3] Type 2 diabetes in adolescents increased ten-fold between 1982 and 1994.[4]

- Prevention, says former U.S. Secretary of Health and Human Services Tommy Thompson, is the key to fighting cardiovascular disease, cancer, type 2 diabetes, and other chronic diseases—and helping students increase physical activity is one way to put prevention into action.[5,6]

Our children are becoming increasingly less physically active.

- Fewer than 1 in 4 children get 20 minutes of vigorous physical activity per day, and less than 1 in 4 get at least 30 minutes of physical activity per day.[7]

- Participation in all types of physical activity declines as age or grade in school increases. By the time they reach their teens, nearly half of America's youth are not vigorously active on a regular basis, and over one third aged 12 to 17 are physically active less than 3 out of 7 days a week.[8]

Many of our children are sedentary at school.

- The vast majority of children (85%) travel to school by car or bus—only 13% of children walk or bike to school.[9]

- Since 1989, many school systems have abolished recess, with only "4.1% of states requir[ing] and 22.4% of states recommend[ing] that elementary schools provide students with regularly scheduled recess."[10]

- In grade 9, 72% of students get regular physical activity, but by the time they reach grade 12, only 55% of them are physically active.[8] Nearly 10% of students in grades 9 to 12 participate in no vigorous or moderate physical activity on a weekly basis.[10]

Emphasis on physical education in the public school system has markedly declined.

- Between 1991 and 1999, the percentage of students who took physical education on a daily basis dropped from 42% to 29%.[11]

- Although most states have some mandate for physical education (78.4% at the elementary school level, 85.7% at the middle school level, and 82.4% at the senior high school level[10]), most states require only that physical education be provided. Local districts have control over content and format.[12]

- No federal law requires physical education to be included in public schools, and Illinois is the only state to enforce daily physical education requirements in grades K-12.[12]

- While a majority of secondary school principal leaders agree that students' level of physical activity is important, for most the issue is a low priority compared to other concerns such as student achievement, teacher quality, school safety, alcohol and drug prevention, and school budgets.[27]

When children are active, their academic performance improves.

- "Nearly 200 studies on the effect of exercise on cognitive functioning suggest that physical activity supports learning."[13]

- Two studies demonstrated that providing more time for physical activity (by reducing class time) can lead to increased test scores, particularly in the area of mathematics,[14,15] and another study linked physical activity programs to stronger academic achievement, increased concentration, and improved math, reading, and writing test scores.[16]

- The California correlation of the SAT-9 with the *Fitnessgram*, says California State Superintendent of Public Instruction Delaine Eastin, "provides compelling evidence that the physical well-being of students has a direct impact on their ability to achieve academically. We now have the proof we've been looking for: students achieve best when they are physically fit. Thousands of years ago, the Greeks understood the importance of improving spirit, mind, and body. The research presented here validates their philosophic approach with scientific validation."[17]

- Children with daily physical education exhibit better attendance, a more positive attitude to school, and superior academic performance.[18]

- From the Comprehensive School Health Program in McComb, Mississippi, to the SPARK Program founded at San Diego State University, school administrators and education researchers are demonstrating again and again that physical education and physical activity may strengthen academic achievement, self-esteem, and mental health—all leading to stronger student performance.[19,20,21,22]

- "Evidence suggests," says the President's Council on Physical Fitness and Sports, "that time spent in physical education does not decrease learning in other subjects. Youth who spend less time in other subjects to allow for regular physical education have been shown to do equally well or better in academic classes."[23]

Our students and their parents join the U.S. Surgeon General, National Association for Sport and Physical Education (NASPE), and the CDC in calling for more opportunities for physical activity and physical education.

- A majority of student leaders (72%) feel schools should make physical activity for all students a priority, with 81% calling for more students to get involved in physical activity and 56% stressing the importance of having more physical education classes.[24]

- The vast majority of parents (95%) think "physical education should be part of a school curriculum for all students in grades K-12."[25]

- David Satcher, the former U.S. Surgeon General and chair of the Action for Healthy Kids Initiative, calls for all students to receive quality physical education on a daily basis.[26]

- The NASPE calls for all students to receive quality physical education as an integral part of K-12 education. All states, says NASPE, should set minimum standards of achievement in physical education and should develop standards for physical education based on the National Standards for Physical Education.[12]

- The Centers for Disease Control (CDC) calls for sequential physical education that helps students develop the skills and knowledge to enjoy and maintain a lifelong physically active lifestyle.[8]

References

1. U.S. Department of Health and Human Services. *The Surgeon General's Call to Action to Prevent and Decrease Overweight and Obesity.* 2001.

2. *JAMA.* 2002;288:1723–1727.

3. Associated Press. Diabetes in children set to soar. MSNBC. June 16, 2003.

4. Pinhas-Harniel, O., et al. Increased incidence of non-insulin-dependent diabetes mellitus among adolescents. *Journal of Pediatrics* 1996; 128: 608–615.

5. Department of Health and Human Services. *Steps to a Healthier US: The Power of Prevention.* 2003.

6. Department of Health and Human Services. *Steps to a Healthier US: Prevention Strategies That Work.* 2003.

7. International Life Sciences Institute. *Improving Children's Health through Physical Activity: A New Opportunity, A Survey of Parents and Children about Physical Activity Patterns.* 1997.

8. Centers for Disease Control and Prevention. *Guidelines for School and Community Programs: Promoting Lifelong Physical Activity.* 1997.

9. Centers for Disease Control and Prevention. Fact sheet. Kids Walk-to-School Program. 2002.

10. Action for Healthy Kids. *National Profile.* 2002.

11. Centers for Disease Control and Prevention. Physical activity and good nutrition: essential elements to prevent chronic diseases and obesity. *At a Glance.* 2003.

12. National Association for Sport and Physical Education (NASPE). *Shape of the Nation Report.* 2001.

13. Etnier, J. L., Salazar, W., Landers, D. M., Petruzzello, S. J., Han, M., & Nowell, P. The influence of physical fitness and exercise upon cognitive functioning: a meta-analysis. *Journal of Sport and Exercise Psychology* (1997); 19(3): 249–277.

14. Shephard, R.J., Volle, M., Lavalee, M., LaBarre, R., Jequier, J.C., Rajic, M. Required physical activity and academic grades: a controlled longitudinal study. In: Limarinen and Valimaki, editors. *Children and Sport.* Berlin: Springer Verlag, 1984. 58–63.

15. Shephard, R.J. Curricular physical activity and academic performance. *Pediatric Exercise Science* 1997; 9: 113–126.

16. Symons, C.W., Cinelli, B., James, T.C., Groff, P. Bridging student health risks and academic achievement through comprehensive school health programs. *Journal of School Health* 1997; 67(6): 220–227.

17. National Association for Sport and Physical Education (NASPE). New study supports physically fit kids perform better academically. 2002.

18. National Association for Sport and Physical Education/Council of Physical Education for Children. Physical education is critical to a complete education. 2001.

19. Cooper, Pat. Our journey to good health. *School Administrator.* January 2003.

20. Sallis, J.F., McKenzie, T.L., Kolody, B., Lewis, M., Marshall, S., and Rosengard, P. Effects of health-related physical education on academic achievement: Project SPARK. *Research Quarterly for Exercise and Sport* 1999; 70:127–134.

21. Keays, J., and Allison, R. The effects of regular moderate to vigorous physical activity on student outcomes: A review. *Canadian Journal of Public Health* 1995; 86: 62–66.

22. Shephard, R.J. Habitual physical activity and academic performance. *Nutrition Reviews* 1996; 54(4 supplement): S32–S36.

23. President's Council on Physical Fitness and Sports. Physical activity promotion and school physical education. *Physical Activity and Fitness Research Digest.* 1999.

24. Action for Healthy Kids. Student Poll. 2002.

25. National Association for Sport and Physical Education (NASPE). Parents' views of children's health and fitness. 2003.

26. Satcher, D. Pound-foolish. *Education Week.* 2002.

27. AFHK/NASSP School Principal Leadership Poll, conducted with state leaders of National Association of Secondary School Principals, 2002.

Section 36.2

More Physical Activity Can Boost Achievement and Schools' Bottom Line

This information adapted from Action for Healthy Kids' Fact Sheet, "Better Nutrition and More Physical Activity Can Boost Achievement and Schools' Bottom Line." Please visit www.actionforhealthykids.org for more information and resources to improve the health environment of schools nationwide.

The excessive rise in poor nutrition, inactivity, and weight problems adversely affect academic achievement and possibly cost schools millions of dollars each year.

It is critical that as schools search for solutions to meet performance outcomes and minimize budget cuts, schools do not further aggravate problems of poor nutrition and inactive lifestyles—in turn it may undermine schools' overall goal to provide high-quality education for all students.

Here are the costs to schools due to problems associated with poor nutrition and physical activity—the root causes of obesity.

Costs in Achievement

- Schools with high percentages of students who did not routinely engage in physical activity or eat well had smaller gains in test scores than other schools.

- Well-nourished students who skip breakfast perform worse on tests and have poor concentration.

- Children not getting adequate nutrients have lower test scores; even transient hunger from missing a meal affects performance.

- Physical activity programs are linked to stronger academic achievement.

- Students participating in daily physical education exhibit better attendance and achievement.

Costs in Dollars

- In states that use attendance to help determine state funding, a single-day absence by just one student can cost a school district anywhere from $9 to $20.

- If children miss just one day per month, this could cost a large school district like New York about $28 million each year, while Chicago would forfeit about $9 million each year in state funds.

- This type of absentee rate is highly probable, and could cost an average size school district from $95,000 to $160,000 annually in important state aid.

The Hidden Costs

- Extra staff time needed for students with low academic performance or behavior problems caused by poor nutrition and physical inactivity.

- Costs associated with time and staff needed to administer medications needed by students with associated health problems.

- Health care costs, absenteeism, and lower productivity due to the effects of poor nutrition, inactivity, and overweight among school employees.

What Can Schools Do?

- Form a school health advisory council and involve students, parents, teachers, health professionals, and other community leaders.

- Develop a comprehensive wellness policy that includes recommendations for increasing physical activity and improving the nutrition environment.

- Offer more after-school programs that provide nutritious snacks, physical activity and nutrition education.

- Encourage staff to model healthy lifestyles.

- Integrate physical activity and nutrition education into the regular school day.

Chapter 37

Fitness for Kids Who Do Not Like Sports

Team sports can help a child gain self-esteem, coordination, and general fitness, and help them learn how to work with other kids and adults. But some kids aren't natural athletes and they may tell you—directly or indirectly—that they just don't like sports. What then?

Why Some Kids Don't Like Teams

Every child doesn't have to join a team, and with enough other activities, kids can be fit without them. But it's a good idea to find out why your child isn't interested. You might be able to help solve any deeper concerns your child might be having, or steer your child toward something else. Talk with your child and let him or her know that you'd like to work on a solution together. That solution might mean making changes and sticking with the team sport or finding a new activity to try.

Here are some reasons why sports might be a turnoff for a child.

Still Developing Basic Skills

Though many sports programs are available for preschoolers, it's not until about age 6 or 7 that most kids have the physical skills, the attention span, and the ability to grasp the rules needed to play organized

This information was provided by KidsHealth, one of the largest resources online for medically reviewed health information written for parents, kids, and teens. For more articles like this one, visit www.KidsHealth.org, or www.Teens Health.org. © 2005 The Nemours Foundation. Reviewed by Barbara P. Homeier, M.D., and Mary L. Gavin, M.D., in August 2005.

sports. If your child hasn't had much practice in a specific sport, it may take a while for him or her to be expected to reliably perform necessary skills such as kicking a soccer ball on the run or hitting a baseball thrown from the pitcher's mound. Trying and failing, especially in a game situation, might frustrate your child and make him or her nervous.

What You Can Do. Practice with your child at home. Whether you're shooting baskets, playing catch, or going for a jog together, you're giving your child an opportunity to build his or her skills and fitness in a safe environment. Your child can freely try—and risk failing—new things without the self-consciousness of being around his or her peers. And you're also getting a good dose of quality together time.

Coach or League Is Too Competitive

A kid who's already a reluctant athlete might feel extra nervous when the coach barks out orders or the league focuses heavily on winning.

What You Can Do. Investigate sports programs before signing your child up for one. Talk with coaches and other parents about the philosophy. Some athletic associations, like the YMCA, have noncompetitive leagues. In some programs, they don't even keep score.

Keep in mind that as kids get older, they can handle more competitive aspects such as keeping score and keeping track of wins and losses for the season. Some kids may be motivated by competitive play, but the average child may not be ready for the increased pressure until he or she is 11 or 12 years old. Remember that even in more competitive leagues, the atmosphere should remain positive and supportive for all the participants.

Stage Fright

If your child isn't a natural athlete, or is a little shy, he or she might be uncomfortable with the pressure of being on a team. More self-conscious kids also might worry about letting their parents, coaches, or teammates down. This is especially true if the child is still working on basic skills and if the league is very competitive.

What You Can Do. Keep your expectations realistic—most kids don't become Olympic medalists or get sports scholarships. Let your child know the goal is to be fit and have fun. If the coach or league doesn't agree, it's probably time to look for something new.

Still Shopping for a Sport

Some kids haven't found the right sport. Maybe your child didn't have the hand-eye coordination for baseball, but he or she has the drive and the build to be a swimmer, a runner, or a cyclist. The idea of an individual sport also can be more appealing to some kids who like to go it alone.

What You Can Do. Be open to your child's interests in other sports or activities. That can be tough if, for instance, you just loved basketball and wanted to continue the legacy. But by exploring other options, you give your child a chance to get invested in something he or she truly enjoys.

Other Barriers

Different kids mature at different rates, so it's common for there to be a wide range of heights, weights, and athletic abilities among kids of the same age group. So if your child is much bigger or smaller than other kids of the same age—or less coordinated or not as strong— he or she may feel self-conscious and uncomfortable competing with them. Your child also may be afraid of getting injured or worried that he or she can't keep up. A child who is overweight might be reluctant to participate in a sport, for example, while a child who has asthma might feel more comfortable with sports that require short outputs of energy, like baseball, football, gymnastics, downhill skiing, and shorter track and field events.

What You Can Do. Give some honest thought to your child's strengths, abilities, and temperament, and find an activity that might be a good match. Some kids are afraid of the ball, so they don't like softball or volleyball, but may enjoy an activity like running. If your child is overweight, he or she might lack the endurance to run, but might enjoy a sport like swimming. Your child may be too short for the basketball team, but may enjoy gymnastics or wrestling.

Keep in mind that some kids just prefer sports that focus on individual performance rather than teamwork. Remember that the goal is to prevent your child from feeling frustrated, wanting to quit, and being turned off from sports and physical activity altogether.

With good communication, you may be able to address your child's concerns. Other issues may naturally fade as your child grows. If you can understand what your child is going through and provide a supportive environment, you can help your child succeed in whatever activity he or she chooses.

341

Ways to Stay Fit Outside of Team Sports

Even kids who once said they hated sports might learn to like team sports as their skills improve, or if they find the right sport or a league with the right level of intensity. But even if team sports never thrill your child, there's plenty a kid can do to get the recommended 60 minutes or more of physical activity each day.

Free play can be very important for a child who doesn't play a team sport. What's free play? It's the activity kids get when they're left to their own devices, like shooting hoops, riding bikes, playing whiffleball, playing tag, jumping rope, or dancing.

Outside of the most common team sports, your child might want to try individual sports or other organized activities that can boost his or her fitness. Here are some ideas:

- swimming
- horseback riding
- dance classes
- in-line skating
- cycling
- cheerleading
- skateboarding
- hiking

- golf
- tennis
- fencing
- gymnastics
- martial arts
- yoga and other fitness classes
- ultimate Frisbee
- running

Note: Before beginning any sport or fitness program, it's a good idea for your child to have a physical examination from the doctor. Kids with undiagnosed medical conditions, vision or hearing problems, or other disorders may have difficulty participating in certain activities.

Supporting Your Kid's Choices

Even if the going's tough, work with your child to find something active that he or she likes. Try to remain open-minded. Maybe your child is interested in an activity that is not offered at his or her school. If your daughter wants to try flag football or ice hockey, for example, help her find a local league or talk to school officials about starting up a new team.

You'll need to be patient if your child has difficulty choosing and sticking to an activity. It often takes several tries before a child finds one that feels like the right fit. But when something clicks, you'll be glad you invested the time and effort. For your child, it's one big step toward developing active habits that can last a lifetime.

Chapter 38

Preparticipation Physical Exams for Young Athletes

What are the goals and objectives of the preparticipation evaluation (PPE)?

The overall goal of the PPE is to help maintain the health and safety of athletes. Its purpose is not to exclude athletes from participation but to promote safe participation. If not cleared, most athletes can be redirected to another sport. This goal is achieved by adhering to the evaluation's three primary objectives. The three secondary objectives take advantage of the doctor-athlete contact.

Primary objectives

* Detect conditions that might predispose the athlete to injury
* Detect conditions that might be life-threatening or disabling
* Meet legal and insurance requirements

Secondary objectives

* Determine general health
* Counsel on health-related issues
* Assess fitness level for specific sports

"Preparticipation Evaluations," © 2003 The Cleveland Clinic Foundation, 9500 Euclid Avenue, Cleveland, OH 44195, www.clevelandclinic.org. Additional information is available from the Cleveland Clinic Health Information Center, 216-444-3771, toll-free 800-223-2273 extension 43771, or at http://www.clevelandclinic.org/health.

What are the appropriate time, setting, and structure of the PPE?

Ideally, the PPE should be performed at least six weeks prior to preseason practice, allowing time for correction or rehabilitation of any identified problems. To avoid potential scheduling difficulties, the PPE might be performed at the end of the previous school year.

Opinions vary regarding how often the young athlete should be evaluated. In some high schools, a full annual evaluation is the norm. Another option, followed primarily at the college level, is a complete evaluation at an entry or new level, followed by an interim annual evaluation.

The two most common settings for performing the PPE are the doctor's office or in a station-based screening environment.

What are the advantages of mass PPEs?

These evaluations are less expensive. Multiple specialists can be involved, such as athletic trainers, physical therapists, orthopaedic surgeons, family doctors, and pediatricians who have a special interest in sports medicine.

What are the advantages of office-based PPEs?

An office-based exam is usually performed by the athlete's primary care doctor. The doctor is familiar with the athlete's medical and family history. The setting is much quieter and allows for the discussion of multiple health issues that are pertinent to adolescents. These include the use of drugs, supplements, and alcohol; sexual activity; and other topics. Immunization history can be reviewed and updated accordingly.

What are the components of the PPE?

The medical history is the cornerstone of any medical evaluation. A complete history will identify about 75 percent of problems affecting athletes. To increase the information obtained, the athlete and parent should complete the history together before the examination. The recommended baseline history includes the following general information:

- Medical conditions and diseases
- Surgeries
- Hospitalizations
- Medicines (prescription, over-the-counter, supplements)

- Allergies (medicines, insects, environmental)
- Immunization status
- Menstrual history
- Psycho- and sociosexual development

Other information about the following should also be included:

- Cardiovascular health
- Pulmonary health
- Neurologic health
- Musculoskeletal health
- Injuries or illness since last exam

The PPE is a screening tool that emphasizes the areas of greatest concern in sports participation and areas identified as problems in the history. The recommended standard components of the PPE include the following:

- Height
- Weight
- Pulse
- Blood pressure
- Eye exam
- Ear/nose/throat exam
- Heart exam
- Abdominal exam
- Genitalia exam
- Skin exam
- Musculoskeletal system exam

What is involved in determining clearance for participation in sports?

The most important and difficult decision in the PPE is determining whether an athlete should be cleared for sports participation. Clearance can be divided into three categories:

- Unrestricted clearance
- Clearance after completion of further evaluation or rehabilitation

- No clearance for certain types of sports or for all sports

When an abnormality or condition is found that might limit an athlete's participation or predispose him or her to further injury, the doctor must consider the following questions:

- Does the problem place the athlete at increased risk for injury?
- Is another participant at risk for injury because of the problem?
- Can the athlete safely participate with treatment?
- Can limited participation be allowed while treatment is being completed?
- If clearance is denied only for certain sports or sports categories, in what activities can the athlete safely participate?

To aid in this decision, sports are classified based on degree or level of contact and strenuousness:

- Contact/collision
- Limited contact
- Strenuous, non-contact
- Moderately strenuous, non-contact
- Non-strenuous, non-contact

What is athletic heart syndrome?

The heart of an athlete undergoes certain functional and morphological changes (physical size and shape) that distinguish it from the heart of non-exercising individuals. These changes represent a normal physiologic response to exercise and not a disease process. The type and degree of change is affected by the type of training—endurance (aerobic) versus strength (isometric). Endurance athletes have an increased left ventricular volume and cardiac output. Strength athletes have an increase in thickness of the heart muscle wall. Endurance athletes have a lower heart rate.

What is the cause of sudden cardiac death syndrome (SCDS)?

Sudden death in the athlete under the age of 35 is most commonly due to congenital heart disease. Usually the athlete is male, has been involved in a variety of sports, and is at the junior high or high school level. Unfortunately, there are usually no preceding symptoms.

How can the athlete at risk for SCDS be identified?

The PPE history is designed to identify athletes at risk, such as those with chest pain or heaviness, palpitations, shortness of breath, fainting spells (syncope), or family history of sudden death. Any athlete with these symptoms requires full evaluation. The PPE physical examination might reveal a murmur. The evaluation might include further testing [electrocardiogram (EKG), chest X-ray, stress test, echocardiography] or consultation with a cardiologist.

Chapter 39

Exercise and Adolescents

Chapter Contents

Section 39.1

Is Exercise Safe for Teens?

This information was provided by TeensHealth, one of the largest resources online for medically reviewed health information written for parents, kids, and teens. For more articles like this one, visit www.Teens Health.org, or www.KidsHealth.org. © 2005 The Nemours Foundation. This article was reviewed by Mary L. Gavin, M.D., February 2005.

If you're an active person, you probably get a lot of exercise, whether you work out at a gym, play football at school, or simply bike to school. Do you ever worry that too much exercise may hurt instead of help your health? Relax—sticking to a routine of regular exercise is one of the best things you can do for your body. In fact, experts recommend that teens get at least 60 minutes of moderate to vigorous activity every day.

Why? Because exercise serves several purposes: It makes your heart and lungs strong, it increases your strength and endurance, and it helps you maintain a healthy weight. In fact, you can actually change your physique through exercise by building or defining certain muscle groups over time. Exercise benefits your body not just in your teen years, but helps you stay healthy throughout adulthood, too.

Although some teens worry that exercise could stunt their growth, when you exercise safely and eat properly, there's no danger that your height or growth pattern will stall out. Exercise can help you alter your body composition, increasing your ratio of muscle to fat. And most people who exercise say that they feel more alert and better in general.

Exercise, though, like most things in life, is best done in moderation. If you overdo it, it is possible to injure yourself. Pain during or after a workout is a clear sign that you are exercising improperly or too often.

Working out too often or for too long can cause added problems for girls, who may experience amenorrhea, which means their periods stop. And some teens who start out with the intention of becoming healthy may begin to feel guilty or anxious if they don't exercise—an unhealthy problem called compulsive exercise. If you have pain after working out, if you stop getting your period, or you feel like you must exercise every day even if you're tired or injured, discuss these things with your doctor.

Your doctor can be a good resource before you start an exercise plan, too. If you are just beginning an exercise program, your doctor can help you decide on the best type of exercise for your individual health needs.

Then consult with someone who understands the mechanics of exercise, like a coach or a fitness expert at a gym, to help you get started. He or she will help you select a program that combines aerobic activity, which focuses on the heart and lungs, with weight training, which concentrates on strengthening and conditioning your muscles. You may also want to learn some stretching exercises to help you increase your flexibility, another important part of fitness.

Once you start, be sure to eat nutritiously by chowing down on a variety of vegetables, fruits, whole grains, low-fat and nonfat dairy products, and lean protein sources. You should also drink plenty of water before, during, and after workouts to make up for fluids lost during exercise. And you'll need plenty of sleep, so your body has time to rest and recover between workouts. You can also take care of your body and improve your performance by avoiding smoking, alcohol, and drugs. Drugs include dietary supplements and anabolic steroids, powerful chemicals that can cause behavior problems, liver problems, and increase your risk for heart attack and stroke.

With a commitment to regular exercise now, you'll be setting the stage for a lifetime of good health.

Section 39.2

Strength Training and Your Child or Teen

This information was provided by KidsHealth, one of the largest resources online for medically reviewed health information written for parents, kids, and teens. For more articles like this one, visit www.KidsHealth.org, or www.TeensHealth.org. © 2005 The Nemours Foundation. This article was updated and reviewed by Barbara P. Homeier, M.D., in May 2005.

Strength training can be a fun way for your child to build healthy muscles, joints, and bones. With a properly designed and supervised program, your child can improve his or her endurance, total fitness level, and sports performance. Strength training can even help prevent injuries and speed up recovery.

What Is Strength Training?

Strength training is the practice of using free weights, weight machines, and rubber resistance bands to build muscles. With resistance the muscles have to work extra hard to move. When the muscles work extra hard, they grow stronger and more efficient.

Strength training can also help fortify the ligaments and tendons that support the muscles and bones and improve bone density, which is the amount of calcium and minerals in the bone. And the benefits may go beyond physical health. Young athletes may feel better about themselves as they get stronger.

The goal of strength training is not to bulk up. It should not be confused with weight lifting, bodybuilding, and powerlifting, which are not recommended for kids and teens. In these sports, people train with very heavy weights and participate in modeling and lifting competitions. Kids and teens who do those sports can risk injuring their growing bones, muscles, and joints.

Age Guidelines on Strength Training

Generally, if your child is ready to participate in organized sports or activities such as baseball, soccer, or gymnastics, it is usually safe to start strength training.

A child's strength-training program shouldn't just be a scaled-down version of an adult's weight training regimen. A trainer who has experience in working with kids should design a program for your child and show your child the proper techniques, safety precautions, and how to properly use the equipment.

Kids as young 6 years old can usually do strength-training activities (such as push-ups and sit-ups) as long as they can perform the exercises safely and follow instructions. These exercises can help kids build a sense of balance, control, and awareness of their bodies.

Typically, it's a good idea for younger kids to stay away from heavier weights. Instead, they should lift small amounts of weight with a high number of repetitions. In general as kids get older and stronger, they can gradually increase the amount of resistance they use. A trained professional can help your child determine what the appropriate weight may be.

Strength-Training Safety

As with any sport, it's a good idea to have your child visit a doctor before beginning a strength-training regimen. If the doctor signs off on the idea, you'll need to make sure that your child will be properly supervised, using safe equipment, and following an age-appropriate routine.

Muscle strains are the most common form of injury, and the lower back is the most commonly injured area. But these injuries usually happen because the child has not used the proper lifting technique or is trying to lift too much weight.

As long as your child is using the proper techniques and lifting an appropriate amount of weight, strength training shouldn't have any effect on your child's growth plates, the layer of cartilage near the end of the bone where most of the bone growth occurs.

Strength training should not involve the use of anabolic steroids. Some young and professional athletes have abused these drugs to build muscles and improve athletic performance and appearance. But these drugs, some of which are illegal, can pose severe risks to physical and psychological health.

A Healthy Routine

In general, kids and teens should tone their muscles using a low amount of weight and a high number of repetitions, instead of trying to lift a heavy load one or two times. The amount of weight will depend on your child's current size and strength level. But in general, your child should be able to lift a weight with proper technique at least 10 to 12 times. If he or she can't lift the weight at least 10 times, it's likely that the weight is too heavy for your child.

Kids shouldn't even consider concentrating on adding muscle bulk until after they have passed through puberty. Even then, it's important to focus on technique so that they can strengthen their muscles safely.

The focus of each training session should be on proper form and technique, and if free weights are used, there should be an adult around to spot your child. The National Strength and Conditioning Association has created the following guidelines for strength-training programs:

- An instructor-to-child ratio of at least 1 to 10 is recommended.

- The instructor should have experience with children and strength training.

- When teaching a new exercise, the trainer should have the child perform the exercise under his or her supervision in a hazard-free, well-lit, and adequately ventilated environment.

- Calisthenics and stretching exercises should be performed before and after strength training.

- Children should begin with one set of 10 to 15 repetitions of six to eight exercises that focus on the major muscle groups of the upper and lower body.

- Children should start with a relatively light weight and a high number of repetitions and increase the load and decrease the repetitions as strength improves. Progression can also be achieved by increasing the number of sets (up to three) or types of exercises.

- Two to three training sessions per week on nonconsecutive days is sufficient.

It's important to remember that strength training should be one part of a total fitness program. It can play a vital role in keeping your child healthy and fit, along with aerobic exercise such as biking and running, which keeps the heart and lungs in shape.

Chapter 40

Staying Active during and after Pregnancy

Chapter Contents

Section 40.1

Guidelines for Safe Exercising during Pregnancy

"Exercising During Pregnancy" was provided by KidsHealth, one of the largest resources online for medically reviewed health information written for parents, kids, and teens. For more articles like this one, visit www.Kids Health.org, or www.TeensHealth.org. © 2004 The Nemours Foundation. This article was updated and reviewed by George A. Macones, M.D., June 2004.

Although you may not feel like running a marathon, most women benefit greatly from exercising throughout their pregnancies. But during that time, you'll need to discuss your exercise plans with your doctor or other health care provider early on and make a few adjustments to your normal exercise routine. The level of exercise recommended will depend, in part, on your level of prepregnancy fitness.

What are the benefits of exercising during pregnancy?

No doubt about it, exercise is a big plus for both you and your baby (if complications don't limit your ability to exercise throughout your pregnancy). It can help you:

- **feel better.** At a time when you wonder if this strange body can possibly be yours, exercise can increase your sense of control and boost your energy level. Not only does it make you feel better by releasing endorphins (naturally occurring chemicals in your brain), appropriate exercise can: relieve backaches and improve your posture by strengthening and toning muscles in your back, butt, and thighs; reduce constipation by accelerating movement in your intestine; prevent wear and tear on your joints (which become loosened during pregnancy due to normal hormonal changes) by activating the lubricating synovial fluid in your joints; and help you sleep better by relieving the stress and anxiety that might make you restless at night.

- **look better.** Exercise increases the blood flow to your skin, giving you a healthy glow.

- **prepare you and your body for birth.** Strong muscles and a fit heart can greatly ease labor and delivery. Gaining control over your breathing can help you manage pain. And in the event of a lengthy labor, increased endurance can be a real help.

- **regain your prepregnancy body more quickly.** You'll gain less fat weight during your pregnancy if you continue to exercise (assuming you exercised before becoming pregnant). But don't expect or try to lose weight by exercising while you're pregnant. For most women, the goal is to maintain their fitness level throughout pregnancy.

What's a safe exercise plan when you're pregnant?

It depends on when you start and whether your pregnancy is complicated. If you exercised regularly before becoming pregnant, continue your program, with modifications as you need them. If you weren't fit before you became pregnant, don't give up! Begin slowly and build gradually as you become stronger. Whatever your fitness level, you should talk to your doctor about exercising while you're pregnant.

Discuss any concerns you have with your doctor. You may need to limit your exercise if you have:

- pregnancy-induced high blood pressure;
- early contractions;
- vaginal bleeding; or
- premature rupture of your membranes, also known as your water (the fluid in the amniotic sac around the fetus) breaking early.

What kinds of exercises can you do?

That depends on what interests you and what your doctor advises. Many women enjoy dancing, swimming, water aerobics, yoga, Pilates, biking, or walking. Swimming is especially appealing, as it gives you welcome buoyancy (floatability or the feeling of weightlessness). Try for a combination of cardio (aerobic), strength, and flexibility exercises, and avoid bouncing.

Many experts recommend walking. It's easy to vary the pace, add hills, and add distance. If you're just starting, begin with a moderately brisk pace for a mile, 3 days a week. Add a couple of minutes every week, pick up the pace a bit, and eventually add hills to your route. Whether you're a pro or a novice, go slowly for the first 5 minutes to warm up and use the last 5 minutes to cool down.

Whatever type of exercise you and your doctor decide on, the key is to listen to your body's warnings. Many women, for example, become dizzy early in their pregnancy, and as the baby grows, their center of gravity changes. So it may be easy for you to lose your balance, especially in the last trimester.

Your energy level may also vary greatly from day to day. And as your baby grows and pushes up on your lungs, you'll notice a decreased ability to breathe in more air (and the oxygen it contains) when you exercise. If your body says, "Stop!"—stop!

Your body is signaling that it's had enough if you feel:

- fatigue;
- dizziness;
- heart palpitations (your heart pounding in your chest);
- shortness of breath; or
- pain in your back or pelvis.

And if you can't talk while you're exercising, you're doing it too strenuously. You should also keep your heart rate below 160 beats per minute.

It also isn't good for your baby if you become overheated because temperatures greater than 102.6 degrees Fahrenheit (39 degrees Celsius) could cause problems with the developing fetus—especially in the first trimester—which can potentially lead to birth defects. So don't overdo exercise on hot days.

When the weather is hot, try to avoid exercising outside during the hottest part of the day (from about 10 AM to 3 PM) or exercise in an air-conditioned place. Also remember that swimming makes it more difficult for you to notice your body heating up because the water makes you feel cooler.

What exercises should you avoid?

Most doctors recommend that pregnant women avoid weight training and sit-ups after the first trimester, especially women who are at risk for preterm labor.

Lifting reduces the blood flow to the kidneys and uterus, and exercises done on your back (including sit-ups and leg lifts) cause your heart rate to drop, also decreasing the flow of oxygenated blood to your body and the baby. It's better to tone your abdominal muscles while on all fours, by relaxing and then tightening your muscles as you exhale.

Unless your doctor tells you otherwise, it's also a good idea to avoid any activities that include:

- bouncing;
- jarring (anything that would cause a lot of up and down movement);
- leaping;
- a sudden change of direction; or
- a risk of abdominal injury.

Typical limitations include contact sports, downhill skiing, scuba diving, and horseback riding because of the risk of injury they pose.

Although some doctors say step aerobics are acceptable if you can lower the height of your step as your pregnancy progresses, others caution that a changing center of gravity makes falls much more likely. If you do choose to do aerobics, just make sure to avoid becoming extremely winded or exercising to the point of exhaustion.

And check with your doctor if you experience any of these warning signs during any type of exercise:

- vaginal bleeding
- unusual pain
- dizziness or lightheadedness
- unusual shortness of breath
- racing heartbeat or chest pain
- fluid leaking from your vagina
- uterine contractions

What are Kegel exercises?

Although the effects of Kegel exercises can't be seen from the outside, some women use them to reduce incontinence (the leakage of urine) caused by the weight of the baby on their bladder. Kegels help to strengthen the "pelvic floor muscles" (the muscles that aid in controlling urination).

Kegels are easy, and you can do them any time you have a few seconds—sitting in your car, at your desk, or standing in line at the store. No one will even know you're doing them!

To find the correct muscles, pretend you're trying to stop urinating. Squeeze those muscles for a few seconds, then relax. You're using the

359

correct muscles if you feel a pull. Or place a finger inside your vagina and feel it tighten when you squeeze. Your doctor can also help you identify the correct muscles.

A few things to keep in mind when you're doing Kegel exercises:

- Don't tighten other muscles (stomach or legs, for example) at the same time. You want to focus on the muscles you're exercising.

- Don't hold your breath while you do them because it's important that your body and muscles continue to receive oxygen while you do any type of exercise.

- Don't regularly do Kegels by stopping and starting your flow of urine while you're actually going to the bathroom, as this can lead to incomplete emptying of your bladder, which increases the risk of urinary tract infections.

Getting Started

Always talk to your doctor before beginning any exercise program. Once you're ready to get going:

- Start gradually. Even 5 minutes a day is a good start if you've been inactive. Add 5 minutes each week until you reach 30 minutes.

- Dress comfortably in loose-fitting clothes and wear a supportive bra to protect your breasts.

- Drink plenty of water to avoid overheating and dehydration.

- Skip your exercises if you're sick.

- Opt for a walk in an air-conditioned mall on hot, humid days.

- Above all, listen to your body.

Section 40.2

Postpartum Exercise Tips

This information is excerpted from the booklet "Fit for Two: Tips for Pregnancy," by the Weight-control Information Network, part of the National Institute of Diabetes & Digestive & Kidney Diseases (NIDDK), September 2002.

Being physically active may help you have a more comfortable 9 months and an easier delivery. Use these ideas and tips to become more physically active before, during, and after your pregnancy. Make changes now, and be a healthy example for your family for a lifetime.

- Go for a walk around the block or through a shopping mall with your spouse or a friend.

- Sign up for a prenatal yoga, aqua aerobics, or fitness class. Make sure you let the instructor know that you are pregnant before beginning.

- Rent or buy an exercise video for pregnant women. Look for videos at your local library, video store, health care provider's office, hospital, or maternity clothing store.

- At your gym, community center, YMCA, or YWCA, sign up for a session with a fitness trainer who knows about physical activity during pregnancy.

- Get up and move around at least once an hour if you sit in a chair most of the day; get up and move around during commercials when watching TV.

What habits should I keep up after my baby is born?

Following healthy eating and physical activity habits after your baby is born may help you return to a healthy weight more quickly, provide you with good nutrition (which you especially need if you are breastfeeding), and give you the energy you need. You can also be a good role model for your growing child. After your baby is born:

- Continue eating well. Eat a variety of foods from the five food groups. If you are not breastfeeding, you will need about 300

361

fewer calories per day than you did while you were pregnant.

- If you are breastfeeding, you will need to eat about 200 more calories a day than you did while you were pregnant. Breastfeeding may help you return to a healthy weight more easily because it requires a great deal of energy. Breastfeeding can also protect your baby from illnesses such as ear infections, colds, and allergies, and may help lower your risk for breast and ovarian cancer.

- When you feel able and your health care provider says it is safe, slowly get back to your routine of regular, moderate physical activity. Wait for 4 to 6 weeks after you have your baby to begin doing higher levels of physical activity. Doing physical activity that is too hard, too soon after delivery, can slow your healing process. Regular, moderate physical activity will not affect your milk supply if you are breastfeeding.

Return to a healthy weight gradually. Lose no more than 1 pound per week through a sound eating plan and regular physical activity after you deliver your baby.

Why should I try to return to a healthy weight after delivery?

After you deliver your baby, your health will be better if you try to return to a healthy weight. Not losing weight after your baby is born may lead to overweight or obesity later in life, which may lead to health problems. Talk to your health care provider about reaching a weight that is healthy for you.

Pregnancy and the time after you deliver your baby can be wonderful, exciting, emotional, stressful, and tiring, all at once. Experiencing this whirlwind of feelings may cause you to overeat, not eat enough, or lose your drive and energy. Being good to yourself can help you to cope with your feelings and to follow eating and physical activity habits for a healthy pregnancy, a healthy baby, and a healthy family after delivery. Here are some ideas for being good to yourself:

- Try to get enough sleep.
- Rent a funny movie and laugh.
- Take pleasure in the miracles of pregnancy and birth.
- Invite people whose company you enjoy to visit your new family member.
- Explore groups that you and your newborn can join, such as new moms groups.

Chapter 41

Physical Activity Later in Life

Chapter Contents

Section 41.1

Staying Active after Menopause

"Exercise after Menopause," by Dixie L. Thompson, Ph.D., FACSM, is from the ACSM Fit Society® Page, Summer 2003, p. 7. Reprinted with permission of the American College of Sports Medicine.

There are many well-recognized reasons for exercise: better heart health, lower risk of type 2 diabetes, and weight management are just a few. Unfortunately, many women fail to make the time to exercise regularly, and subsequently miss the benefits that come from an active lifestyle. Some women believe that exercise is more important for men, while others confuse being busy with getting adequate exercise. Some older women also mistakenly believe that it is too late to begin an exercise program after menopause. However, a recent study showed that women 65 or older who increased their physical activity lowered their risk of death during the follow-up period by almost 50 percent! In fact, there are many well-documented benefits that can be gained by postmenopausal women when they exercise regularly.

One of the benefits to regular exercise is cardiovascular health. Regular aerobic exercise reduces the risk of dying from heart disease, lowers blood pressure, and helps control cholesterol levels. According to data from the Women's Health Study, women who walk two or more hours per week reduce their risk of coronary heart disease by two-thirds. One of the reasons that heart disease risk climbs in women after menopause is the tendency for blood pressure to increase with age. Researchers at the University of Tennessee at Knoxville studied previously sedentary, postmenopausal women with elevated blood pressure and found they were able to lower their systolic blood pressure by walking approximately two miles per day. This reduction in blood pressure translates into an approximate 20 percent lower risk of coronary heart disease.

Bone health is a particular concern for many postmenopausal women because of the decline in bone density after menopause. Approximately eight million American women have osteoporosis, and more than 30 million more have low bone density, although not clinically low enough to be diagnosed as osteoporosis. It is estimated that one-half of all women over the age of 50 will have an osteoporosis-related fracture. Exercise and a healthy diet across the lifespan are two ways to maximize bone health. Once menopause is reached, it appears that regular weight-bearing exercise can help minimize bone loss. According to data from the Nurses Health Study, the risk of hip fracture in postmenopausal women declines by six percent for every hour per week spent walking. Strength training, as a supplement to aerobic exercise, can also be useful in maintaining bone.

A common complaint among postmenopausal women is weight gain. In addition to weight gain, there are other unhealthy menopause-related body composition changes, such as a decrease in muscle mass and an increase in abdominal fat. Although some of these changes may be inevitable, the magnitude of these changes can be controlled. A large number of studies have found that exercise during the time around menopause is critical in minimizing fat accumulation. Post-menopausal women who exercise regularly are much less likely to be obese than their sedentary counterparts. In addition to maintaining regular exercise, it is important that women recognize that a decrease in resting metabolism occurs with age. In order to prevent body fat gain, this decrease in metabolic rate must be matched by a decrease in caloric intake.

So, how much exercise is enough to experience the benefits that have been described? From a public health standpoint, the Centers for Disease Control and Prevention, the American College of Sports Medicine, and the Surgeon General agree that 30 minutes of moderate aerobic exercise on most, if not all, days of the week will provide health benefits. It is important to note, however, that this is a minimal recommendation and greater benefits, particularly in controlling weight, can be achieved with additional exercise. The specific type of exercise (walking, swimming, cycling, etc.) seems less important than the fact that the exercise is performed regularly. Find a type of exercise that you enjoy and that best suits your individual needs.

Here are a few tips if you are a postmenopausal woman and just beginning an exercise program.

- Make a commitment to exercise regularly. Have contingency plans when time conflicts, travel, weather issues, or other unexpected issues arise. Even if illness or emergencies force you out of your routine, return to your plan as quickly as possible. Keeping a daily journal of your exercise can be useful in helping you monitor your commitment to exercise.

- Find an exercise support system. For some women this will mean enlisting an exercise buddy to work out with you. For others it may mean finding someone to talk with about the struggles and successes that are encountered with leading an active lifestyle. People are much more likely to continue exercising regularly when they have supportive people around them.

- Start out slowly and progress naturally. Too many people begin exercise programs that are either too intense or too long in duration. This often leads to frustration and/or injury. Listen to your body—it will tell you if you are being too aggressive in your approach. After a workout, you may be slightly tired but should recover in an hour.

- Get regular medical checkups. Most doctors now encourage their patients to exercise regularly. When you visit your physician, be sure to inform him or her about any changes in your exercise routine and ask questions as needed. Be sure to inform your physician immediately if you experience chest pain, have severe difficulty breathing, or injure a muscle or joint.

There are a number of resources for information about exercise for the postmenopausal woman. An excellent source of information is the website for the National Institute of Aging (www.nia.nih.gov). Their booklet, "Exercise: A Guide from the National Institute of Aging" has specific information about how to design your exercise program and forms that can be helpful in tracking your progress.

Section 41.2

Lifelong Fitness: Exercise Recommendations for Seniors

From the *AgePage* article titled "Exercise: Getting Fit For Life,"
from the National Institute on Aging (www.nia.nih.gov), May 2004.

"I don't have time."

"I'm too old—I might hurt myself."

"I'd be too embarrassed at a gym with all those fit young people around."

Sound familiar? Maybe one of these is the reason you aren't physically active or exercising. But, in fact, scientists now know that it's usually more dangerous to not exercise, no matter how old you are. And you don't need to buy fancy clothes or belong to a gym to become more active.

Most older people don't get enough physical activity. Here are some reasons why they should:

- Lack of physical activity and not eating the right foods, taken together, are the second greatest underlying cause of death in the United States. (Smoking is the #1 cause.)

- Exercise can help older people feel better and enjoy life more. No one is too old or too out of shape to be more active.

- Regular exercise can prevent or delay some diseases like cancer, heart disease, or diabetes. It can also perk up your mood and help depression, too.

- Being active can help older people to stay independent and able to keep doing things like getting around or dressing themselves.

So, make physical activity a part of your everyday life. Find things you enjoy. Go for brisk walks. Ride a bike. Dance. Work around the house and in the yard. Take care of your garden. Climb stairs. Rake leaves. Do a mix of things that keep you moving and active.

Four Types of Exercise

There are four types of exercises you need to do to have the right mixture of physical activities.

- **Be sure to get at least 30 minutes of activity that makes you breathe harder on most or all days of the week.** That's called endurance activity, because it builds your energy or staying power. You don't have to be active for 30 minutes all at once. Ten minutes of endurance activity at a time is fine. Just make sure those 10-minute sessions add up to a total of 30 minutes most days. How hard do you need to push yourself? One doctor describes the right level of effort this way: If you can talk without any trouble at all, you're not working hard enough. If you can't talk at all, it's too hard.

- **Keep using your muscles.** When muscles aren't used, they waste away at any age. How important is it to have enough muscle? Very! When you have enough muscle, you can get up from a chair by yourself. When you don't—you have to wait for someone to help you. When you have enough muscle, you can walk through the park with your grandchildren. When you don't—you have to stay home. That's true for younger adults as well as for people age 90 and older. Keeping your muscles in shape can help prevent another serious problem in older people—falls that cause problems like broken hips. When the leg and hip muscles that support you are strong, you're less likely to fall. Even if you do fall, you will be more likely to be able to get up on your own. And using your muscles may make your bones stronger, too.

- **Do things to help your balance.** For example, stand on one foot, then the other. If you can, don't hold on to anything for support. Stand up from sitting in a chair without using your hands or arms. Every now and then walk heel-to-toe. When you walk this way, the toes of the foot in back should almost touch the heel of the foot in front.

- **Stretch.** Stretching can help keep you flexible. You will be able to move more freely. Stretch when your muscles are warmed up. Never stretch so far that it hurts.

Who Should Exercise?

Almost anyone, at any age, can improve his or her health by doing some type of activity. But, check with your doctor first if you plan to do strenuous activity (the kind that makes you breathe hard and sweat) and you are a man over 40 or a woman over 50. Your doctor might be able to give you a go-ahead over the phone, or he or she might ask you to come in for a visit.

You can still exercise even if you have a long-term condition like heart disease or diabetes. In fact, physical activity may help your illness, but only if it's done during times when your condition is under control. During flare-ups, exercise could be harmful. If you have any of the following problems, it's important to check with your doctor before starting an exercise program:

- a chronic disease, or a high risk of getting one—for example, if you smoke, if you are obese, or if you have a family history of a long-term disease
- any new symptom you haven't talked about with your doctor
- chest pain
- shortness of breath
- the feeling that your heart is skipping, racing, or fluttering
- blood clots
- infections or fever
- unplanned weight loss
- foot or ankle sores that won't heal
- joint swelling
- pain or trouble walking after you've fallen
- a bleeding or detached retina, eye surgery, or laser treatment
- a hernia
- hip surgery

Safety Tips

Here are some things you can do to make sure you are exercising safely:

- Start slowly. Little by little build up your activities and how hard you work at them. Doing too much, too soon, can hurt you, especially if you have not been active.
- Don't hold your breath while straining—when using your muscles, for example. That could cause changes in your blood

369

pressure. It may seem strange at first, but the rule is to breathe out while your muscle is working, breathe in when it relaxes. For example, if you are lifting something, breathe out as you lift; breathe in when you stop.

- If you are taking any medicines or have any illnesses that change your natural heart rate, don't use your pulse rate as a way of judging how hard you should exercise. One example of this kind of medicine is a type of blood pressure drug known as a beta blocker.

- Use safety equipment to keep you from getting hurt. That means, for example, a helmet for bike riding or the right shoes for walking or jogging.

- Unless your doctor has asked you to limit fluids, be sure to drink plenty when you are doing activities that make you sweat. Many older people tend to be low on fluid much of the time, even when not exercising.

- Always bend forward from the hips, not the waist. If you keep your back straight, you're probably bending the right way. If your back "humps," that's probably wrong.

- Warm up your muscles before you stretch. For example, do a little easy biking or walking and light arm pumping first.

- Exercises should not hurt or make you feel really tired. You might feel some soreness, a little discomfort, or a bit weary, but you should not feel pain. In fact, in many ways, being physically active will probably make you feel better.

How to Find out More

Local gyms, universities, or hospitals might be able to help you find a teacher or program that works for you. You can also check with nearby churches or synagogues, senior and civic centers, parks, recreation associations, YMCAs, YWCAs, or even area shopping malls for exercise, wellness, or walking programs.

Section 41.3

Overcoming Exercise Obstacles: Suggestions for Seniors

Excerpted from chapter 2 of the book *Exercise: A Guide from the National Institute on Aging,* published by the National Institute on Aging (www.nia .nih.gov), part of the National Institutes of Health, May 2004.

Dr. Andrew Puckett is a busy man with an impressive list of titles after his name. The 60-year-old associate dean for medical education at Duke University, in Durham, North Carolina, has a Ph.D. in adult education and a minor in clinical psychology, and he has been a counselor for years. He also has Parkinson's disease, a chronic condition that causes muscles to tremble and become rigid. He was diagnosed with it a few years ago.

Has his chronic condition slowed down his activities? It doesn't appear that way. In addition to his regular activities, 2 years ago, Dr. Puckett volunteered to take part in a study of how stretching exercises affect people with Parkinson's disease. He enjoyed the feeling of stretching so much that he kept doing the exercises after the 10-week study ended, and now does them at least 3 days a week for 40 minutes at a time.

It's not yet clear whether or not stretching exercises have an effect on Parkinson's disease specifically, but it's very clear to Dr. Puckett that they have helped him feel better overall.

"I literally feel so much better from doing the exercises," he told us. "I'm more flexible than I've been in 20 years. Stretching has given me so much ease of movement. It's a fluid feeling," he said. In addition, Dr. Puckett finds that stretching exercises give him a sense of well-being. He likens it to the "runner's high" that some joggers experience.

Dr. Puckett noted another positive aspect of his stretching exercises: the feeling that he is nurturing himself. He described it as a secure feeling; a feeling that he is doing something good for himself.

Another motivator for keeping up with his stretching exercises is "the fear of being stiff and rigid; bent over. I want to keep that from happening," he told us.

371

Besides working at the university, Dr. Puckett splits his own firewood, plays tennis, gardens, mows his lawn with a push mower, and walks a mile or more at least 3 days a week.

"But people shouldn't feel that physical activity has to be some super-human or highly disciplined effort," he said. "I don't want them to be scared off from the idea of exercising. I think once they experience how much better they feel, they'll want to keep on doing it. It has so many built-in benefits."

Is It Safe for Me to Exercise?

"Too old" and "too frail" are not, in and of themselves, reasons to prohibit physical activity. In fact, there aren't very many health reasons to keep older adults from becoming more active.

Most older people think they need their doctor's approval to start exercising. That's a good idea for some people. Your doctor can talk to you not only about whether it's all right for you to exercise but also about what can be gained from exercise.

Chronic Diseases: Not Necessarily a Barrier

Chronic diseases can't be cured, but usually they can be controlled with medications and other treatments throughout a person's life. They are common among older adults, and include diabetes, cardiovascular disease (such as high blood pressure), and arthritis, among many others.

Traditionally, exercise has been discouraged in people with certain chronic conditions. But researchers have found that exercise can actually improve some chronic conditions in most older people, as long as it's done when the condition is under control.

Congestive heart failure (CHF) is an example of a serious chronic condition common in older adults. In people with CHF, the heart can't empty its load of blood with each beat, resulting in a backup of fluid throughout the body, including the lungs. Disturbances in heart rhythm also are common in CHF. Older adults are hospitalized more often for this disease than for any other.

No one is sure why, but muscles tend to waste away badly in people with CHF, leaving them weak, sometimes to the point that they can't perform everyday tasks. No medicine has a direct muscle-strengthening effect in people with CHF, but muscle-building exercises (lifting weights, for example) can help them improve muscle strength.

Having a chronic disease like CHF probably doesn't mean you can't exercise. But it does mean that keeping in touch with your doctor is important if you do exercise. For example, some studies suggest that endurance exercises, like brisk walking, may improve how well the heart and lungs work in people with CHF, but only in people who are in a stable phase of the disease. People with CHF, like those with most chronic diseases, have periods when their disease gets better, then worse, then better again, off and on. The same endurance exercises that might help people in a stable phase of CHF could be very harmful to people who are in an unstable phase; that is, when they have fluid in their lungs or an irregular heart rhythm.

If you have a chronic condition, you need to know how you can tell whether your disease is stable; that is, when exercise would be OK for you and when it wouldn't.

Chances are good that, if you have a chronic disease, you see a doctor regularly (if you don't, you should, for many reasons). Talk with your doctor about symptoms that mean trouble—a flare-up, or what doctors call an acute phase or exacerbation of your disease. If you have CHF, you know by now that the acute phase of this disease should be taken very, very seriously. You should not exercise when warning symptoms of the acute phase of CHF, or any other chronic disease, appear. It could be dangerous.

But you and your doctor also should discuss how you feel when you are free of those symptoms—in other words, stable or under control. This is the time to exercise.

Diabetes is another chronic condition common among older people. Too much sugar in the blood is a hallmark of diabetes. It can cause damage throughout the body. Exercise can help your body "use up" some of the damaging sugar.

The most common form of diabetes is linked to physical inactivity. In other words, you are less likely to get it in the first place, if you stay physically active.

If you do have diabetes and it has caused changes in your body—cardiovascular disease, eye disease, or changes in your nervous system, for example—check with your doctor to find out what exercises will help you and whether you should avoid certain activities. If you take insulin or a pill that helps lower your blood sugar, your doctor might need to adjust your dose so that your blood sugar doesn't get too low.

Your doctor might find that you don't have to modify your exercises at all, if you are in the earlier stages of diabetes or if your condition is stable.

If you are a man over 40 or a woman over 50, check with your doctor first if you plan to start doing vigorous, as opposed to moderate, physical activities. Vigorous activity could be a problem for people who have "hidden" heart disease—that is, people who have heart disease but don't know it because they don't have any symptoms.

How can you tell if the activity you plan to do is vigorous? There are a couple of ways. If the activity makes you breathe hard and sweat hard (if you tend to sweat, that is), you can consider it vigorous.

If you have had a heart attack recently, your doctor or cardiac rehabilitation therapist should have given you specific exercises to do. Research has shown that exercises done as part of a cardiac rehabilitation program can improve fitness and even reduce your risk of dying. If you didn't get instructions, call your doctor to discuss exercise before you begin increasing your physical activity.

For some conditions, vigorous exercise is dangerous and should not be done, even in the absence of symptoms. Be sure to check with your physician before beginning any kind of exercise program if you have:

- **abdominal aortic aneurysm**, a weakness in the wall of the heart's major outgoing artery (unless it has been surgically repaired or is so small that your doctor tells you that you can exercise vigorously)

- **critical aortic stenosis**, a narrowing of one of the valves of the heart.

Most older adults, regardless of age or condition, will do just fine in increasing their physical activity. You might want to show your doctor this information, to open the door to discussions about exercise.

Checkpoints

You have already read about precautions you should take if you have a chronic condition. Other circumstances require caution, too. You shouldn't exercise until checking with a doctor if you have:

- chest pain;
- irregular, rapid, or fluttery heartbeat;
- severe shortness of breath;
- significant, ongoing weight loss that hasn't been diagnosed;
- infections, such as pneumonia, accompanied by fever;

- fever, which can cause dehydration and a rapid heartbeat;
- acute deep-vein thrombosis (blood clot);
- a hernia that is causing symptoms;
- foot or ankle sores that won't heal;
- joint swelling;
- persistent pain or a problem walking after you have fallen; or
- certain eye conditions, such as bleeding in the retina or detached retina. Before you exercise after a cataract or lens implant, or after laser treatment or other eye surgery, check with your physician.

Part Five

Physical Activity for People with Health Concerns

Chapter 42

Exercise Tips for Overweight or Obese Adults

Chapter Contents

Section 42.1

Active at Any Size

From the booklet by the Weight-control Information Network, part of the National Institute of Diabetes and Digestive and Kidney Diseases (NIDDK, www.niddk.nih.gov), NIH Publication No. 04-4352, May 2004.

Do you feel that you can barely do any activity at all? That you cannot exercise, play sports, or become more fit?

Very large people face special challenges in trying to be active. You may not be able to bend or move in the same way that other people can. It may be hard to find clothes and equipment for exercising. You may feel self-conscious being physically active around other people.

Facing these challenges is hard—but it can be done. The information in this chapter may help you start being more active and healthier—no matter what your size.

How do I get started?

Appreciate yourself. If you cannot do an activity, don't be hard on yourself. Feel good about what you can do. Be proud of pushing yourself up out of a chair or walking a short distance.

Pat yourself on the back for trying even if you can't do it the first time. It may be easier the next time.

To start being more active and keep at it:

- **Start slowly.** Your body needs time to get used to your new activity.

- **Warm up.** Warmups get your body ready for action. Shrug your shoulders, tap your toes, swing your arms, or march in place. You should spend a few minutes warming up for any physical activity—even walking. Walk more slowly for the first few minutes.

- **Cool down.** Slow down little by little. If you have been walking fast, walk slowly or stretch for a few minutes to cool down. Cooling down may protect your heart, relax your muscles, and keep you from getting hurt.

- **Set goals.** Set short-term and long-term goals. A short-term goal may be to walk 5 minutes on at least 3 days for 1 week. It may not seem like a lot, but any activity is better than none. A long-term goal may be to walk 30 minutes on most days of the week by the end of 6 months.

- **Get support.** Get a family member or friend to be physically active with you. It may be more fun, and your buddy can cheer you on.

- **Track progress.** Keep a journal of your physical activity. You may not feel like you are making progress but when you look back at where you started, you may be pleasantly surprised!

Have fun! Try different activities to find the ones you really enjoy.

What physical activities can a very large person do? Do I need to see my health care provider before I start being physically active?

You should talk to your health care provider if you:

- have a chronic health problem such as diabetes, heart disease, asthma, or arthritis;

- have high blood pressure, high cholesterol, or personal or family history of heart disease; or

- are a woman over age 50 or a man over age 40.

Gentle physical activity is healthy. You do not have to push yourself to benefit from physical activity. Thirty minutes of gentle physical activity (like walking) can be just as healthy as 15 minutes of intense physical activity (like fast dancing).

Most very large people can do some or all of the physical activities in this chapter. You do not need special skills or a lot of equipment. You can do:

- **weight-bearing activities**, like walking and golfing, which involve lifting or pushing your own body weight.

- **non-weight-bearing activities**, like swimming and water workouts, which put less stress on your joints because you do not have to lift or push your own weight. If your feet or joints hurt when you stand, non-weight-bearing activities may be best for you.

- **lifestyle activities**, like gardening, which do not have to be planned.

Physical activity does not have to be hard or boring to be good for you. Anything that gets you moving around—even for only a few minutes a day—is a healthy start to getting more fit.

Chances are your health care provider will be pleased with your decision to start an activity program. It is unlikely that you will need a complete medical exam before you go out for a short walk.

Walking (Weight-Bearing)

The walking that you do during the day (like doing chores around the house or in the yard) can help you be more fit. But regular, steady walking that makes you breathe heavier can help you to be healthier. It will give your heart and lungs—as well as your leg muscles—a good workout.

If you are not active now, start slowly. Try to walk 5 minutes a day for the first week. Walk 8 minutes the next week. Stay at 8-minute walks until you feel comfortable. Then increase your walks to 11 minutes. Slowly lengthen each walk by 3 minutes—or walk faster.

Tips for walking:

- Wear comfortable walking shoes with a lot of support. If you walk often, you may need to buy new shoes every 6 to 8 months.

- Wear garments that prevent inner thigh chafing, such as tights or spandex shorts.

- Make walking fun. Walk with a friend or pet. Walk in places you enjoy, like a park or shopping mall.

Dancing (Weight-Bearing or Non-Weight-Bearing)

Dancing may help:

- tone your muscles;
- improve your flexibility;
- make your heart stronger; and
- make your lungs work better.

You can dance in a health club, in a nightclub, or at home. To dance at home, just move your body to some lively music.

Dancing on your feet is a weight-bearing activity. Dancing while seated lets you move your arms and legs to music while taking the weight off your feet. This may be a good choice if you can't stand on your feet very long.

Water Workouts (Non-Weight-Bearing)

Exercising in water helps you feel:

- flexible. You can bend and move your body in water in ways you cannot on land.

- strong. Working against the water will help your body get stronger.

- at less risk of injury. Water makes your body float. This keeps your joints from being pounded or jarred and helps prevent sore muscles and injury.

- refreshed. You can keep cooler in water—even when you are working hard.

You do not need to know how to swim to work out in water—you can do shallow-water or deep-water exercises without swimming.

For shallow-water exercise, the water level should be between your waist and your chest. If the water is too shallow, it will be hard to move your arms underwater. If the water is deeper than chest height, it will be hard to keep your feet touching the pool bottom.

For deep-water exercise, most of your body is underwater. This means that your whole body will get a good workout. For safety and comfort, wear a foam belt or life jacket.

Many swim centers offer classes in water workouts. Check with the pools in your area to find the best water workout for you.

Weight Training (Weight-Bearing or Non-Weight-Bearing)

Weight training builds strong muscles and bones. Getting stronger can also help prepare you for other kinds of physical activity. You can weight train at home or at a fitness center.

You do not need benches or bars to begin weight training at home. You can use a pair of hand weights or even two soup cans.

Make sure you know the correct posture and that your movements are slow and controlled. Here is a weight training rule of thumb: If you cannot lift a weight 6 times in a row, the weight you are lifting is too heavy. If you can easily lift a weight 15 times in a row, your weight is too light.

Before you buy a home gym, check its weight rating (the number of pounds it can support) to make sure it is safe for your size. If you want to join a fitness center where you can use weights, shop around for one where you feel at ease.

Bicycling (Non-Weight-Bearing)

You can bicycle indoors on a stationary bike or outdoors on a road bike. Biking does not stress any one part of the body—your weight is spread between your arms, back, and hips.

You may want to use a recumbent bike. On this type of bike, you sit low to the ground with your legs reaching forward to the pedals. This may feel better than sitting upright. The seat on a recumbent bike is also wider than the seat on an upright bike.

For biking outdoors, you may want to try a mountain bike. These bikes have wider tires and are heavy. You can also buy a larger seat to put on your bike.

Make sure the bike you buy has a weight rating at least as high as your own weight.

Stretching (Weight-Bearing or Non-Weight-Bearing)

Stretching may help you:

- be more flexible;
- feel more relaxed;
- improve your blood flow; and
- keep your muscles from getting tight after doing other physical activities.

You do not have to set aside a special time or place to stretch. At home or at work, stand up, push your arms toward the ceiling, and stretch. Stretch slowly and only enough to feel tightness—not until you feel pain. Hold the stretch, without bouncing, for about 30 seconds. Do not stretch cold muscles.

Yoga and tai chi are types of stretching. They help you breathe deeply, relax, and get rid of stress.

Your local fitness center may offer yoga, tai chi, or other stretching classes. You may want to start with "gentle" classes, like those aimed at seniors.

If you can do only a few or none of these activities, it's OK. Remember to appreciate what you can do, even if you think it's a small amount. Just moving any part of your body—even for a short time—can make you healthier.

Where to Work Out

You can do many activities in your home. But there are other fun ways to be active in health clubs, in recreation centers, or outdoors. It may be hard to be physically active around other people. Keep in mind that you have just as much right to be healthy and active as anyone else.

Questions to ask when choosing a fitness center:

- Can the treadmills or benches support people who are large?
- Do the fitness staff know how to work with people of larger sizes?
- Can I take time to see how I like the center before I sign up?
- Is the aim to have fun and get healthy—not to lose weight?

Lifestyle Activities

Lifestyle physical activities do not have to be planned. You can make small changes to make your day more physically active and improve your health. For example:

- Take 2- to 3-minute walking breaks at work a few times a day.
- Put away the TV remote control—get up to change the channel.
- March in place during TV commercials.
- Sit in a rocking chair and push off the floor with your feet.
- Take the stairs instead of the elevator.

Doing chores like lawn mowing, leaf raking, gardening, and housework may also improve your health.

Safety Tips

Stop your activity right away if you:

- have pain, tightness, or pressure in your chest or left neck, shoulder, or arm;

- feel dizzy or sick;

- break out in a cold sweat;

- have muscle cramps; or

- feel pain in your joints, feet, ankles, or legs. You could hurt yourself if you ignore the pain.

Ask your health care provider what to do if you have any of these symptoms.

Here are some other tips:

- Slow down if you feel out of breath. You should be able to talk during your activity, without gasping for breath.

- Drink lots of water before, during, and after physical activity (even water workouts) to replace the water you lose by sweating.

- Do not do hard exercise for 2 hours after a big meal (but taking a walk is OK). If you eat small meals, you can be physically active more often.

- Wear the right clothes:

  - Wear lightweight, loose-fitting tops so you can move easily.

  - Wear clothes made of fabrics that absorb sweat and remove it from your skin.

  - Never wear rubber or plastic suits. Plastic suits could hold the sweat on your skin and make your body overheat.

  - Women should wear a good support bra.

  - Wear supportive athletic shoes for weight-bearing activities.

  - Wear a knit hat to keep you warm when you are physically active outdoors in cold weather. Wear a tightly woven, wide-brimmed hat in hot weather to help keep you cool and protect you from the sun.

- Wear sunscreen when you are physically active outdoors.

Healthy, fit bodies come in all sizes. Whatever your size or shape, get physically active now and keep moving for a healthier life!

Section 42.2

Choosing a Safe and Successful Weight-Loss Program

Excerpted from the booklet by the Weight-control Information Network, part of the National Institute of Diabetes and Digestive and Kidney Diseases (NIDDK), NIH Publication No. 03-3700, February 2006.

Choosing a weight-loss program may be a difficult task. You may not know what to look for in a weight-loss program or what questions to ask. This chapter can help you talk to your health care professional about weight loss and get the best information before choosing a program.

Talk with Your Health Care Professional

If your health care provider tells you that you should lose weight and you want to find a weight-loss program to help you, look for one that is based on regular physical activity and an eating plan that is balanced, healthy, and easy to follow.

You may want to talk with your doctor or other health care professional about controlling your weight before you decide on a weight-loss program. Even if you feel uncomfortable talking about your weight with your doctor, remember that he or she is there to help you improve your health. Here are some tips:

- Tell your provider that you would like to talk about your weight. Share your concerns about any medical conditions you have or medicines you are taking.

- Write down your questions in advance.

- Bring pen and paper to take notes.

- Bring a friend or family member along for support if this will make you feel more comfortable.

- Make sure you understand what your health care provider is saying. Ask questions if there is something you do not understand.

- Ask for other sources of information like brochures or websites.

- If you want more support, ask for a referral to a registered dietitian, a support group, or a commercial weight-loss program.

- Call your provider after your visit if you have more questions or need help.

A Responsible and Safe Weight-loss Program

If your health care provider tells you that you should lose weight and you want to find a weight-loss program to help you, look for one that is based on regular physical activity and an eating plan that is balanced, healthy, and easy to follow. Weight-loss programs should encourage healthy behaviors that help you lose weight and that you can stick with every day. Safe and effective weight-loss programs should include:

- Healthy eating plans that reduce calories but do not forbid specific foods or food groups.

- Tips to increase moderate-intensity physical activity.

- Tips on healthy behavior changes that also keep your cultural needs in mind.

- Slow and steady weight loss. Depending on your starting weight, experts recommend losing weight at a rate of ½ to 2 pounds per week. Weight loss may be faster at the start of a program.

- Medical care if you are planning to lose weight by following a special formula diet, such as a very low-calorie diet.

- A plan to keep the weight off after you have lost it.

Get Familiar With the Program

Gather as much information as you can before deciding to join a program. Professionals working for weight-loss programs should be able to answer the questions listed below.

What does the weight-loss program consist of?

- Does the program offer one-on-one counseling or group classes?

- Do you have to follow a specific meal plan or keep food records?

- Do you have to purchase special food, drugs, or supplements?

- Does the program help you be more physically active, follow a specific physical activity plan, or provide exercise instruction?

- Does the program teach you to make positive and healthy behavior changes?
- Is the program sensitive to your lifestyle and cultural needs?

What are the staff qualifications?

- Who supervises the program?
- What type of weight management training, experience, education, and certifications do the staff have?

Does the product or program carry any risks?

- Could the program hurt you?
- Could the recommended drugs or supplements harm your health?
- Do participants talk with a doctor?
- Does a doctor run the program?
- Will the program's doctors work with your personal doctor if you have a medical condition such as high blood pressure or are taking prescribed drugs?

How much does the program cost?

- What is the total cost of the program?
- Are there other costs, such as weekly attendance fees, food and supplement purchases, etc.?
- Are there fees for a follow-up program after you lose weight?
- Are there other fees for medical tests?

What results do participants typically have?

- How much weight does an average participant lose and how long does he or she keep the weight off?
- Does the program offer publications or materials that describe what results participants typically have?

If you are interested in finding a weight-loss program near you, ask your health care provider for a referral or contact your local hospital.

Chapter 43

Physical Activity and Diabetes

How can I take care of my diabetes?

Diabetes means that your blood glucose (also called blood sugar) is too high. Your body uses glucose for energy. But having too much glucose in your blood can hurt you. When you take care of your diabetes, you'll feel better. You'll reduce your risk for problems with your kidneys, eyes, nerves, feet and legs, and teeth. You'll also lower your risk for a heart attack or a stroke. You can take care of your diabetes by:

- being physically active;
- following a healthy meal plan; and
- taking medicines (if prescribed by your doctor).

What can a physically active lifestyle do for me?

Research has shown that physical activity can:

- lower your blood glucose and your blood pressure;
- lower your bad cholesterol and raise your good cholesterol;
- improve your body's ability to use insulin;
- lower your risk for heart disease and stroke;

From "What I Need to Know about Physical Activity and Diabetes," by the National Diabetes Information Clearinghouse, part of the National Institute of Diabetes and Digestive and Kidney Diseases (www.niddk.nih.gov), June 2004.

- keep your heart and bones strong;
- keep your joints flexible;
- lower your risk of falling;
- help you lose weight;
- reduce your body fat;
- give you more energy; and
- reduce your stress.

Physical activity also plays an important part in preventing type 2 diabetes. A major government study, the Diabetes Prevention Program (DPP), showed that a healthy diet and a moderate exercise program resulting in a 5 to 7 percent weight loss can delay and possibly prevent type 2 diabetes.

What kinds of physical activity can help me?

Four kinds of activity can help. You can try:

- being extra active every day;
- doing aerobic exercise;
- doing strength training; and
- stretching.

Be Extra Active Every Day

Being extra active can increase the number of calories you burn. There are many ways to be extra active.

- Walk around while you talk on the phone.
- Play with the kids.
- Take the dog for a walk.
- Get up to change the TV channel instead of using the remote control.
- Work in the garden or rake leaves.
- Clean the house.
- Wash the car.
- Stretch out your chores. For example, make two trips to take the laundry downstairs instead of one.

- Park at the far end of the shopping center lot and walk to the store.
- At the grocery store, walk down every aisle.
- At work, walk over to see a coworker instead of calling or e-mailing.
- Take the stairs instead of the elevator.
- Stretch or walk around instead of taking a coffee break and eating.
- During your lunch break, walk to the post office or do other errands.

Do Aerobic Exercise

Aerobic exercise is activity that requires the use of large muscles and makes your heart beat faster. You will also breathe harder during aerobic exercise. Doing aerobic exercise for 30 minutes a day, most days of the week, provides many benefits. You can even split up those 30 minutes into several parts. For example, you can take three brisk 10-minute walks, one after each meal.

If you haven't exercised lately, see your doctor first to make sure it's OK for you to increase your level of physical activity. Talk with your doctor about how to warm up and stretch before exercise and how to cool down after exercise. Then start slowly with 5 to 10 minutes a day. Add a little more time each week, aiming for 150 to 200 minutes per week. Try:

- walking briskly;
- hiking;
- climbing stairs;
- swimming or taking a water-aerobics class;
- dancing;
- riding a bicycle outdoors or a stationary bicycle indoors;
- taking an aerobics class;
- playing basketball, volleyball, or other sports;
- in-line skating, ice skating, or skate boarding;
- playing tennis; or
- cross-country skiing.

Do Strength Training

Doing exercises with hand weights, elastic bands, or weight machines two or three times a week builds muscle. When you have more muscle and less fat, you'll burn more calories because muscle burns more calories than fat, even between exercise sessions. Strength training can help make daily chores easier, improving your balance and coordination, as well as your bones' health. You can do strength training at home, at a fitness center, or in a class. Your health care team can tell you more about strength training and what kind is best for you.

Stretch

Stretching increases your flexibility, lowers stress, and helps prevent muscle soreness after other types of exercise. Your health care team can tell you what kind of stretching is best for you.

Can I exercise any time I want?

Ask your health care team about the best time of day for you to exercise. Consider your daily schedule, your meal plan, and your diabetes medications in deciding when to exercise.

If you exercise when your blood glucose is above 300, your level can go even higher. It's best not to exercise until your blood glucose is lower. Also, exercise is not recommended if your fasting blood glucose is above 250 and you have ketones in your urine.

Are there any types of physical activity I shouldn't do?

If you have diabetes complications, some exercises can make your problems worse. For example, activities that increase the pressure in the blood vessels of your eyes, such as lifting heavy weights, can make diabetic eye problems worse. If nerve damage from diabetes has made your feet numb, your doctor may suggest that you try swimming instead of walking for aerobic exercise.

Numbness means that you may not feel any pain from sores or blisters on your feet and so may not notice them. Then they can get worse and lead to more serious problems. Make sure you exercise in cotton socks and comfortable, well-fitting shoes that are designed for the activity you are doing. After you exercise, check your feet for cuts, sores, bumps, or redness. Call your doctor if any foot problems develop.

Can physical activity cause low blood glucose?

Physical activity can cause hypoglycemia (low blood glucose) in people who take insulin or certain diabetes pills, including sulfonylureas and meglitinides. Ask your health care team whether your diabetes pills can cause hypoglycemia. Some types of diabetes pills do not.

Hypoglycemia can happen while you exercise, right afterward, or even up to a day later. It can make you feel shaky, weak, confused, irritable, hungry, or tired. You may sweat a lot or get a headache. If your blood glucose drops too low, you could pass out or have a seizure.

However, you should still be physically active. These steps can help you be prepared for hypoglycemia.

Before Exercise

- Be careful about exercising if you have skipped a recent meal. Check your blood glucose. If it's below 100, have a small snack.

- If you take insulin, ask your health care team whether you should change your dosage before you exercise.

During Exercise

- Wear your medical identification or other ID.

- Always carry food or glucose tablets so that you'll be ready to treat hypoglycemia.

- If you'll be exercising for more than an hour, check your blood glucose at regular intervals. You may need snacks before you finish.

After Exercise

- Check to see how exercise affected your blood glucose level.

Treating Hypoglycemia

If your blood glucose is 70 or lower, have one of the following right away:

- 2 or 3 glucose tablets
- ½ cup (4 ounces) of any fruit juice
- ½ cup (4 ounces) of a regular (not diet) soft drink

- 1 cup (8 ounces) of milk
- 5 or 6 pieces of hard candy
- 1 or 2 teaspoons of sugar or honey

After 15 minutes, check your blood glucose again. If it's still too low, have another serving. Repeat until your blood glucose is 70 or higher. If it will be an hour or more before your next meal, have a snack as well.

What should I do first?

- **Check with your doctor.** Always talk with your doctor before you start a new physical activity program. Ask about your medications—prescription and over-the-counter—and whether you should change the amount you take before you exercise. If you have heart disease, kidney disease, eye problems, or foot problems, ask which types of physical activity are safe for you.

- **Decide exactly what you'll do and set some goals.** Choose:
  - the type of physical activity you want to do
  - the clothes and items you'll need to get ready
  - the days and times you'll add activity
  - the length of each session
  - your warmup and cooldown plan for each session
  - alternatives, such as where you'll walk if the weather is bad
  - your measures of progress

- **Find an exercise buddy.** Many people find that they are more likely to do something active if a friend joins them. If you and a friend plan to walk together, for example, you may be more likely to do it.

- **Keep track of your physical activity.** Write down when you exercise and for how long in your blood glucose record book. You'll be able to track your progress and to see how physical activity affects your blood glucose.

- **Decide how you'll reward yourself.** Do something nice for yourself when you reach your activity goals. For example, treat yourself to a movie or buy a new plant for the garden.

What can I do to make sure I stay active?

One of the keys to staying on track is finding some activities you like to do. If you keep finding excuses not to exercise, think about why. Are your goals realistic? Do you need a change in activity? Would another time be more convenient? Keep trying until you find a routine that works for you. Once you make physical activity a habit, you'll wonder how you lived without it.

Chapter 44

Lung Conditions and Exercise

Chapter Contents

Section 44.1

How Smoking Affects Physical Activity

This section includes "Facts on Youth Smoking, Health, and Performance" and "Facts on Sports and Smoke-free Youth," both from the Office on Smoking and Health, National Center For Chronic Disease Prevention and Health Promotion, part of the Centers for Disease Control and Prevention, January 2005. For references, see http://www.cdc.gov/tobacco.

Facts on Youth Smoking, Health, and Performance

Among young people, the short-term health effects of smoking include damage to the respiratory system, addiction to nicotine, and the associated risk of other drug use. Long-term health consequences of youth smoking are reinforced by the fact that most young people who smoke regularly continue to smoke throughout adulthood.

- Smoking hurts young people's physical fitness in terms of both performance and endurance—even among young people trained in competitive running.

- Smoking among youth can hamper the rate of lung growth and the level of maximum lung function.

- The resting heart rates of young adult smokers are two to three beats per minute faster than those of nonsmokers.

- Among young people, regular smoking is responsible for cough and increased frequency and severity of respiratory illnesses.

- The younger people start smoking cigarettes, the more likely they are to become strongly addicted to nicotine.

- Teens who smoke are three times more likely than nonsmokers to use alcohol, eight times more likely to use marijuana, and 22 times more likely to use cocaine. Smoking is associated with a host of other risky behaviors, such as fighting and engaging in unprotected sex.

- Smoking is associated with poor overall health and a variety of short-term adverse health effects in young people and may also be a marker for underlying mental health problems, such as depression, among adolescents. High school seniors who are regular smokers and began smoking by grade nine are:

- 2.4 times more likely than their nonsmoking peers to report poorer overall health;
- 2.4 to 2.7 times more likely to report cough with phlegm or blood, shortness of breath when not exercising, and wheezing or gasping; and
- 3.0 times more likely to have seen a doctor or other health professional for an emotional or psychological complaint.

Facts on Sports and Smoke-Free Youth

Research has shown that students who participate in interscholastic sports are less likely to be regular and heavy smokers. Students who play at least one sport are 40% less likely to be regular smokers and 50% less likely to be heavy smokers. Regular and heavy smoking decreases substantially with an increase in the number of sports played.

The lower rates of smoking for student athletes may be related to a number of factors:

- greater self-confidence gained from sports participation;
- additional counseling from coaching staff about smoking;
- reduced peer influences about smoking;
- perceptions about reduced sports performance because of smoking; and
- greater awareness about the health consequences of smoking.

Special Benefits for Girls

Smoking becomes a way for preteen and teen women to build a sense of self and stay connected with peers in the face of enormous pressures to be beautiful, successful, sophisticated, thin, independent, and popular—seductive images that are reinforced in movies, music videos, and advertising.

Sports and physical activity are positive, viable alternatives to smoking in the lives of young women. They can give adolescent women the very benefits they perceive in smoking: independence, status with their peers, a chance to make friends, relaxation, weight management, and a more positive sense of self.

- Girls who play sports have higher levels of self-esteem and lower levels of depression than girls who do not play sports.

- Girls who play sports have a more positive body image and experience higher states of psychological well-being than girls and women who do not play sports.

- Girls who play sports learn about teamwork, goal-setting, the experience of success, the pursuit of excellence in performance, how to deal with failures, and other positive behaviors—all of which are important skills for the workplace and life.

Section 44.2

Asthma and Exercise

Exercise can make asthma symptoms worse. This is called exercise-induced asthma. Exercise can cause asthma symptoms in up to 80 percent of people with asthma. Treatment and monitoring can allow people with exercise-induced asthma to participate fully in the physical activity or exercise of their choice.

How will I know if I have exercise-induced asthma?

For some people, exercise-induced asthma occurs within three to eight minutes of starting activity or exercise. For others, exercise-induced asthma occurs after stopping exercise. Often the exercise-induced asthma starts during exercise and worsens when exercise stops. The most common symptoms of exercise-induced asthma are:

- coughing
- wheezing
- shortness of breath
- chest tightness

Some people are not aware of these symptoms but know they tire easily and have a hard time keeping up with others. It is important to recognize the difference between poor conditioning and exercise-induced asthma. In well-conditioned athletes, symptoms of exercise-induced asthma may only occur with the most vigorous activity or exercise.

Think about how you feel when you exercise. Do you tire easily or cough and wheeze? Share this information with your health care provider. Your health care provider will ask you questions about your asthma and do a physical exam. He or she may also order a test called an exercise induced bronchoconstriction to help diagnose exercise-induced asthma. An exercise challenge may be done in your doctor's office or the hospital. During an exercise challenge, you will walk or run on a treadmill or ride an exercise bicycle and perform repeated breathing tests. Using this information, your health care provider will be able to understand if exercise can make your asthma symptoms worse.

How is exercise-induced asthma treated?

There is a simple and effective way of treating exercise-induced asthma. Your health care provider may prescribe a "pre-treatment." A pre-treatment is a medicine that is inhaled before exercise. By using a prescribed pre-treatment, people with asthma are often able to participate safely and successfully in the exercise they enjoy. A pre-treatment can prevent asthma symptoms during and after exercise. Examples of inhaled medicines often used as a pre-treatment include:

- Proventil®, Proventil HFA®, Ventolin® (albuterol)
- Maxair® (pirbuterol)
- Xopenex® (levalbuterol)

These medicines are often prescribed 10 to 15 minutes before exercise and quickly open the airways to prevent asthma symptoms. Discuss the use of a pre-treatment with your health care provider.

Some people with exercise-induced asthma respond well to other medications. Healthcare providers may recommend using Intal® (cromolyn sodium) or Tilade® (nedocromil sodium) as a pre-treatment. In all cases, work with your health care provider to decide the pre-treatment that is right for you.

Regardless of which inhaled medicine you use, it is important to use good technique. Good technique helps you get the full dosage and benefit from the medicine. Using a spacer device with your metered-dose-inhaler can improve delivery of the medicine to your airways. Review your inhaled medicine technique with your health care provider at your next visit.

If your asthma symptoms are occurring more often with exercise or are more severe, talk with your health care provider. Your health care provider may increase the medicine you take every day (long-term control medicine) to get your asthma under better control.

How is exercise-induced asthma monitored?

Monitor your asthma while you exercise by watching for asthma symptoms. The peak flow meter can also be useful in monitoring your asthma. A peak flow meter is a portable, handheld device that measures how fast you blow air out. When the airways are narrowed by asthma, the peak flow number will drop. A significant drop in your peak flow number and/or asthma symptoms is a signal that you need extra medicine or maybe a short rest during exercise. Ask your health care provider about a written asthma action plan. It will help you know what to do if you are getting worse while you exercise.

A peak flow meter can be an objective way to make decisions about participation in sports, gym class, recess, or other activities. In many situations physical education teachers, coaches, and employers may be confused about asthma and exercise or physical activity. Some may prohibit people from participation while others may push those with asthma to keep up with their peers without proper monitoring or treatment. A peak flow meter combined with monitoring asthma symptoms can help take the confusion out of this situation.

What sports are best for people with exercise-induced asthma?

Sports or activities with bursts of activity are least likely to cause asthma symptoms. Activities followed by brief rest periods can allow the person to regain control of their breathing. Activities such as baseball, softball, volleyball, tennis, downhill skiing, golf, and some track and field events all have brief rest periods.

Sports that require continuous activity like swimming, cycling, distance running, and soccer also can be enjoyed by people with exercise-induced asthma. Participation in any sport often requires use of a pre-treatment before exercise and close monitoring. Along with appropriate treatment and close monitoring, a good warmup and cooldown period are often helpful.

Research shows everyone can benefit greatly from exercise physically and in terms of self-esteem and stress relief. When asthma is well controlled people with exercise-induced asthma should be able to participate in any sport. In fact, it is estimated that exercise-induced asthma affects one in ten athletes. At the 1984 summer Olympic games in Los Angeles, 67 of the 597 members (or 11%) of the American team tested positive for exercise-induced asthma. These 67 athletes won a total of 41 medals.

Chapter 45

Exercise Your Way to Lower Blood Pressure

What Are High Blood Pressure and Prehypertension?

Blood pressure is the force of blood against the walls of arteries. Blood pressure rises and falls throughout the day. When blood pressure stays elevated over time, it's called high blood pressure.

The medical term for high blood pressure is hypertension. High blood pressure is dangerous because it makes the heart work too hard and contributes to atherosclerosis (hardening of the arteries). It increases the risk of heart disease and stroke, which are the first- and third-leading causes of death among Americans. High blood pressure also can result in other conditions, such as congestive heart failure, kidney disease, and blindness.

Risk Factors for Heart Disease

Risk factors are conditions or behaviors that increase your chances of developing a disease. When you have more than one risk factor for heart disease, your risk of developing heart disease greatly multiplies. So if you have high blood pressure, you need to take action. Fortunately, you can control most heart disease risk factors.

Risk factors you can control:

• High blood pressure

Excerpted from the brochure "Your Guide to Lowering High Blood Pressure," by the National Heart, Lung and Blood Institute (NHLBI, www.nhlbi.nih.gov), part of the National Institutes of Health, May 2003.

- Abnormal cholesterol
- Tobacco use
- Diabetes
- Overweight
- Physical inactivity

Risk factors beyond your control:

- Age (55 or older for men; 65 or older for women)
- Family history of early heart disease (having a father or brother diagnosed with heart disease before age 55 or having a mother or sister diagnosed before age 65)

A blood pressure level of 140/90 mmHg or higher is considered high. About two-thirds of people over age 65 have high blood pressure. If your blood pressure is between 120/80 mmHg and 139/89 mmHg, then you have prehypertension. This means that you don't have high blood pressure now but are likely to develop it in the future unless you adopt the healthy lifestyle changes described in this brochure.

People who do not have high blood pressure at age 55 face a 90 percent chance of developing it during their lifetimes. So high blood pressure is a condition that most people will have at some point in their lives.

Both numbers in a blood pressure test are important, but for people who are age 50 or older, systolic pressure gives the most accurate diagnosis of high blood pressure. Systolic pressure is the top number in a blood pressure reading. It is high if it is 140 mmHg or above.

How Can You Prevent or Control High Blood Pressure?

If you have high blood pressure, you and your health care provider need to work together as a team to reduce it. The two of you need to agree on your blood pressure goal. Together, you should come up with a plan and timetable for reaching your goal.

Blood pressure is usually measured in millimeters of mercury (mmHg) and is recorded as two numbers—systolic pressure (as the heart beats) "over" diastolic pressure (as the heart relaxes between beats)—for example, 130/80 mmHg. Ask your doctor to write down your blood pressure numbers and your blood pressure goal level for you.

Monitoring your blood pressure at home between visits to your doctor can be helpful. You also may want to bring a family member with you when you visit your doctor. Having a family member who knows that you have high blood pressure and who understands what you need to do to lower your blood pressure often makes it easier to make the changes that will help you reach your goal.

The steps that follow will help lower your blood pressure. If you have normal blood pressure or prehypertension, following these steps will help prevent you from developing high blood pressure. If you have high blood pressure, following these steps will help you control your blood pressure.

Lower Your Blood Pressure by Being Active

Being physically active is one of the most important things you can do to prevent or control high blood pressure. It also helps to reduce your risk of heart disease.

It doesn't take a lot of effort to become physically active. All you need is 30 minutes of moderate-level physical activity on most days

Table 45.1. Blood Pressure Levels for Adults

Category	Systolic[1] (mmHg)[2]		Diastolic[1] (mmHg)[2]	Result
Normal	less than 120	*and*	less than 80	Good for you!
Prehypertension	120-139	*or*	80 to 89	Your blood pressure could be a problem. Make changes in what you eat and drink, be physically active, and lose extra weight. If you also have diabetes, see your doctor.
Hypertension	140 or higher	*or*	90 or higher	You have high blood pressure. Ask your doctor or nurse how to control it.

Note: These levels apply to adults ages 18 and older who are not on medicine for high blood pressure and do not have a short-term serious illness. Source: The Seventh Report of the Joint National Committee on Prevention, Detection, Evaluation, and Treatment of High Blood Pressure; NIH Publication No. 03-5230, National High Blood Pressure Education Program, May 2003.

[1]If systolic and diastolic pressures fall into different categories, overall status is the higher category.

[2]Millimeters of mercury.

of the week. Examples of such activities are brisk walking, bicycling, raking leaves, and gardening. For more examples, see Table 45.2.

Table 45.2. Examples of Moderate-Level Physical Activities

Common Chores	Sporting Activities
Washing and waxing a car for 45-60 minutes	Playing volleyball for 45-60 minutes
	Playing touch football for 45 minutes
Washing windows or floors for 45-60 minutes	Walking 2 miles in 30 minutes (1 mile in 15 minutes)
Gardening for 30-45 minutes	Shooting baskets for 30 minutes
Wheeling self in wheelchair for 30-40 minutes	Bicycling 5 miles in 30 minutes
	Dancing fast (social) for 30 minutes
Pushing a stroller 1 1/2 miles in 30 minutes	Performing water aerobics for 30 minutes
	Swimming laps for 20 minutes
Raking leaves for 30 minutes	Playing basketball for 15-20 minutes
Shoveling snow for 15 minutes	Jumping rope for 15 minutes
Stair walking for 15 minutes	Running 1½ miles in 15 minutes (1 mile in 10 minutes)

You can even divide the 30 minutes into shorter periods of at least 10 minutes each. For instance: Use stairs instead of an elevator, get off a bus one or two stops early, or park your car at the far end of the lot at work. If you already engage in 30 minutes of moderate-level physical activity a day, you can get added benefits by doing more. Engage in a moderate-level activity for a longer period each day or engage in a more vigorous activity.

Most people don't need to see a doctor before they start a moderate-level physical activity. You should check first with your doctor if you have heart trouble or have had a heart attack, if you're over age 50 and are not used to moderate-level physical activity, if you have a family history of heart disease at an early age, or if you have any other serious health problem.

Chapter 46

Physical Activity and the Heart

Chapter Contents

Section 46.1

Reducing Your Risk of Heart Disease with Physical Activity

Excerpted from the brochure "Your Guide to a Healthy Heart," published by the National Heart, Lung and Blood Institute (NHLBI, www.nhlbi.nih .gov), part of the National Institutes of Health, December 2005.

What Is Heart Disease?

Coronary heart disease—often simply called heart disease—occurs when the arteries that supply blood to the heart muscle become hardened and narrowed due to a buildup of plaque on the arteries' inner walls. Plaque is the accumulation of fat, cholesterol, and other substances. As plaque continues to build up in the arteries, blood flow to the heart is reduced.

Heart disease can lead to a heart attack. A heart attack happens when an artery becomes totally blocked with plaque, preventing vital oxygen and nutrients from getting to the heart. A heart attack can cause permanent damage to the heart muscle.

Heart disease is one of several cardiovascular diseases, which are disorders of the heart and blood vessel system. Other cardiovascular diseases include stroke, high blood pressure, and rheumatic heart disease.

Some people aren't too concerned about heart disease because they think it can be "cured" with surgery. This is a myth. Heart disease is a lifelong condition: Once you get it, you'll always have it. It's true that procedures such as angioplasty and bypass surgery can help blood and oxygen flow more easily to the heart. But the arteries remain damaged, which means you are still more likely to have a heart attack. What's more, the condition of your blood vessels will steadily worsen unless you make changes in your daily habits and control your risk factors. Many people die of complications from heart disease, or become permanently disabled. That's why it is so vital to take action to prevent this disease.

Risk Factors for Heart Disease: Physical Inactivity

"I'd love to take a walk—tomorrow."

"I can't wait to start yoga—if I can find a class."

"I'm going to start lifting weights—as soon as I get the time."

Many of us put off getting regular physical activity, and hope that our bodies will understand. But our bodies don't understand, and sooner or later they rebel. Even if a person has no other risk factors, being physically inactive greatly boosts the chances of developing heart-related problems. It also increases the likelihood of developing other heart disease risk factors, such as high blood pressure, diabetes, and overweight. Lack of physical activity also leads to more visits to the doctor, more hospitalizations, and more use of medicines for a variety of illnesses.

Despite these risks, most Americans aren't getting enough physical activity. According to the CDC, nearly 40 percent of Americans are not active at all during their free time. Overall, women tend to be less physically active than men, and older people are less likely to be active than younger individuals. But young people need to get moving, too. Forty percent of high school-aged girls and 27 percent of high school-aged boys don't get enough physical activity to protect their health.

Fortunately, research shows that as little as 30 minutes of moderate-intensity physical activity on most, and preferably all, days of the week helps to protect heart health. This level of activity can reduce your risk of heart disease as well as lower your chances of having a stroke, colon cancer, high blood pressure, diabetes, and other medical problems.

Examples of moderate activity are taking a brisk walk, light weight lifting, dancing, raking leaves, washing a car, house cleaning, or gardening. If you prefer, you can divide your 30-minute activity into shorter periods of at least 10 minutes each.

Get Moving

Regular physical activity is a powerful way to reduce your risk of heart disease. Physical activity directly helps prevent heart problems. Staying active also helps prevent and control high blood pressure, keep cholesterol levels healthy, and prevent and control diabetes. Plus, regular physical activity is a great way to help take off extra pounds—and keep them off.

Regular physical activity has a host of other health benefits. It may help prevent cancers of the breast, uterus, and colon. Staying active also strengthens the lungs, tones the muscles, keeps the joints in good condition, improves balance, and may slow bone loss. It also helps many people sleep better, feel less depressed, cope better with stress and anxiety, and generally feel more relaxed and energetic.

You can benefit from physical activity at any age. In fact, staying active can help prevent, delay, or improve many age-related health problems. As you grow older, weightbearing activities can be particularly helpful for strengthening bones and muscles, improving balance, and lowering the risk for serious falls. Good weightbearing activities include carrying groceries, walking, jogging, and lifting weights. (Start with 1- to 3-pound hand weights and gradually progress to heavier weights.)

Activities that promote balance and flexibility are also important. Practices such as tai chi and yoga can improve both balance and flexibility and can be done alternately with heart-healthy physical activities. Check with your health insurance plan, local recreation center, YWCA or YMCA, or adult education program for low-cost classes in your area.

A Little Activity Goes a Long Way

The good news is that to reap benefits from physical activity, you don't have to run a marathon—or anything close to it. To reduce the risk of disease, you only need to do about 30 minutes of moderate intensity physical activity on most, and preferably all, days of the week. If you're trying to manage your weight and prevent gradual, unhealthy weight gain, try to boost that level to approximately 60 minutes of moderate- to vigorous-intensity physical activity on most days of the week.

Brisk walking (3 to 4 miles per hour) is an easy way to help keep your heart healthy. One study, for example, showed that regular, brisk walking reduced the risk of heart attack by the same amount as more vigorous exercise, such as jogging. To make physical activity a pleasure rather than a chore, choose activities you enjoy. Ride a bike. Go hiking. Dance. Play ball. Swim. Keep doing physical tasks around the house and yard. Rake leaves. Climb stairs. Mulch your garden. Paint a room.

You can do an activity for 30 minutes at one time, or choose shorter periods of at least 10 minutes each. For example, you could spend 10 minutes walking on your lunch break, another 10 minutes raking leaves in the backyard, and another 10 minutes lifting weights. The important thing is to total about 30 minutes of activity each day. (To avoid weight gain, try to total about 60 minutes per day.)

414

No Sweat

Getting regular physical activity can be easy—especially if you take advantage of everyday opportunities to move around. For example:

- Use stairs—both up and down—instead of elevators. Start with one flight of stairs and gradually build up to more.

- Park a few blocks from the office or store and walk the rest of the way. If you take public transportation, get off a stop or two early and walk a few blocks.

- Instead of eating that rich dessert or extra snack, take a brisk stroll around the neighborhood.

- Do housework or yard work at a more vigorous pace.

- When you travel, walk around the train station, bus station, or airport rather than sitting and waiting.

- Keep moving while you watch TV. Lift hand weights, do some gentle yoga stretches, or pedal an exercise bike.

- Spend less time watching TV and using the computer.

Safe Moves

Some people should get medical advice before starting regular physical activity. Check with your doctor if you:

- are over 50 years old and not used to moderately energetic activity;

- currently have heart trouble or have had a heart attack;

- have a parent or sibling who developed heart disease at an early age; or

- have a chronic health problem, such as high blood pressure, diabetes, osteoporosis, or obesity.

Once you get started, keep these guidelines in mind:

Go slow. Before each activity session, allow a 5-minute period of slow-to-moderate movement to give your body a chance to limber up and get ready for more exercise. At the end of the warmup period, gradually increase your pace. Toward the end of your activity, take another 5 minutes to cool down with a slower, less energetic pace.

415

It's best to wait until after your activity to do stretching exercises. Listen to your body. A certain amount of stiffness is normal at first. But if you hurt a joint or pull a muscle, stop the activity for several days to avoid more serious injury. Rest and over-the-counter painkillers can heal most minor muscle and joint problems.

Check the weather report. Dress appropriately for hot, humid days and for cold days. In all weather, drink lots of water before, during, and after physical activity.

Pay attention to warning signals. While physical activity can strengthen your heart, some types of activity may worsen existing heart problems. Warning signals include sudden dizziness, cold sweat, paleness, fainting, or pain or pressure in your upper body just after doing a physical activity. If you notice any of these signs, call your doctor right away.

Use caution. If you're concerned about the safety of your surroundings, pair up with a buddy for outdoor activities. Walk, bike, or jog during daylight hours.

Stay the course. Unless you have to stop your activity for a health reason, stick with it. If you feel like giving up because you think you're not going as fast or as far as you should, set smaller, short-term goals for yourself. If you find yourself becoming bored, try doing an activity with a friend. Or switch to another activity. The tremendous health benefits of regular, moderate-intensity physical activity are well worth the effort.

Section 46.2

What You Can Do to Exercise If Heart Disease Has Slowed You Down

"Getting Real about How Much to Exercise: What You Can Do If Heart Disease Has Slowed You Down" is reprinted with permission from The Cleveland Clinic Heart Center, http://www.clevelandclinic.org/heartcenter. © 2004 The Cleveland Clinic Foundation, revised May 2006. All rights reserved. Reviewed by Dr. Gordon Blackburn, Program Director of Cardiac Rehabilitation, Section of Preventive Cardiology.

You probably are aware of the benefits that regular exercise has for the heart. Many studies show that exercise positively affects heart rate, blood pressure, and the body's oxygen use, reducing fatal and non-fatal heart attacks as well as other cardiac problems such as arrhythmias (heart-rhythm disturbances) and thrombosis (clotting). Sound, scientific research shows us that exercise's health benefits include better control of diabetes, obesity, and cholesterol levels. Regular aerobic physical activity has repeatedly been shown to reduce the risk of future heart attacks in both those with and without documented heart disease.

Based on such convincing data, the American Heart Association (AHA) has reached a consensus on what constitutes a healthful amount of exercise. The guidelines call for a minimum of 30 minutes (ideally 60 minutes) of aerobic physical activity performed at moderate intensity, either in one continuous period or in intervals of at least 10-minutes duration on most—preferably all—days of the week. This is the amount called for to reduce the risk of coronary disease. It is equivalent to briskly walking at least 1.5 miles per day or raking leaves for half an hour. Although any increase in activity level imparts benefit, recent research suggests that a significant cardiovascular protection is achieved when at least 1,000 calories are expended in exercise per week (equivalent of walking approximately 10 miles a week). Greater cardiovascular protection is gained if the caloric expenditure increases up to 2,000 kcal /week (equivalent of walking approximately 20 miles/week = 4 miles a day/5 times a week or 3 miles a day, 6 to 7

417

days a week). Beyond this level the cardioprotective benefit of exercise plateaus.

Such guidelines may seem daunting, particularly if you have already been diagnosed with heart disease. Even without a specific health challenge, many of us are so busy that it's hard to fit the recommended amount of exercise into our day. But Cleveland Clinic exercise physiologist Gordon Blackburn, Ph.D., says giving up is not the answer. "Even if you can't meet the AHA requirements, exercising still will give you benefits," he notes. "Exercising a little bit each day is better than not exercising at all."

"In a way, it's kind of the same situation as with smoking," Dr. Blackburn continues. "For example, if you must smoke, smoking three cigarettes a day is better than smoking three packs a day, even though the best thing for your health would be to quit completely." If you are unable to follow the AHA guidelines because of cardiac problems, Dr. Blackburn suggests getting what's called an "exercise prescription." Exercise can be—in fact should be—tailored to your own individual situation, just like other health programs. After all, a patient with a low-density-lipoprotein (LDL) cholesterol of 140 mg/dl is not prescribed the same medication dose as someone with an LDL cholesterol of 180 mg/dl.

You can get an exercise prescription from a cardiac rehabilitation specialist, usually an exercise physiologist. He or she, in consultation with your cardiologist, can put together a highly individualized program that takes into consideration your specific cardiac problem, your age, and stage of recovery. For example, someone who has mild-to-moderate heart failure may be advised to start a walking program but to walk only a few blocks or just a few minutes and repeat the activity several times a day. Someone else who had bypass surgery a couple years ago and participated in a cardiac rehabilitation program afterward and continues to do well may be advised to perform a more vigorous activity program of longer duration.

"We try to set exercise prescriptions based on accepted guidelines," Dr. Blackburn explains, "but at the same time, we work with the patient to help get them to their optimal activity level over time. The patients find that, as they follow their prescription, they get stronger and feel better as a result of the exercise. This allows us to increase the amount and duration of exercise as their health improves."

Don't let poor health or lack of time rob you of a plan for physical exercise. The improvements you'll experience—in physical, mental, and emotional health—are well worth the effort.

418

Chapter 47

Physical Activity Recommendations for Stroke Survivors

Exercises and Recommendations

The ability to move around is basic to the level of independence you can achieve and maintain after a stroke. Walking, bending, and stretching are forms of exercise that can help strengthen your body and keep it flexible.

Types of Exercise

Mild exercise, which should be undertaken every day, can take the form of a short walk or a simple activity like sweeping the floor. Stretching exercises, such as extending the arms or bending the torso, should be done regularly. Moving weakened or paralyzed parts can be done while seated or lying down. Swimming is another beneficial exercise if the pool is accessible and a helper is available.

A physical or occupational therapist can help with such problems as muscle tightness, low endurance, or the inability to sit up from a lying position. The exercise program should be written down, with illustrations and guidelines for a helper as necessary.

Fatigue

Fatigue while exercising is to be expected. Like everyone else, you will have "good" and "bad" days. You can modify these programs to accommodate for fatigue or other conditions. Avoid overexertion and pain. However, it may be necessary to tolerate some discomfort to make progress.

Sample Exercise Programs

There are two exercise programs on the following pages. The first is for the person whose physical abilities have been mildly affected by the stroke. The second is for those with greater limitations. If you're not sure which one is appropriate, consult the profile that precedes each program.

All of the exercises may be performed alone if you are able to do so safely. However, for many stroke survivors, it is advisable for someone to stand nearby while an exercise session is in progress. Your caregiver should watch for errors in judgment that could affect safety. For instance, some stroke survivors are not aware that their balance is unsteady, nor can they tell left from right. Others may have lost the ability to read the exercise instructions, or may need assistance to remember a full sequence of movements.

In general, each exercise is performed five to ten times daily, unless otherwise directed. The exercise session should be scheduled for a time of day when you feel alert and well, not at a "down" time when you have less energy. You might have these ups and downs frequently. If the exercises are too tiring, divide them into two sessions—perhaps once in the morning and again in the afternoon.

Because the effects of stroke vary, it is impossible to devise a single exercise program suitable for everyone. The two programs detailed here are general and are intended to serve as a guide. You should consult an occupational therapist and/or physical therapist, who can help in selecting the specific exercises that will benefit you, and who will provide instruction for both you and your caregiver.

For referral to an occupational or physical therapist, consult your physician or contact a home health agency, a family service agency, or the physical therapy department in your community hospital. You may also try contacting the American Occupational Therapy Association or the American Physical Therapy Association for a referral in your area.

As with any exercise program, consult with your physician and/or therapist before beginning this program. If any exercises are too difficult and cause pain or increased stiffness in your limbs, do not do them.

Exercise Program 1: For Those Mildly Affected by Stroke

If you were mildly affected by stroke, you may still have some degree of weakness in the affected arm and leg, but generally have some ability to control your movements. Some obvious stiffness or muscle spasms may be evident, particularly with fatigue or stress.

You may be able to walk without assistance from a person, but may use a walker, cane, or brace. For managing longer distances or uneven terrain, you may require some minimal assistance from another person, a more supportive walking aid, or a wheelchair.

Abnormalities may be present when you walk, but may be corrected by exercise and by fitting shoes with lifts or wedges. A prescription for these shoe modifications can be obtained from a physician following evaluation by a physical therapist. You can usually negotiate stairs with or without handrails, with a helper close by or with very minimal assistance. The following exercises can help you:

- require less assistance for stair climbing;
- move more steadily when you walk;
- improve balance and endurance;
- strengthen and refine movement patterns; and
- improve the coordination and speed of movement necessary for fine motor skills, such as fastening buttons or tying shoelaces.

Clothing that does not restrict movement is appropriate for exercising. It is not necessary to wear shorts. Leisure clothing such as sweat suits or jogging suits is appropriate. Sturdy, well-constructed shoes with non-skid soles, such as athletic shoes, are recommended at all times. It is important that your foot on the affected side be checked periodically for reddened areas, pressure marks, swelling, or blisters—especially when there is poor sensation or a lack of sensation. Reddened areas and pressure marks should be reported to a physician or physical therapist.

The exercises can be performed on the floor, on a firm mattress, or on any appropriate supportive surface.

Exercise 1: To strengthen the muscles that stabilize the shoulder.

1. Lie on your back with your arms resting at your sides.

2. Keeping your elbow straight, lift your affected arm to shoulder level with your hand pointing to the ceiling.

3. Raise your hand toward the ceiling, lifting your shoulder blade from the floor.

4. Hold for three to five seconds, and then relax, allowing your shoulder blade to return to the floor.

5. Slowly repeat the reaching motion several times.

6. Lower your arm to rest by your side.

Exercise 2: To strengthen the shoulder muscles as well as those which straighten the elbow.

1. Lying on your back, grasp one end of an elasticized band in each hand with enough tension to provide light resistance to the exercise, but without causing undue strain.

2. To start, place both hands alongside the unaffected hip, keeping your elbows as straight as possible.

3. Move your affected arm upward in a diagonal direction, reaching out to the side, above your head, keeping your elbow straight. Your unaffected arm should remain at your side throughout the exercise. If it is too difficult to keep the elbow straight, the exercise can be done with the elbow bent.

4. During the exercise, stretch the band so that it provides resistance.

Elasticized bands are marketed as Thera-band®. They are available in varying strengths (color-coded) to provide progressive resistance. Initially, a three- or four-foot length band—perhaps with the ends knotted together to improve grip—is sufficient for the exercise. To increase resistance as strength improves, the next density of Thera-Band can be purchased, or two or more bands of the original density can be used at once. Thera-Band can be obtained from a surgical supply house. Similar elastic bands or cords are also available at many sporting goods stores where exercise equipment is sold.

Exercise 3: To strengthen the muscles which straighten the elbow.

1. Lie on your back with your arms resting at your sides and a rolled towel under the affected elbow.

2. Bend affected elbow and move your hand up toward your shoulder. Keep your elbow resting on the towel.

3. Hold for a few seconds.

4. Straighten your elbow and hold.

5. Slowly repeat several times.

Exercise 4: To improve hip control in preparation for walking activities.

1. Start with your unaffected leg flat on the floor and your affected leg bent.

2. Lift your affected foot and cross your affected leg over the other leg.

3. Lift your affected foot and uncross, resuming the position of step 2.

4. Repeat the crossing and uncrossing motion several times.

Exercise 5 : To enhance hip and knee control.

1. Start with your knees bent, feet resting on the floor.

2. Slowly slide the heel of your affected leg down so that the leg straightens.

3. Slowly bring the heel of your affected leg along the floor, returning to the starting position. Keep your heel in contact with the floor throughout the exercise.

4. Your foot will slide more smoothly if you do this exercise without shoes.

Exercise 6: To improve control of knee motions for walking.

1. Lie on your unaffected side with the bottom knee bent for stability and your affected arm placed in front for support.

2. Starting with your affected leg straight, bend your affected knee, bringing the heel toward your buttocks, then return to the straightened position.

3. Concentrate on bending and straightening your knee while keeping your hip straight.

Exercise 7: To improve weight shift and control for proper walking technique.

1. Start with your knees bent, feet flat on the floor and knees close together.

2. Lift your hips from the floor and keep them raised in the air.

3. Slowly twist your hips side to side. Return to center and lower your hips to the floor.

4. Rest. Repeat motion.

Note: This exercise may be difficult for some stroke survivors and it may aggravate back problems. Do not do it if you experience pain.

Exercise 8: To improve balance, weight shift, and control to prepare for walking activities.

1. The starting position is on your hands and knees. Weight should be evenly distributed on both arms and both legs.

2. Rock in a diagonal direction back toward your right heel as far as possible, then as far forward toward your left hand as possible.

3. Repeat motion several times, slowly rocking as far as possible in each direction.

4. Return to center.

5. Rock in a diagonal direction back toward your left heel and forward toward your right hand. Move as far as possible in each direction slowly.

Note: For safety, an assistant may be nearby to prevent loss of balance. This position may not be appropriate or safe for elderly stroke survivors. Consult your doctor and/or physical therapist before attempting this exercise.

Exercise 9: To simulate proper weight shift and knee control necessary for walking.

1. Stand with your unaffected side next to a countertop or other firm surface. Rest your unaffected arm on the surface for support.

2. Lift your unaffected foot from the floor so that you are standing on your affected leg.

3. Slowly bend and straighten the leg on which you are standing through a small range of motion. Try to move smoothly, not allowing your knee to buckle when you bend, or to snap back when you straighten.

4. Repeat the knee bending and straightening several times, slowly.

Exercise 10: To simulate proper weight shift while strengthening hip and pelvis muscles.

1. Stand facing a countertop or other firm surface with both hands on the surface for support.

2. Shift your weight onto your right leg and lift your left leg out to the side. Keep your back and knee straight.

3. Return to center with both feet on the floor.

4. Shift your weight onto your left leg and lift your right leg out to the side, keeping your back and knee straight.

5. Repeat several times, alternating lifts.

Exercise Program 2: For the Person Moderately Affected by Stroke

If you were moderately affected by your stroke, you may use a wheelchair most of the time. You are probably able to walk—at least around the house—with the aid of another person or by using a walking aid. A short leg brace may be needed to help control foot drop or inward turning of the foot. A sling may be used to help support the arm and aid in shoulder positioning for controlling pain. Your affected arm and leg may be stiff or may assume a spastic posture that is difficult to control. The toe may turn inward or the foot may drag. When walking, you may lead with the unaffected side, leaving the other side behind. Often there are balance problems and difficulty shifting weight toward the affected side.

The purpose of this exercise program is to:

*   promote flexibility and relaxation of muscles on the affected side;

*   help return to more normal movement;

- improve balance and coordination;
- decrease pain and stiffness; and
- maintain range of motion in the affected arm and leg.

For the Stroke Survivor

Begin with exercises done lying on your back, then move on to those performed lying on your unaffected side, then sitting, then standing. Make sure that the surface on which you lie is firm and provides good support. Take your time when you exercise. Don't rush the movements or strain to complete them.

Note: The exercises can be performed on the floor, on a firm mattress, or on any appropriate supporting surface.

For the Helper

There may be no need to assist the stroke survivor in the exercises, but you should be nearby during the exercise session. If the stroke survivor has difficulty reading or remembering the sequence of movements, you can hold the illustration up to where it can be seen or repeat the instructions one by one. You can also offer physical assistance and encouragement when needed.

Any clothing that does not restrict movement is appropriate for exercising. It is not necessary to wear shorts. Leisure clothing such as sweat suits or jogging suits are appropriate. Sturdy, well-constructed athletic shoes with non-skid rubber soles are recommended at all times. It is important that the stroke survivor's foot on the affected side be checked periodically for reddened areas, pressure marks, swelling, or blisters—especially when there is poor sensation or a lack of sensation. Reddened areas and pressure marks should be reported to a physician or physical therapist.

Exercise 1: To enhance shoulder motion and possibly prevent shoulder pain.

1. Lie on your back on a firm bed. Interlace your fingers with your hands resting on your stomach.

2. Slowly raise your arms to shoulder level, keeping your elbows straight.

3. Return your hands to resting position on your stomach. If pain occurs, it may be reduced by working within the range of motion

that is relatively pain-free, then going up to the point where pain is felt. The arm should not be forced if pain is excessive, but effort should be made to daily increase the range of pain-free motion.

Exercise 2: To maintain shoulder motion (may be useful for someone who has difficulty rolling over in bed).

1. Lie on your back on a firm bed. Interlace your fingers, with your hands resting on your stomach.

2. Slowly raise your hands directly over your chest, straightening your elbows.

3. Slowly move your hands to one side and then the other.

4. When all repetitions have been completed, bend your elbows and return your hands to resting position on your stomach.

If shoulder pain occurs, move only to the point where it begins to hurt. If the pain persists, don't do this exercise.

Exercise 3: To promote motion in the pelvis, hip, and knee (can help to reduce stiffness and is also useful for rolling over and moving in bed).

1. Lie on your back on a firm bed. Keep your interlaced fingers resting on your stomach.

2. Bend your knees and put your feet flat on the bed.

3. Holding your knees tightly together, slowly move them as far to the right as possible. Return to center.

4. Slowly move your knees as far as possible to the left, still keeping them together. Return to center. The helper may provide assistance or verbal cues to help you keep your knees together during this exercise.

Exercise 4: To improve motion at the hip and knee, simulating the movements needed for walking (can be useful when moving toward the edge of the bed before coming to a sitting position).

1. Lie on your unaffected side, with your legs together.

2. Bend and move your affected knee as far as possible toward your chest. You may need your helper's assistance to support the leg you're exercising.

3. Return to starting position.

Exercise 5: To strengthen the muscles that straighten the elbow (necessary for getting up from a lying position).

1. Sitting on a firm mattress or sofa, put your affected forearm flat on the surface with your palm facing down if possible. You may want to place a firm pillow under your elbow.

2. Slowly lean your weight onto your bent elbow. You may need your helper's assistance to maintain your balance.

3. Push your hand down against the support surface, straightening your elbow and sitting more upright. (Assistance may be required to prevent sudden elbow collapse.)

4. Slowly allow your elbow to bend, returning your forearm to the support surface.

5. Work back and forth between the two extremes (completely bent or completely straight) in a slow, rhythmical manner.

Note: This exercise should not be performed if your shoulder is not yet stable and/or will not support your upper body weight. Consult your doctor and/or physical therapist before attempting this exercise.

Exercise 6: To reduce stiffness in the trunk and promote the body rotation needed for walking.

1. Sit on a firm straight chair with both feet flat on the floor. If necessary, a firm mattress, sofa, or wheelchair may be used.

2. Interlace your fingers.

3. Bend forward and reach with your hands toward the outside of your right foot, rotating your trunk. Only individuals with good balance who can sit fairly independently should do this exercise. If balance is impaired, an assistant may stand in front, guiding the arms through the motions.

4. Move your hands upward in a diagonal direction toward your left shoulder, keeping your elbows as straight as possible.

Only individuals with good balance who can sit fairly independently should do this exercise. If balance is impaired, an assistant may stand in front, guiding the arms through the motions.

5. Repeat the motions, moving your hands from your left foot to your right shoulder.

Exercise 7: Movements needed to rise from a sitting position.

1. Sit on a firm chair that has been placed against the wall to prevent slipping.

2. Interlace your fingers. Reach forward with your hands.

3. With your feet slightly apart and your hips at the edge of the seat, lean forward, lifting your hips up slightly from the seat. In a progression of the exercise, try to rise to a complete standing position and return to sitting. However, this should only be done by someone with good balance who can come to a standing position safely.

4. Slowly return to sitting.

Exercise 8: To maintain the ankle motion needed for walking (also maintains motion at the wrist and elbow).

1. Stand at arm's length from the wall, knees straight, feet planted slightly apart and flat on the floor with equal weight on both feet.

2. With your unaffected hand, hold your affected hand in place against the wall at chest level.

3. Slowly bend your elbows, leaning into the wall. This places a stretch on the back of your lower legs. Keep your heels on the floor.

4. Straighten your elbows, pushing your body away from the wall.

Note: If the stroke survivor's affected arm is very involved, he or she may find this exercise too difficult. Consult your doctor and/or physical therapist before attempting this exercise.

Walking Aids

There are four types of walking aids, which might be helpful for someone who has had a stroke. Recommendations for the appropriate device and the progression to less supportive equipment should be made by a physical therapist. Training in safety procedures and proper technique for use is essential.

The walker, which provides the most support, requires the use of two hands. It can be fitted with wheels if it is too difficult to lift between steps.

The hemi-walker, less supportive than the walker, is used with one hand on the unaffected side of the body. It has a strong base of support and is quite stable, but requires a large, open walking space for maneuvering around objects.

The quad cane, a four-footed device, provides a broad base of support, although less than either the walker or the hemi-walker. It is recommended for individuals with fairly good balance and weight-shifting ability who require additional stability.

The standard cane provides minimal support for the person who needs only occasional assistance with balance, or while walking on uneven terrain, or when fatigued.

Getting up from a Fall

Before attempting to help a person stand up after a fall, make sure they have not been injured. If there are any cuts, bruises, or painful areas, make the person comfortable on the floor while you get help. Do not attempt to move the individual until help arrives.

Most falls, however, do not result in injury. The steps that follow outline a recommended method for getting from the floor onto a chair. The individual who has fallen may need assistance, but should be able to rise using this technique.

1. Assume a side-sitting position with the unaffected side close to a heavy chair or other object that will not move.

2. Place the unaffected forearm on the seat of the chair and lean on the elbow or hand. Shift weight forward onto your knees and lift your hips until you are in a kneeling position.

3. Supporting yourself with your unaffected arm, bring your unaffected foot forward and place it flat on the floor. Some assistance may be required to keep the affected limb in the kneeling position while placing the unaffected one in the position illustrated.

4. Lift yourself up by pushing with your unaffected arm and leg. Twist your hips toward the chair and sit on the seat.

Chapter 48

Questions and Answers about Arthritis, Joint Problems, and Exercise

This chapter answers general questions about arthritis and exercise. The amount and form of exercise recommended for each individual will vary depending on which joints are involved, the amount of inflammation, how stable the joints are, and whether a joint replacement procedure has been done. A skilled physician who is knowledgeable about the medical and rehabilitation needs of people with arthritis, working with a physical therapist also familiar with the needs of people with arthritis, can design an exercise plan for each patient.

What is arthritis?

There are over 100 forms of arthritis and other rheumatic diseases. These diseases may cause pain, stiffness, and swelling in joints and other supporting structures of the body such as muscles, tendons, ligaments, and bones. Some forms can also affect other parts of the body, including various internal organs.

Many people use the word arthritis to refer to all rheumatic diseases. However, the word literally means joint inflammation; that is, swelling, redness, heat, and pain caused by tissue injury or disease in the joint. The many different kinds of arthritis comprise just a portion of the rheumatic diseases. Some rheumatic diseases are described as

From the booklet "Questions and Answers about Arthritis and Exercise," by the National Institute of Arthritis and Musculoskeletal and Skin Diseases (NIAMS, www.niams.nih.gov), NIH Publication No. 01-4855, May 2001. Reviewed by David A. Cooke, MD, on June 12, 2006.

connective tissue diseases because they affect the body's connective tissue—the supporting framework of the body and its internal organs. Others are known as autoimmune diseases because they are caused by a problem in which the immune system harms the body's own healthy tissues. Examples of some rheumatic diseases are:

- osteoarthritis;
- rheumatoid arthritis;
- fibromyalgia;
- systemic lupus erythematosus;
- scleroderma;
- juvenile rheumatoid arthritis;
- ankylosing spondylitis; and
- gout.

In this chapter, the term arthritis will be used as a general term to refer to arthritis and other rheumatic diseases.

Should people with arthritis exercise?

Yes. Studies have shown that exercise helps people with arthritis in many ways. Exercise reduces joint pain and stiffness and increases flexibility, muscle strength, cardiac fitness, and endurance. It also helps with weight reduction and contributes to an improved sense of well-being.

How does exercise fit into a treatment plan for people with arthritis?

Exercise is one part of a comprehensive arthritis treatment plan. Treatment plans also may include rest and relaxation, proper diet, medication, and instruction about proper use of joints and ways to conserve energy (that is, not waste motion) as well as the use of pain relief methods.

What types of exercise are most suitable for someone with arthritis?

Three types of exercise are best for people with arthritis:

- **Range-of-motion exercises** (e.g., dance) help maintain normal joint movement and relieve stiffness. This type of exercise helps maintain or increase flexibility.

- **Strengthening exercises** (e.g., weight training) help keep or increase muscle strength. Strong muscles help support and protect joints affected by arthritis.

- **Aerobic or endurance exercises** (e.g., bicycle riding) improve cardiovascular fitness, help control weight, and improve overall function. Weight control can be important to people who have arthritis because extra weight puts extra pressure on many joints. Some studies show that aerobic exercise can reduce inflammation in some joints.

Most health clubs and community centers offer exercise programs for people with physical limitations.

How does a person with arthritis start an exercise program?

People with arthritis should discuss exercise options with their doctors and other health care providers. Most doctors recommend exercise for their patients. Many people with arthritis begin with easy, range-of-motion exercises and low-impact aerobics. People with arthritis can participate in a variety of, but not all, sports and exercise programs. The doctor will know which, if any, sports are off-limits.

The doctor may have suggestions about how to get started or may refer the patient to a physical therapist. It is best to find a physical therapist who has experience working with people who have arthritis. The therapist will design an appropriate home exercise program and teach clients about pain-relief methods, proper body mechanics (placement of the body for a given task, such as lifting a heavy box), joint protection, and conserving energy.

What are some tips on getting started?

- Discuss exercise plans with your doctor.
- Start with supervision from a physical therapist or qualified athletic trainer.
- Apply heat to sore joints (optional; many people with arthritis start their exercise program this way).
- Stretch and warm up with range-of-motion exercises.
- Start strengthening exercises slowly with small weights (a 1- or 2-pound weight can make a big difference).
- Progress slowly.

- Use cold packs after exercising (optional; many people with arthritis complete their exercise routine this way).

- Add aerobic exercise.

- Consider appropriate recreational exercise (after doing range-of-motion, strengthening, and aerobic exercise). Fewer injuries to joints affected by arthritis occur during recreational exercise if it is preceded by range-of-motion, strengthening, and aerobic exercise that gets your body in the best condition possible.

- Ease off if joints become painful, inflamed, or red, and work with your doctor to find the cause and eliminate it.

- Choose the exercise program you enjoy most and make it a habit.

What are some pain relief methods for people with arthritis?

There are known methods to help stop pain for short periods of time. This temporary relief can make it easier for people who have arthritis to exercise. The doctor or physical therapist can suggest a method that is best for each patient. The following methods have worked for many people:

- **Moist heat** supplied by warm towels, hot packs, a bath, or a shower can be used at home for 15 to 20 minutes three times a day to relieve symptoms. A health professional can use short waves, microwaves, and ultrasound to deliver deep heat to non-inflamed joint areas. Deep heat is not recommended for patients with acutely inflamed joints. Deep heat is often used around the shoulder to relax tight tendons prior to stretching exercises.

- **Cold** supplied by a bag of ice or frozen vegetables wrapped in a towel helps to stop pain and reduce swelling when used for 10 to 15 minutes at a time. It is often used for acutely inflamed joints. People who have Raynaud phenomenon should not use this method.

- **Hydrotherapy (water therapy)** can decrease pain and stiffness. Exercising in a large pool may be easier because water takes some weight off painful joints. Community centers, YMCAs, and YWCAs have water exercise classes developed for people with arthritis. Some patients also find relief from the heat and movement provided by a whirlpool.

- **Mobilization therapies** include traction (gentle, steady pulling), massage, and manipulation (using the hands to restore normal movement to stiff joints). When done by a trained professional, these methods can help control pain and increase joint motion and muscle and tendon flexibility.

- **TENS (transcutaneous electrical nerve stimulation) and biofeedback** are two additional methods that may provide some pain relief, but many patients find that they cost too much money and take too much time. In TENS, an electrical shock is transmitted through electrodes placed on the skin's surface. TENS machines cost between $80 and $800. The inexpensive units are fine. Patients can wear them during the day and turn them off and on as needed for pain control.

- **Relaxation therapy** also helps reduce pain. Patients can learn to release the tension in their muscles to relieve pain. Physical therapists may be able to teach relaxation techniques. The Arthritis Foundation has a self-help course that includes relaxation therapy. Health spas and vacation resorts sometimes have special relaxation courses.

- **Acupuncture** is a traditional Chinese method of pain relief. A medically qualified acupuncturist places needles in certain sites. Researchers believe that the needles stimulate deep sensory nerves that tell the brain to release natural painkillers (endorphins). Acupressure is similar to acupuncture, but pressure is applied to the acupuncture sites instead of using needles.

How often should people with arthritis exercise?

- Range-of-motion exercises can be done daily and should be done at least every other day.

- Strengthening exercises should be done every other day unless you have severe pain or swelling in your joints.

- Endurance exercises should be done for 20 to 30 minutes three times a week unless you have severe pain or swelling in your joints. According to the American College of Rheumatology, 20- to 30-minute exercise routines can be performed in increments of 10 minutes over the course of a day.

What type of strengthening program is best?

This varies depending on personal preference, the type of arthritis involved, and how active the inflammation is. Strengthening one's muscles can help take the burden off painful joints. Strength training can be done with small free weights, exercise machines, isometrics, elastic bands, and resistive water exercises. Correct positioning is critical, because if done incorrectly, strengthening exercises can cause muscle tears, more pain, and more joint swelling.

Are there different exercises for people with different types of arthritis?

There are many types of arthritis. Experienced doctors, physical therapists, and occupational therapists can recommend exercises that are particularly helpful for a specific type of arthritis. Doctors and therapists also know specific exercises for particularly painful joints.

There may be exercises that are off-limits for people with a particular type of arthritis or when joints are swollen and inflamed. People with arthritis should discuss their exercise plans with a doctor. Doctors who treat people with arthritis include rheumatologists, orthopaedic surgeons, general practitioners, family doctors, internists, and rehabilitation specialists (physiatrists).

How much exercise is too much?

Most experts agree that if exercise causes pain that lasts for more than 1 hour, it is too strenuous. People with arthritis should work with their physical therapist or doctor to adjust their exercise program when they notice any of the following signs of strenuous exercise:

- unusual or persistent fatigue
- increased weakness
- decreased range of motion
- increased joint swelling
- continuing pain (pain that lasts more than 1 hour after exercising)

Should someone with rheumatoid arthritis continue to exercise during a general flare? How about during a local joint flare?

It is appropriate to put joints gently through their full range of motion once a day, with periods of rest, during acute systemic flares or local joint flares. Patients can talk to their doctor about how much rest is best during general or joint flares.

Chapter 49

Fitness Information for People with Chronic Pain and Fatigue

Chapter Contents

Section 49.1

Starting an Exercise Program with Fibromyalgia

Reprinted with permission from the National Fibromyalgia Association, http://www.fmaware.com. This document is undated; accessed August 15, 2006.

When you suffer from fibromyalgia (FM) or an overlapping condition, just the thought of physical fitness may be an exercise in frustration and pain. Your muscles already hurt and you feel exhausted. How can you even consider exercise when just getting out of bed feels like climbing a mountain? The answer is: very carefully. But exercise is possible for many patients if it is begun correctly. And the benefits may be greater than you thought possible.

In her essay, "Fibromyalgia: Improving through Fitness," Deborah Barrett writes of a doctor with fibromyalgia who once told her: "You can have weak muscles that hurt, or strong muscles that hurt." Although exercise is in no way a cure for the pain and fatigue of fibromyalgia, strengthening our muscles and increasing our endurance may actually allow us to do more and feel better.

Research has repeatedly shown that FM sufferers who exercise experience a decrease in their symptoms. This data should not be used as evidence that FM is "all in the head," or to imply that if FM patients would only get up and get moving, then they wouldn't be ill. Exercise can easily be damaging for some patients, if it is done without gradually building up tolerance. Especially in people with chronic fatigue syndrome, for whom the diagnosis is in fact defined in part by a difficulty to exercise (i.e. post-exertional malaise), any physical activity must be approached extremely cautiously, and for some patients may be contraindicated.

But for many of us, gentle exercise can be helpful. Starting an exercise program should be done under supervision of a doctor who is familiar with FM and can monitor your condition, noting any exacerbation. Nevertheless, you are the one who will have the most essential role in keeping track of your progress and adjusting your program.

So where do we begin? Following are some essential strategies in starting a successful exercise program.

Start Slowly

With fibromyalgia, you cannot start too small. For a healthy person, the recommended fitness program is at least 20 minutes of aerobic activity three times a week. For many people with FM, 20 minutes might as well be 20 hours. Although many of us have memories of what it felt like to "get in shape" before we were sick, FM makes the process completely different. There is no reason to feel ashamed of starting slowly; remember that you are limited not by laziness or a lack of desire, but by a disease that is severely debilitating. Make sure that your expectations are realistic. One physical therapist once told me, "anything is better than nothing." If you're moving more today than yesterday, that's progress! For some of you, it may be a workout to walk to the mailbox. That's a great place to start; after doing that for a few days, try walking a few steps past it.

Walking is a great form of exercise because it requires no special equipment, and it is easy to alter the length and intensity of the exercise. Start with a level you know you can tolerate without an exacerbation in your symptoms. If you know you can walk for five minutes, but any longer is pushing it, then start there. After you are consistently successful for several days, you can slowly increase the length of the exercise session—add a minute to your walk. Resist the temptation to increase too quickly; the goal is to do some exercise while minimizing any flare in your symptoms. According to Barrett, "The golden rule is to moderate your activity so you can exercise again two days later. If you hurt too much, cut back!" The most important thing is to listen to your body.

Tracking Your Progress

Create a personalized report sheet to keep track of your exercise program and your reactions to it. It's helpful to include other factors that might be affecting how you feel, such as medications or quality of sleep. Be sure to note the exercise you're doing and how you feel both during and afterward. It's quite common to feel fine while exercising but then be completely wiped out a day or two later. If this happens, try cutting back. Careful record keeping will make it possible for you to adjust your program and monitor your progress. As the weeks and months pass, long-term improvements will show how much you've accomplished and help keep you motivated.

Coping with the Pain and Fatigue

Even healthy people who have not exercised in a long time experience muscle soreness when beginning an exercise program. Initially, you are likely to hurt more than the average healthy person and that pain may last longer. In one article about exercising with a chronic pain condition, it said "No matter what you do, you're going to be in pain." But the article went on to say that while the pain may increase at first, in the long term it's worth it if it allows us to participate more fully in our lives and/or experience an ultimate decrease in symptoms.

Since increased muscle soreness can be excruciating to FM sufferers with already high levels of pain, it's essential to avail yourself of any available strategies to make yourself feel more comfortable and make it possible to keep going. Make sure you stretch your muscles before and after exercise, which can decrease the likelihood of muscle soreness. Applying heat, using muscle relaxants and analgesics, warm baths or hot-tub soaks, and relaxation exercises may be helpful tools in relieving pain. Barrett points out that you should "keep in mind that although our muscles may hurt, using them will not injure them. Post-exercise soreness will decrease over time, especially if you respond to your body's signals and pace yourself."

Getting extra rest can also help make exercise possible. I find that it is impossible for me to exercise if my general activity level is too high. But if I'm resting during the day, I find that some exercise is tolerable.

Most of all, remember that each of us is different. Our experience with exercise will vary according to age and severity of symptoms. Listen to your body, and keep adjusting until you find something that works for you. As Deborah Barrett writes, "In the worst case, you will be stronger, in better shape, and look better . . . and still hurt. Most likely, however, physical fitness will decrease your pain and increase your abilities. It has for me."

Section 49.2

Chronic Fatigue: Exercise for Energy

Chronic fatigue is more than just feeling tired all the time. For those who suffer from this mysterious syndrome, it can be a constant battle simply to get out of bed in the morning.

Symptoms of chronic fatigue syndrome (CFS) include unexplained fatigue lasting 30 days or more; flu-like symptoms such as a sore throat, generalized muscle pains, headaches, and swollen lymph nodes; difficulty concentrating; and sensitivity to bright light.

CFS was dubbed the yuppie flu in the 1980s and, despite the fact that it has been recognized as a legitimate, often debilitating illness, it is still met with scorn and disbelief.

There is no cure for CFS. For some people, it simply goes away, while others are debilitated by it for many years. Because the cause is largely unexplainable, treatment for CFS focuses primarily on relieving symptoms.

Low Blood Pressure Can Bring You Down

One of the latest theories proposed to explain CFS is that individuals who suffer from this condition also may have extremely low blood pressure. Researchers at Johns Hopkins University found that 22 of 23 CFS patients also had a disorder called neurally mediated hypotension (NMH). People with NMH get dizzy from standing up too quickly or from standing for extended periods of time, signaling that not enough blood is reaching the brain.

When treated for NMH for six months (either with medication or by increasing salt and fluid intake), nine of the 22 CFS patients said that all or nearly all of their CFS symptoms had disappeared; another seven said that their symptoms had improved.

441

A Novel Approach

But what about those who have normal blood pressure, but still fight persistent fatigue? Here's an interesting proposition: Is it possible to treat chronic fatigue with exercise?

Some researchers think so. A recent review of existing research on CFS explored the possibility of using physical activity programs to treat this puzzling condition. The findings are intriguing, if not conclusive.

Many people with CFS claim that they are too tired to exercise. Measurements of strength, exercise capacity, and muscle function, however, suggest that CFS patients are not much weaker than the controls (people without CFS) they are compared to in research studies. This suggests that their capacity to exercise is greater than they may perceive. But telling someone who feels unable to get out of bed to exercise is probably an exercise in futility.

Exercise for Energy

Still, physicians such as Dr. Neil Gordon, author of *Chronic Fatigue: Your Complete Exercise Guide,* view exercise as a form of medication and an integral part of rehabilitation from CFS. Exercise programs for people with CFS are not much different than any other comprehensive exercise program: Cardiovascular, strengthening, and range-of-motion training should all be addressed.

The primary difference is the pace and degree of progression: CFS patients need time to build their strength and adapt to the increased demands of exercise. And, as with any other physical condition, CFS patients should consult with their physicians before beginning an exercise program.

Exercise Your Options

People with CFS feel limited by their condition to enjoy the benefits of an active life. But as anyone who exercises will tell you, expending energy brings about increased energy in return. The same may hold true for individuals who are plagued by the unexplained tiredness of CFS.

Chapter 50

Exercise and Cancer

Chapter Contents

Section 50.1

Physical Activity and the Risk of Cancer

Excerpted from "Questions and Answers: Physical Activity and Cancer,"
a National Cancer Institute (NCI) Fact Sheet, March 29, 2004.

Researchers are learning that physical activity can also affect the
risk of cancer. There is convincing evidence that physical activity is
associated with a reduced risk of cancers of the colon and breast. Several studies also have reported links between physical activity and a
reduced risk of cancers of the prostate, lung and lining of the uterus
(endometrial cancer). Despite these health benefits, recent studies
have shown that more than 60 percent of Americans do not engage
in enough regular physical activity.

What is the relationship between physical activity and colon cancer risk?

Individuals who are physically active can reduce their risk of developing colon cancer by 40 percent to 50 percent, with the greatest
reduction in risk among those who are most active. A decreased risk of
colon cancer has been consistently reported for physically active men.
Many studies have reported a reduction in colon cancer risk for physically active women. The relationship between physical activity and risk
in women, however, has been less consistent. Physical activity most
likely influences the development of colon cancer through multiple,
perhaps overlapping, biological pathways. Many researchers believe
physical activity aids in regular bowel movements, which may decrease
the time the colon is exposed to potential carcinogens. Increased physical activity also causes changes in insulin resistance, metabolism, and
hormone levels, which may help prevent tumor development. Physical
activity has also been found to alter a number of inflammatory and
immune factors, some of which may influence colon cancer risk.

How can physical activity reduce breast cancer risk?

Physically active women have up to a 40 percent reduced risk of
developing breast cancer. Most evidence suggests that physical activity

reduces breast cancer risk in both premenopausal and postmenopausal women. Although a lifetime of regular, vigorous activity is thought to be of greatest benefit, women who occasionally engage in physical activity also experience a reduced risk compared to inactive women. A number of studies also suggest that the effect of physical activity may be different across levels of BMI, with the greatest benefit seen in women in the normal weight range (generally a BMI under 25 kg/m-squared). For example, a recent major report from the Women's Health Initiative found that among postmenopausal women, walking 30 minutes per day was associated with a 20 percent reduction in breast cancer risk. The health benefits of physical activity were greatest among women who were of normal weight; they experienced a 37 percent decrease in risk. The protective effect of physical activity was not found among overweight or obese women. Researchers have proposed several biological mechanisms that may explain the relationship between physical activity and breast cancer development. Physical activity causes changes in hormone metabolism, body mass, and immune function, which may prevent tumor development.

How might physical activity reduce prostate cancer risk?

Physical activity probably reduces men's risk for prostate cancer by 10 percent to 30 percent. The likely association between physical activity and prostate cancer is based on a small number of studies that evaluated the role of physical activity in men who developed prostate cancer. Most of these studies indicate that inactive men have higher rates of prostate cancer compared to men who are very physically active. While it is probable that men who are physically active experience a reduction in risk for prostate cancer, the potential biological mechanisms that may explain this association are unknown.

How might physical activity reduce endometrial cancer risk?

Studies also suggest that women who are physically active have a 30 percent to 40 percent reduced risk of endometrial cancer, with the greatest reduction in risk among those who are most active. The possible association between physical activity and endometrial cancer is based on a limited number of studies, some of which indicate that inactive women have higher rates of endometrial cancer compared to physically active women. Changes in body mass and alterations in level and metabolism of sex hormones, such as estrogen, are the major biological mechanisms thought to explain the association between physical activity and endometrial cancer. A few studies have examined whether the effect of physical activity varies according to the weight of the woman, but the results have been inconsistent.

How might physical activity reduce lung cancer risk?

It is possible that individuals who are physically active have a 30 percent to 40 percent reduced risk of developing lung cancer. The possible link between physical activity and lung cancer is based on a limited number of studies that have found higher rates of lung cancer among those who are physically inactive compared to those who are active, after accounting for smoking status. The relationship between physical activity and lung cancer risk is less clear for women than it is for men.

However, the results of many of these studies are difficult to interpret because smokers who are able to engage in physical activity may have much better lung function. Investigators hypothesize that improvements in pulmonary function and ventilation in active, compared to inactive individuals, may explain the possible association between lung cancer and reduced physical activity.

Section 50.2

Exercising after Cancer Treatment

Excerpted from "Life After Cancer Treatment," part of the
Facing Forward Series, published by the National Cancer Institute
(www.cancer.gov), April 1, 2002.

What Is Normal after Cancer Treatment?

Congratulations on finishing your cancer treatment! Ending cancer treatment can be both exciting and challenging. Most people are relieved to be finished with the demands of treatment, but many also feel sadness and worry. Many are concerned about whether the cancer will come back and what they should do after treatment.

When treatment ends, people often expect life to return to the way it was before they were diagnosed with cancer. This rarely happens. You may have permanent scars on your body, or you may not be able to do some things you once did easily. Others may think of you—or you may view yourself—as being somehow different.

One of the hardest things after treatment is not knowing what happens next. "Because the doctors and nurses never told me the range of what to expect, I had expectations of wellness that were absolutely unrealistic," one woman said, "and so did my family and friends. This . . . led to a great deal of worry."

What is "normal" after cancer treatment? Those who have lived through treatment talk about the first few months as a time of change. It is not so much "getting back to normal" as it is finding out what is normal for you now. You can also expect things to keep changing as you begin your recovery. As one man put it, "I thought when I had finished treatment—when they looked at my tests and they said it looked good—I thought, 'OK, this is done'. . . [but] it is not over."

Your new normal may include making changes in the way you eat, the activities you do, and your sources of support, all of which are discussed here.

Exercise after Cancer Treatment

Few studies have been done to find out whether physical activity affects survival after cancer treatment. More research is needed to answer this question, but studies have shown that moderate exercise (walking, biking, swimming) for about 30 minutes every—or almost every—day can:

- reduce anxiety and depression;
- improve mood;
- boost self-esteem; and
- reduce symptoms of fatigue, nausea, pain, and diarrhea.

During recovery, it is important to start an exercise program slowly and increase activity over time, working with your doctor or a specialist (such as a physical therapist) if needed. If you need to stay in bed during your recovery, even small activities—like moving your arms or legs around—can help you stay flexible, relieve muscle tension, and help you feel better. Some survivors may need to take special care in exercising. Talk with your doctor before you begin any exercise program.

Practicing Relaxation to Relieve Pain and Stress

Relaxation can help you feel better—both mentally and physically. For most of us, though, it is not easy to "just relax." Relaxation is a skill, and it needs to be practiced just like any other skill.

Many people wait until they are in a lot of pain or feel a lot of stress before they try to relax, when it can be hardest to succeed. Then they might try to relax by overeating, smoking, or drinking—activities that are not helpful and might even be harmful.

Take the time to learn helpful relaxation skills and practice them often. You can try the following exercises, take a class, or buy a relaxation tape or CD.

Relaxation Exercises

Many people with cancer have found that practicing deep relaxation has helped relieve their pain or reduced their stress. The exercises that follow may not be right for everyone. Ask your doctor or nurse if these exercises can help you. Before trying Exercise 1, first practice steps 1 through 5, so you can get used to deep breathing and muscle relaxation.

Exercise 1

1. Find a quiet place where you can rest undisturbed for 20 minutes. Let others know you need this time for yourself.

2. Make sure the setting is relaxing. For example, dim the lights if you like, and find a comfortable chair or couch.

3. Get into a comfortable position where you can relax your muscles. Close your eyes and clear your mind of distractions.

4. Breathe deeply, at a slow and relaxing pace. People usually breathe shallowly, high in their chests. Concentrate on breathing deeply and slowly, raising your belly, rather than just your chest, with each breath.

5. Next, go through each of your major muscle groups, tensing (squeezing) them for 10 seconds and then relaxing. If tensing any particular muscle group is painful, skip the tensing step and concentrate just on relaxing. Focus completely on releasing all the tension from your muscles and notice the differences you feel when they are relaxed. Focus on the pleasant feeling of relaxation. In turn, tense, hold, and relax your:

- **right and left arms.** Make a fist and bring it up to your shoulder, tightening your arm.

- **lips, eyes, and forehead.** Scowl, raise your eyebrows, pucker your lips, and then grin.

- **jaws and neck.** Clench your teeth and relax, then tilt your chin down toward your chest.

- **shoulders.** Shrug your shoulders upward toward your ears.

- **chest.** Push out your chest.

- **stomach.** Suck in your stomach.

- **lower back.** Stretch your lower back so that it forms a gentle arch, with your stomach pushed outward. Make sure to do this gently, as these muscles are often tight.

- **buttocks.** Squeeze buttocks together.

- **thighs.** Press thighs together.

- **calves.** Point your toes up, toward your knees.

- **feet.** Point your toes down, like a ballet dancer's.

You may find that your mind wanders. When you notice yourself thinking of something else, gently direct your attention back to your deepening relaxation. Be sure to maintain your deep breathing.

6. Review these parts of your body again, and release any tension that remains. Be sure to maintain your deep breathing.

7. Now that you are relaxed, imagine a calming scene. Choose a spot that is particularly pleasant to you. It may be a favorite comfortable room, a sandy beach, a chair in front of a fireplace, or any other relaxing place. Concentrate on the details:

   - What can you see around you?

   - What do you smell?

   - What are the sounds that you hear? For example, if you are on the beach, how does the sand feel on your feet, how do the waves sound, and how does the air smell?

   - Can you taste anything?

Continue to breathe deeply, as you imagine yourself relaxing in your safe, comfortable place.

8. Some people find it helpful at this point to focus on thoughts that enhance their relaxation. For example: "My arms and legs are very comfortable. I can just sink into this chair and focus only on the relaxation."

9. Spend a few more minutes enjoying the feeling of comfort and relaxation.

10. When you are ready, start gently moving your hands and feet and bringing yourself back to reality. Open your eyes, and spend a few minutes becoming more alert. Notice how you feel now that you have completed the relaxation exercise, and try to carry these feelings with you into the rest of your day.

Exercise 2

1. Sit comfortably. Loosen any tight clothes. Close your eyes. Clear your mind and relax your muscles using steps 4 and 5 above.

2. Focus your mind on your right arm. Repeat to yourself, "My right arm feels heavy and warm." Stick with it until your arm does feel heavy and warm.

3. Repeat with the rest of your muscles until you are fully relaxed.

Keep in Mind

These exercises don't work right away for everyone. It can take some time to feel these exercises are working, so practicing may help. If any of these steps makes you feel uncomfortable, feel free to leave it out. Ask your doctor or nurse about other ways to relax if these exercises don't work for you.

Chapter 51

Why Exercise Is Important for People with HIV

Why is exercise important?

Exercise helps many people with HIV disease feel better and might strengthen your immune system. Exercise cannot control or fight HIV disease, but it may help you feel better and fight many of the side effects of HIV disease and HIV medications.

What are the advantages of exercise?

Regular, moderate exercise has many of the same advantages for people with HIV disease as it does for most people. Exercise can:

- improve muscle mass, strength, and endurance;
- improve heart and lung endurance;
- improve your energy level so you feel less tired;
- reduce stress;
- enhance your sense of well-being;
- help stabilize or prevent declines in CD4 cell counts;
- increase bone strength;
- decrease cholesterol and triglycerides;

"Exercise and HIV," Fact Sheet 802, © 2006 AIDS InfoNet. Reprinted with permission. Fact Sheets are regularly updated. Check http://www.aidsinfonet .org for the most recent information.

- decrease fat in the abdomen;
- improve appetite;
- improve sleep; and
- improve the way the body uses and controls blood sugar (glucose).

What are the risks of exercise?

- You can get dehydrated (lose too much water) if you do not drink enough liquids to keep up your fluid levels.
- Injuries may take more time to heal.
- You can lose lean body mass if you exercise too much. Serious cases can lead to AIDS wasting.
- You can injure yourself if you use the wrong form in exercises
- Exercise can help those with heart disease, but talk to your doctor to make sure that you are able to exercise safely.

What are exercise guidelines for people with HIV?

Don't overdo it.

A moderate exercise program will help your body turn your food into muscle. Take it easy, and work exercise into your daily activities.

Work up to a schedule of at least 20 minutes, at least three times per week as long as you are feeling better. This can lead to significant improvements in your fitness level and you may feel better.

People with HIV can improve their fitness levels through training like those who do not have HIV. However, people with HIV may find it harder to continue with a training program because of fatigue.

Start exercising while you are still healthy. This can help you hold off symptoms of HIV that make you feel bad. Keep your exercise fresh. Find new ways to keep yourself motivated to maintain your exercise program.

Your fitness level may be different than it used to be. It is very important that you work your way into an exercise program to avoid injury.

Eat and drink correctly.

Drinking enough liquids is very important when you exercise. Extra water can help you replace the fluids you lose. Remember that drinking tea, coffee, colas, chocolate, or alcohol can actually make you lose body liquid.

Don't eat when you exercise. In fact, it's best to wait up to 2 hours after a full meal before an exercise session. Also, wait about an hour after a workout before you eat your next meal.

Proper nutrition is also important. With increased activity you may need to eat more calories to avoid losing weight.

Choose something you enjoy.

Choose activities that you like. Whether it is yoga, running, bicycling, or another sport, doing something you like will encourage you to maintain your program. Don't get into a rut! Change your activities if you need to so that you stay motivated.

If your fitness level is good, you can compete in competitive sports. Taking part in competitive or team sports does not pose a risk of spreading HIV to other athletes or coaches.

If you get hurt and you're bleeding, the risk of HIV being spread to other people is very small. However, if you bleed during a sport, you should get out of the game and cover your injuries before returning to the game.

Exercise with weights.

Weight training (resistance exercise) is one of the best ways to increase lean body mass that may be lost through HIV disease and aging. Working out three times a week for an hour should be enough if done well. Combining weight training with 30 minutes of cardiovascular exercise may be the best way to improve body composition and keep your blood lipids and sugar down. Cardiovascular exercise means working large muscle groups continuously for at least 30 minutes. Activities such as brisk walking, jogging, bicycling, or swimming can be cardiovascular exercise.

The Bottom Line

Exercise can improve strength, fight fatigue and depression, improve endurance, increase cardiovascular fitness, help to reduce stress, and promote muscle strength. It may also help the immune system work better.

Chapter 52

People with Disabilities Benefit from Physical Activity

I'm in a wheelchair. It's too difficult to play sports.

I can't think of a physical activity that I would enjoy.

Sports equipment and health clubs are for able-bodied people.

Why should I bother to exercise? It won't help me.

I don't have the time and energy to take care of myself and exercise.

Sound familiar? Maybe you think that you can't enjoy sports or other forms of physical activity either. But, you couldn't be more wrong.

Physical activity can be a part of everyone's life, regardless of your physical limitations. You don't have to be an athlete. The key is to keep your body moving. Start out by keeping it simple—do regular stretching exercises, housework, raised-bed gardening, play catch with kids, or swim. Keeping active means you will feel physically, emotionally, and socially healthy. Here's how you can get started:

1. Choose a physical activity that you can enjoy and that you'll stick with. This chapter contains a wide range of possibilities.

"Fit for Life" is reprinted with permission of the New York State Department of Health. This publication was supported by Cooperative Agreement Number U59/CCU20335. Its contents are solely the responsibility of the authors and do not necessarily represent the official views of the CDC.

2. Be sure that the activity is sustained (15 to 20 minutes per session), and regular (at least three times per week).

3. See your doctor before starting any physical activity program.

4. Start slowly, and increase the amount or duration of activity gradually.

5. Join with others (friends, family, coworkers) to get and give support.

6. Keep a record of your activity (distances, number of times per week, etc.) so you can measure your progress.

"I can't imagine my life without physical activity. It's a great equalizer! I'm healthier and my body responds better to problems presented by my disability." —Donna Ponessa

Tailor Activities to Fit Your Needs and Abilities

Just about any form of physical activity, even sports, can be tailored to meet your needs and abilities. Increasing numbers of exercise programs, sports, and sporting equipment are being designed or adapted for people with disabilities.

More health clubs are becoming accessible, and organizations such as independent living centers can provide information about accessibility and advocacy. But you don't have to join a club or buy expensive equipment. There are many activities that you can do on your own and that are low-cost, if not totally free.

Physical Fitness = Better Health

Staying fit is especially important for people with disabilities, many of whom live sedentary lifestyles. When you're physically active, you're less likely to develop additional health problems, like heart disease, high blood pressure, osteoporosis, or arthritis; to gain excess weight; or become depressed. Physical activity can be good for your body:

• It energizes and increases stamina and strength.

• It enhances mobility.

• It helps prevent pressure sores.

• It may reduce spasticity.

• It may strengthen bones.

- It helps control weight by burning extra calories.
- It improves both appetite and digestion.
- It tones and strengthens muscles.
- It keeps joints, tendons, and ligaments flexible for easy, unrestricted movement.
- It improves heart and lung functions.
- It strengthens the heart and improves circulation.
- It improves blood pressure readings and glucose levels.
- It helps balance and agility.

Physical Activity Is Also Good for Your Mind

- It improves self-image and self-confidence.
- It stimulates self-reliance.
- It relaxes and relieves stress and tension.
- It improves intellectual alertness and concentration skills.
- It fosters an overall feeling of health and well-being.
- It results in a sense of accomplishment and new skills.
- It increases your chances of meeting new people.

Physical activity can ultimately increase your independence and give you more energy to enjoy life. It is fun. It can be done almost anywhere, by anyone (alone or in a group), and is not expensive (unless you want it to be).

"I feel good! Being on a swim team has taught me camaraderie, and I get a lot of support from my teammates. Swimming gives me a sense of accomplishment and self-esteem. Also, competing gives me something physical in which I can excel!" —Judy Goldberg

"Maintaining an exercise routine seems to be easier if you're a disabled 'jock'. I'm more of a 'couch potato' and I'm not inclined to view exercise as fun. But my disability demands that I find some activity that I can enjoy and stick to it. Wheelchair aerobics at home work for me; aquatic exercise is also good but demands more planning. As more adaptive equipment becomes available, I'm sure that I'll find more ways to keep fit." —Dot Nary

Certain Activities Improve Certain Functions.

Besides being enjoyable and healthful, certain activities contribute to specific physical improvements.

Ball games, such as seated volleyball, wheelchair softball, and "beep" baseball for the blind and visually impaired, can help tone or improve upper body strength. Adapted cross-country skiing and aquatics are good for synchronizing arm-leg movements, overall toning, and improved circulation. Even miniature golf can help, by improving grasping and releasing skills and hand-eye coordination.

> "Sports have always been a part of my life. After my injury, I thought that part of my life was over. Then I started playing (chair) tennis, and recently joined a basketball team. I'm again enjoying the feeling of competition—winning and losing, but always trying my hardest. I have made many friends during tournaments and have traveled to many wonderful places. Most importantly, I have regained a sense of myself as a competent, capable person." —Eric Emerick

It's Your Choice

Team sports or individual physical activities? Join a club, or work independently? It's your choice. To find out about the options and opportunities that are available in your community, call local community centers, the YMCA/YWCA, an Independent Living Center, or health clubs. Or you can create a workout or exercise corner right in your own home.

Remember, special equipment can be purchased to adapt activities to your needs, whether it's a flotation device for water aerobics or special gardening tools. But, again, no one says you have spend a lot of money to become physically fit.

Here are some activities for you to consider. Those for which adaptive equipment is available are starred (*):

Sports

- wheelchair basketball, tennis, football, and softball*
- seated volleyball*
- "beep" baseball*
- curling*
- bowling*

- martial arts
- shooting
- table tennis*
- weight lifting
- wrestling
- golf*
- hockey*
- archery

Other Physical Activities

- passive standing*
- walking
- hiking*
- cycling*
- horseback riding*
- orienteering (map reading and survival skills)
- racing
- running and jogging
- rowing
- scuba diving*
- water skiing*
- ice skating*
- cross-country and downhill skiing*
- dancing
- aerobics and seat aerobics
- jumping events
- gardening
- sailing

Make It Even More Enjoyable

Is there a friend or family member you'd like to have join you? A buddy system works well for many activities. With a partner, you'll have companionship as well as shared encouragement and accomplishments.

"There is much enjoyment and benefit to getting back into physical activity or sport. The rules may vary, you may need special equipment, but it's worth it! I have three boys and getting back into sports gives us something to do and enjoy together, as a family. It shows my sons that being in a chair doesn't make you disabled. They get around on foot; I get around on wheels."
—Sandy Koon

Play Safely

Remember, physical activity is not a substitute for any prescribed physical or occupational therapy. It may improve your performance in therapy, but cannot replace the therapy itself. Also, before starting any physical activity, talk to your doctor to make sure that it's the right one for you. And, make sure to follow the safety guidelines for the sport or leisure activity you choose (i.e., wearing a bicycle helmet, strapping yourself to exercise equipment for additional support, and other safety measures).

Once you decide on a physical fitness activity, let your physical therapist know about your choice. She or he can share ways in which you can benefit the most from your efforts.

Kids Need Physical Activity, Too

Many children of all abilities just don't get enough exercise. Yet all kids need to be active. They need something that will help improve endurance, balance, and coordination. Besides the physical and mental benefits, physical activity, especially team sports, can help kids learn social skills, to share and to take turns. So, if you have a child with, or without a disability, encourage physical activity. And, join them. That way, everybody benefits.

For More Information

Contact local health or fitness programs in your area, your Independent Living Center, health care provider, or physical therapist for more ideas or the location of appropriate programs near you, as well as specialty catalogs for adaptive equipment.

Part Six

Exercise-Related Injuries

Chapter 53

Childhood Sports Injuries and Their Prevention: A Guide for Parents

Preventing Injuries

Childhood sports injuries may be inevitable, but there are some things you can do to help prevent them:

- Enroll your child in organized sports through schools, community clubs, and recreation areas where there may be adults who are certified athletic trainers (ATC). An ATC is also trained in the prevention, recognition, and immediate care of athletic injuries.

- Make sure your child uses the proper protective gear for a particular sport. This may lessen the chances of being injured.

- Warmup exercises, such as stretching and light jogging, can help minimize the chance of muscle strain or other soft tissue injury during sports. Warmup exercises make the body's tissues warmer and more flexible. Cooling down exercises loosen the body's muscles that have tightened during exercise. Make warmups and cooldowns part of your child's routine before and after sports participation.

Excerpted from "Childhood Sports Injuries and Their Prevention: A Guide for Parents with Ideas for Kids," by the National Institute of Arthritis and Musculoskeletal and Skin Diseases (NIAMS, www.niams.nih.gov), June 2001. Reviewed by David A. Cooke, MD, on June 12, 2006. Additional information from the American Academy of Orthopaedic Surgeons is cited separately within the chapter.

And don't forget to include sunscreen and a hat (where possible) to reduce the chance of sunburn, which is actually an injury to the skin. Sun protection may also decrease the chances of malignant melanoma—a potentially deadly skin cancer—or other skin cancers that can occur later in life. It is also very important that your child has access to water or a sports drink to stay properly hydrated while playing.

Treat Injuries with RICE

If your child receives a soft tissue injury, commonly known as a sprain or a strain, or a bone injury, the best immediate treatment is easy to remember: RICE (Rest, Ice, Compression, and Elevation). Get professional treatment if any injury is severe. A severe injury means having an obvious fracture or dislocation of a joint, prolonged swelling, or prolonged or severe pain.

RICE involves:

- **Rest:** Reduce or stop using the injured area for 48 hours. If you have a leg injury, you may need to stay off of it completely.

- **Ice:** Put an ice pack on the injured area for 20 minutes at a time, 4 to 8 times per day. Use a cold pack, ice bag, or a plastic bag filled with crushed ice that has been wrapped in a towel.

- **Compression:** Compression of an injured ankle, knee, or wrist may help reduce the swelling. These include bandages such as elastic wraps, special boots, air casts and splints. Ask your doctor which one is best.

- **Elevation:** Keep the injured area elevated above the level of the heart. Use a pillow to help elevate an injured limb.

Sprains and Strains

A sprain is an injury to a ligament—a stretching or a tearing. One or more ligaments can be injured during a sprain. A ligament is a band of tough, fibrous tissue that connects two or more bones at a joint and prevents excessive movement of the joint. Ankle sprains are the most common injury in the United States and often occur during sports or recreational activities. Approximately 1 million ankle injuries occur each year and 85 percent of these are sprains.

A strain is an injury to either a muscle or a tendon. A muscle is a tissue composed of bundles of specialized cells that, when stimulated by nerve impulses, contract and produce movement. A tendon is a tough, fibrous cord of tissue that connects muscle to bone.

Growth Plate Injuries

In some sports accidents and injuries, the growth plate may be injured. The growth plate is the area of developing tissues at the end of the long bones in growing children and adolescents. When growth is complete, some time during adolescence, the growth plate is replaced by solid bone. The long bones in the body are the long bones of the fingers, the outer bone of the forearm, the collarbone, the hip, the bone of the upper leg, the lower leg bones, the ankle, and the foot. If any of these areas become injured, seek professional help from a doctor who specializes in bone injuries in children and adolescents (this type of doctor is called a pediatric orthopaedist).

Repetitive Motion Injuries

Painful injuries such as stress fractures (where the ligament pulls off small pieces of bone) and tendonitis (inflammation of a tendon) can occur from overuse of muscles and tendons. These injuries don't always show up on x-rays, but they do cause pain and discomfort. The injured area usually responds to rest. Other treatments include RICE, crutches, cast immobilization, or physical therapy.

Heat and Hydration

Playing rigorous sports in the heat requires close monitoring of both body and weather conditions. Heat injuries are always dangerous and can be fatal. Children perspire less than adults and require a higher core body temperature to trigger sweating. Heat-related illnesses include dehydration (deficit in body fluids), heat exhaustion (nausea, dizziness, weakness, headache, pale and moist skin, heavy perspiration, normal or low body temperature, weak pulse, dilated pupils, disorientation, fainting spells), and heat stroke (headache, dizziness, confusion, and hot dry skin, possibly leading to vascular collapse, coma, and death). These injuries can be prevented.

Exercise Is Beneficial

Exercise may reduce the chances of obesity, which is becoming more common in children. It may also lessen his risk of diabetes, a disease that is sometimes associated with a lack of exercise and poor eating habits.

As a parent, it is important for you to match your children to the sport, and not push him or her too hard into an activity that he or she may not like or be capable of doing. Sports also helps children build social skills and provides them with a general sense of well-being. Sports participation is an important part of learning how to build team skills.

Sports Injury and Prevention

It is important it is to know which sports are more likely to cause injury than others. In addition, you should check the condition of the athletic area where the sports are to be played to make sure it is properly maintained.

The following "sports scorecard" shows winning ways to help prevent an injury from occurring.

Football

- This popular sport leads the pack in the number of injuries, especially in boys, in organized sports.

- Common injuries and locations: Bruises, sprains, strains, pulled muscles, soft tissue tears such as ligaments, broken bones, internal injuries (bruised or damaged organs), back injuries, sunburn. Knees and ankles are the most common injury sites.

- Safest playing with: Helmet; mouth guard; shoulder pads; athletic supporters for males; chest/rib pads; forearm, elbow, and thigh pads; shin guards; proper shoes; sunscreen; water.

- Prevention: Proper use of safety equipment, warmup exercises, proper coaching and conditioning.

Basketball

- This popular sport has the highest rate of knee injuries requiring surgery among girls.

- Common injuries and locations: Sprains, strains, bruises, fractures, scrapes, dislocation, cuts, dental injuries, ankles, knees (injury rates are higher in girls, especially for the anterior cruciate ligament, the wide ligament that limits rotation and forward movement of the shin bone), and shoulder (rotator cuff strains and tears, where tendons at the end of muscles attach to the upper arm and shoulder bones).

- Safest playing with: Eye protection, elbow and knee pads, mouth guard, athletic supporters for males, proper shoes, water. If playing outdoors, add a hat and sunscreen.

- Prevention: Strength training (particularly knees and shoulders), aerobics (exercises that develop the strength and endurance of heart and lungs), warmup exercises, proper coaching, and use of safety equipment.

Soccer

- This sport has dramatically increased in popularity in the past two decades in the United States.

- Common injuries: Bruises, cuts and scrapes, headaches, sunburn.

- Safest playing with: Shin guards, athletic supporters for males, cleats, sunscreen, water.

- Prevention: Aerobic conditioning and warmups, and proper training in heading the ball. (Heading is using the head to strike or make a play with the ball.)

Baseball and Softball

- Sometimes called America's favorite pastime.

- Common injuries: Soft tissue strains, impact injuries that include fractures due to sliding and being hit by a ball, sunburn.

- Safest playing with: Batting helmet, shin guards, elbow guards, athletic supporters for males, mouth guard, sunscreen, cleats, hat, breakaway bases.

- Prevention: Proper conditioning and warmups.

Gymnastics

- The performance of systematic exercises.

- Common injuries: Sprains and strains of soft tissues.

- Safest playing with: Athletic supporters for males, safety harness, joint supports (such as neoprene wraps), water.

- Prevention: Proper conditioning and warmups.

Track and Field

- Competing at running, walking, jumping, throwing, or pushing events.

- Common injuries: Strains, sprains, scrapes from falls.

- Safest playing with: Proper shoes, athletic supporters for males, sunscreen, water.

- Prevention: Proper conditioning and coaching.

How Your Child Can Prevent Sports Injuries

The following information is adapted and reproduced with permission from Play It Safe, a Guide to Safety for Young Athletes, in Johnson TR, (ed): *Your Orthopaedic Connection, Rosemont*, IL, American Academy of Orthopaedic Surgeons. Available at http://orthoinfo.aaos.org.

- Be in proper physical condition to play the sport.

- Know and abide by the rules of the sport.

- Wear appropriate protective gear (for example, shin guards for soccer, a hard-shell helmet when facing a baseball or softball pitcher, a helmet and body padding for ice hockey).

- Know how to use athletic equipment.

- Always warm up before playing.

- Avoid playing when very tired or in pain.

- Get a preseason physical examination.

- Make sure there is adequate water or other liquids to maintain proper hydration.

Chapter 54

Overview of Acute and Chronic Sports Injuries and Their Treatment

What Are Sports Injuries?

The term sports injury, in the broadest sense, refers to the kinds of injuries that most commonly occur during sports or exercise. Some sports injuries result from accidents; others are due to poor training practices, improper equipment, lack of conditioning, or insufficient warmup and stretching.

Although virtually any part of your body can be injured during sports or exercise, the term is usually reserved for injuries that involve the musculoskeletal system, which includes the muscles, bones, and associated tissues like cartilage. Following are some of the most common sports injuries.

Sprains and Strains

A sprain is a stretch or tear of a ligament, the band of connective tissues that joins the end of one bone with another. Sprains are caused by trauma such as a fall or blow to the body that knocks a joint out of position and, in the worst case, ruptures the supporting ligaments. Sprains can range from first degree (minimally stretched ligament) to third degree (a complete tear). Areas of the body most vulnerable

---

Excerpted from the brochure "Handout on Health: Sports Injuries," by the National Institute of Arthritis and Musculoskeletal and Skin Diseases (NIAMS), April 2004.

to sprains are ankles, knees, and wrists. Signs of a sprain include varying degrees of tenderness or pain; bruising; inflammation; swelling;
inability to move a limb or joint; or joint looseness, laxity, or instability.

A strain is a twist, pull, or tear of a muscle or tendon, a cord of tissue connecting muscle to bone. It is an acute, noncontact injury that
results from overstretching or overcontraction. Symptoms of a strain
include pain, muscle spasm, and loss of strength. While it's hard to
tell the difference between mild and moderate strains, severe strains
not treated professionally can cause damage and loss of function.

Knee Injuries

Because of its complex structure and weight-bearing capacity, the
knee is the most commonly injured joint. Each year, more than 5.5
million people visit orthopaedic surgeons for knee problems.

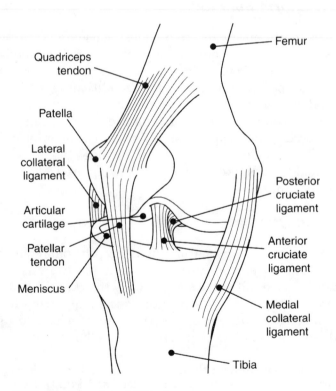

Figure 54.1. The structure of the knee

Knee injuries can range from mild to severe. Some of the less severe, yet still painful and functionally limiting, knee problems are runner's knee (pain or tenderness close to or under the knee cap at the front or side of the knee), iliotibial band syndrome (pain on the outer side of the knee), and tendonitis, also called tendinosis (marked by degeneration within a tendon, usually where it joins the bone). More severe injuries include bone bruises or damage to the cartilage or ligaments. There are two types of cartilage in the knee. One is the meniscus, a crescent-shaped disk that absorbs shock between the thigh (femur) and lower leg bones (tibia and fibula). The other is a surface-coating (or articular) cartilage. It covers the ends of the bones where they meet, allowing them to glide against one another. The four major ligaments that support the knee are the anterior cruciate ligament (ACL), the posterior cruciate ligament (PCL), the medial collateral ligament (MCL), and the lateral collateral ligament (LCL).

Knee injuries can result from a blow to or twist of the knee; from improper landing after a jump; or from running too hard, too much, or without proper warmup.

Compartment Syndrome

In many parts of the body, muscles (along with the nerves and blood vessels that run alongside and through them) are enclosed in a "compartment" formed of a tough membrane called fascia. When muscles become swollen, they can fill the compartment to capacity, causing interference with nerves and blood vessels as well as damage to the muscles themselves. The resulting painful condition is referred to as compartment syndrome.

Compartment syndrome may be caused by a one-time traumatic injury (acute compartment syndrome), such as a fractured bone or a hard blow to the thigh, by repeated hard blows (depending upon the sport), or by ongoing overuse (chronic exertional compartment syndrome), which may occur, for example, in long-distance running.

Shin Splints

While the term "shin splints" has been widely used to describe any sort of leg pain associated with exercise, the term actually refers to pain along the tibia or shin bone, the large bone in the front of the lower leg. This pain can occur at the front outside part of the lower leg, including the foot and ankle (anterior shin splints) or at the inner edge of the bone where it meets the calf muscles (medial shin splints).

Shin splints are primarily seen in runners, particularly those just starting a running program. Risk factors for shin splints include overuse or incorrect use of the lower leg; improper stretching, warmup, or exercise technique; overtraining; running or jumping on hard surfaces; and running in shoes that don't have enough support. These injuries are often associated with flat (overpronated) feet.

Achilles Tendon Injuries

A stretch, tear, or irritation to the tendon connecting the calf muscle to the back of the heel, Achilles tendon injuries can be so sudden and agonizing that they have been known to bring down charging professional football players in shocking fashion.

The most common cause of Achilles tendon tears is a problem called tendonitis, a degenerative condition caused by aging or overuse. When a tendon is weakened, trauma can cause it to rupture.

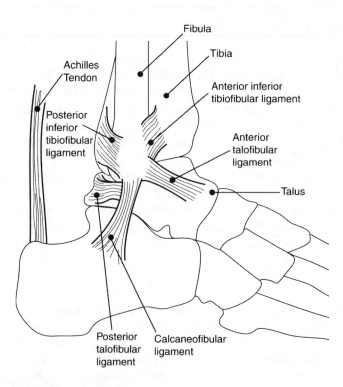

Figure 54.2. *The structure of the ankle.*

Achilles tendon injuries are common in middle-aged "weekend warriors" who may not exercise regularly or take time to stretch properly before an activity. Among professional athletes, most Achilles injuries seem to occur in quick-acceleration, jumping sports like football and basketball, and almost always end the season's competition for the athlete.

Fractures

A fracture is a break in the bone that can occur from either a quick, one-time injury to the bone (acute fracture) or from repeated stress to the bone over time (stress fracture).

Acute fractures can be simple (a clean break with little damage to the surrounding tissue) or compound (a break in which the bone pierces the skin with little damage to the surrounding tissue). Most acute fractures are emergencies. One that breaks the skin is especially dangerous because there is a high risk of infection.

Stress fractures occur largely in the feet and legs and are common in sports that require repetitive impact, primarily running/jumping sports such as gymnastics or track and field. Running creates forces two to three times a person's body weight on the lower limbs.

The most common symptom of a stress fracture is pain at the site that worsens with weight-bearing activity. Tenderness and swelling often accompany the pain.

Dislocations

When the two bones that come together to form a joint become separated, the joint is described as being dislocated. Contact sports such as football and basketball, as well as high-impact sports and sports that can result in excessive stretching or falling, cause the majority of dislocations. A dislocated joint is an emergency situation that requires medical treatment.

The joints most likely to be dislocated are some of the hand joints. Aside from these joints, the joint most frequently dislocated is the shoulder. Dislocations of the knees, hips, and elbows are uncommon.

What's the Difference between Acute and Chronic Injuries?

Regardless of the specific structure affected, sports injuries can generally be classified in one of two ways: acute or chronic.

Acute Injuries

Acute injuries, such as a sprained ankle, strained back, or fractured hand, occur suddenly during activity. Signs of an acute injury include the following:

- Sudden, severe pain
- Swelling
- Inability to place weight on a lower limb
- Extreme tenderness in an upper limb
- Inability to move a joint through its full range of motion
- Extreme limb weakness
- Visible dislocation or break of a bone

Chronic Injuries

Chronic injuries usually result from overusing one area of the body while playing a sport or exercising over a long period. The following are signs of a chronic injury:

- Pain when performing an activity
- A dull ache when at rest
- Swelling

What Should I Do If I Suffer an Injury?

Whether an injury is acute or chronic, there is never a good reason to try to "work through" the pain of an injury. When you have pain from a particular movement or activity, STOP! Continuing the activity only causes further harm.

Some injuries require prompt medical attention, whereas others can be self-treated. Here's what you need to know about both types.

When to Seek Medical Treatment

You should call a health professional if:

- the injury causes severe pain, swelling, or numbness;
- you can't tolerate any weight on the area; or
- the pain or dull ache of an old injury is accompanied by increased swelling or joint abnormality or instability.

When and How to Treat at Home

If you don't have any of the above symptoms, it's probably safe to treat the injury at home—at least at first. If pain or other symptoms worsen, it's best to check with your health care provider. Use the RICE method to relieve pain and inflammation and speed healing. Follow these four steps immediately after injury and continue for at least 48 hours:

- **Rest.** Reduce regular exercise or activities of daily living as needed. If you cannot put weight on an ankle or knee, crutches may help. If you use a cane or one crutch for an ankle injury, use it on the uninjured side to help you lean away and relieve weight on the injured ankle.

- **Ice.** Apply an ice pack to the injured area for 20 minutes at a time, four to eight times a day. A cold pack, ice bag, or plastic bag filled with crushed ice and wrapped in a towel can be used. To avoid cold injury and frostbite, do not apply the ice for more than 20 minutes. (Note: Do not use heat immediately after an injury. This tends to increase internal bleeding or swelling. Heat can be used later on to relieve muscle tension and promote relaxation.)

- **Compression.** Compression of the injured area may help reduce swelling. Compression can be achieved with elastic wraps, special boots, air casts, and splints. Ask your health care provider for advice on which one to use.

- **Elevation.** If possible, keep the injured ankle, knee, elbow, or wrist elevated on a pillow, above the level of the heart, to help decrease swelling.

The Body's Healing Process

From the moment a bone breaks or a ligament tears, your body goes to work to repair the damage. Here's what happens at each stage of the healing process:

- **At the moment of injury:** Chemicals are released from damaged cells, triggering a process called inflammation. Blood vessels at the injury site become dilated; blood flow increases to carry nutrients to the site of tissue damage.

- **Within hours of injury:** White blood cells (leukocytes) travel down the bloodstream to the injury site where they begin to tear down and remove damaged tissue, allowing other specialized cells to start developing scar tissue.

- **Within days of injury:** Scar tissue is formed on the skin or inside the body. The amount of scarring may be proportional to the amount of swelling, inflammation, or bleeding within. In the next few weeks, the damaged area will regain a great deal of strength as scar tissue continues to form.

- **Within a month of injury:** Scar tissue may start to shrink, bringing damaged, torn, or separated tissues back together. However, it may be several months or more before the injury is completely healed.

Who Should I See for My Injury?

Although severe injuries will need to be seen immediately in an emergency room, particularly if they occur on the weekend or after office hours, most sports injuries can be evaluated and, in many cases, treated by your primary health care provider.

Depending on your preference and the severity of your injury or the likelihood that your injury may cause ongoing, long-term problems, you may want to see, or have your primary health care professional refer you to, one of the following:

- **Orthopaedic surgeon:** A doctor specializing in the diagnosis and treatment of the musculoskeletal system, which includes bones, joints, ligaments, tendons, muscles, and nerves.

- **Physical therapist/physiotherapist:** A health care professional who can develop a rehabilitation program. Your primary care physician may refer you to a physical therapist after you begin to recover from your injury to help strengthen muscles and joints and prevent further injury.

How Are Sports Injuries Treated?

Although using the RICE technique described previously can be helpful for any sports injury, RICE is often just a starting point. Here are some other treatments your doctor or other health care provider may administer, recommend, or prescribe to help your injury heal.

Nonsteroidal Anti-Inflammatory Drugs (NSAIDs)

The moment you are injured, chemicals are released from damaged tissue cells. This triggers the first stage of healing: inflammation. Inflammation causes tissues to become swollen, tender, and painful.

Although inflammation is needed for healing, it can actually slow the healing process if left unchecked.

To reduce inflammation and pain, doctors and other health care providers often recommend taking an over-the-counter (OTC) nonsteroidal anti-inflammatory drug (NSAID) such as aspirin, ibuprofen (Advil, Motrin IB, Nuprin), ketoprofen (Actron, Orudis KT), or naproxen sodium (Aleve). For more severe pain and inflammation, doctors may prescribe one of several dozen NSAIDs available in prescription strength.

Notes about NSAIDs: Brand names included in this chapter are provided as examples only, and their inclusion does not mean that these products are endorsed by the National Institutes of Health or any other Government agency. Also, if a particular brand name is not mentioned, this does not mean or imply that the product is unsatisfactory. In addition, like all medications, NSAIDs can have side effects. The list of possible adverse effects is long, but major problems are few. The intestinal tract heads the list with nausea, abdominal pain, vomiting, and diarrhea. Changes in liver function frequently occur in children (but not in adults) who use aspirin. Changes in liver function are rare in children using the other NSAIDs. Questions about the appropriate use of NSAIDs should be directed toward your health care provider or pharmacist.

Though not an NSAID, another commonly used OTC medication, acetaminophen (Tylenol), may relieve pain. It has no effect on inflammation, however.

Immobilization

Immobilization is a common treatment for sports injuries that may be done immediately by a trainer or paramedic. Immobilization involves reducing movement in the area to prevent further damage. By enabling the blood supply to flow more directly to the injury (or the site of surgery to repair damage from an injury), immobilization reduces pain, swelling, and muscle spasm and helps the healing process begin. Following are some devices used for immobilization:

- Slings, to immobilize the upper body, including the arms and shoulders.

- Splints and casts, to support and protect injured bones and soft tissue. Casts can be made from plaster or fiberglass. Splints can be custom made or ready made. Standard splints come in a variety of shapes and sizes and have Velcro straps that make them easy to put on and take off or adjust. Splints generally offer less support and protection than a cast, and therefore may not always be a treatment option.

• Leg immobilizers, to keep the knee from bending after injury or surgery. Made from foam rubber covered with fabric, leg immobilizers enclose the entire leg, fastening with Velcro straps.

Surgery

In some cases, surgery is needed to repair torn connective tissues or to realign bones with compound fractures. The majority of sports injuries, however, do not require surgery.

Rehabilitation (Exercise)

A key part of rehabilitation from sports injuries is a graduated exercise program designed to return the injured body part to a normal level of function.

With most injuries, early mobilization—getting the part moving as soon as possible—will speed healing. Generally, early mobilization starts with gentle range-of-motion exercises and then moves on to stretching and strengthening exercise when you can without increasing pain. For example, if you have a sprained ankle, you may be able to work on range of motion for the first day or two after the sprain by gently tracing letters with your big toe. Once your range of motion is fairly good, you can start doing gentle stretching and strengthening exercises. When you are ready, weights may be added to your exercise routine to further strengthen the injured area. The key is to avoid movement that causes pain.

As damaged tissue heals, scar tissue forms, which shrinks and brings torn or separated tissues back together. As a result, the injury site becomes tight or stiff, and damaged tissues are at risk of reinjury. That's why stretching and strengthening exercises are so important. You should continue to stretch the muscles daily and as the first part of your warmup before exercising.

When planning your rehabilitation program with a health care professional, remember that progression is the key principle. Start with just a few exercises, do them often, and then gradually increase how much you do. A complete rehabilitation program should include exercises for flexibility, endurance, and strength; instruction in balance and proper body mechanics related to the sport; and a planned return to full participation.

Throughout the rehabilitation process, avoid painful activities and concentrate on those exercises that will improve function in the injured part. Don't resume your sport until you are sure you can stretch the injured tissues without any pain, swelling, or restricted movement, and monitor any other symptoms. When you do return to your sport, start slowly and gradually build up to full participation.

Rest

Although it is important to get moving as soon as possible, you must also take time to rest following an injury. All injuries need time to heal; proper rest will help the process. Your health care professional can guide you regarding the proper balance between rest and rehabilitation.

Other Therapies

Other therapies commonly used in rehabilitating sports injuries include:

- **Electrostimulation:** Mild electrical current provides pain relief by preventing nerve cells from sending pain impulses to the brain. Electrostimulation may also be used to decrease swelling, and to make muscles in immobilized limbs contract, thus preventing muscle atrophy and maintaining or increasing muscle strength.

- **Cold/cryotherapy:** Ice packs reduce inflammation by constricting blood vessels and limiting blood flow to the injured tissues. Cryotherapy eases pain by numbing the injured area. It is generally used for only the first 48 hours after injury.

- **Heat/thermotherapy:** Heat, in the form of hot compresses, heat lamps, or heating pads, causes the blood vessels to dilate and increase blood flow to the injury site. Increased blood flow aids the healing process by removing cell debris from damaged tissues and carrying healing nutrients to the injury site. Heat also helps to reduce pain. It should not be applied within the first 48 hours after an injury.

- **Ultrasound:** High-frequency sound waves produce deep heat that is applied directly to an injured area. Ultrasound stimulates blood flow to promote healing.

- **Massage:** Manual pressing, rubbing, and manipulation soothe tense muscles and increase blood flow to the injury site.

Most of these therapies are administered or supervised by a licensed health care professional.

Who Is at Greatest Risk for Sports Injuries?

If a professional athlete dislocates a joint or tears a ligament, it makes the news. But anyone who plays sports can be injured. Three groups—children and adolescents, middle-aged athletes, and women—are particularly vulnerable.

Children and Adolescents

While playing sports can improve children's fitness, self-esteem, coordination, and self-discipline, it can also put them at risk for sports injuries: some minor, some serious, and still others that may result in lifelong medical problems.

Young athletes are not small adults. Their bones, muscles, tendons, and ligaments are still growing and that makes them more prone to injury. Growth plates—the areas of developing cartilage where bone growth occurs in growing children—are weaker than the nearby ligaments and tendons. As a result, what is often a bruise or sprain in an adult can be a potentially serious growth-plate injury in a child. Also, a trauma that would tear a muscle or ligament in an adult would be far more likely to break a child's bone.

Because young athletes of the same age can differ greatly in size and physical maturity, some may try to perform at levels beyond their ability in order to keep up with their peers.

Contact sports have inherent dangers that put young athletes at special risk for severe injuries. Even with rigorous training and proper

Table 54.1. Injuries in Kids, by Sport

Children aged 5 through 14 sustained an estimated 2.38 million sports and recreational injuries annually from 1997 through 1999. By sport, this number includes the following:

Pedal cycling	332,000 injuries
Basketball	261,000 injuries
Football	243,000 injuries
Playground equipment	219,000 injuries
Baseball/softball	185,000 injuries

Source: National Health Interview Survey

safety equipment, youngsters are still at risk for severe injuries to the neck, spinal cord, and growth plates. Evaluating potential sports injuries on the field in very young children can involve its own special issues for concerned parents and coaches.

Adult Athletes

More adults than ever are participating in sports. Many factors contribute to sports injuries as the body grows older. The main one is that adults may not be as agile and resilient as they were when they were younger. It is also possible that some injuries occur when a person tries to move from inactive to a more active lifestyle too quickly.

Women

More women of all ages are participating in sports than ever before. In women's sports, the action is now faster and more aggressive and powerful than in the past. As a result, women are sustaining many more injuries, and the injuries tend to be sport specific.

Female athletes have higher injury rates than men in many sports, particularly basketball, soccer, alpine skiing, volleyball, and gymnastics. Female college basketball players are about six times more likely to suffer a tear of the knee's anterior cruciate ligament (ACL) than men are, according to a study of 11,780 high school and college players. Information on injuries collected since 1982 by the National Collegiate Athletic Association shows that female basketball and soccer players have a much higher incidence of ACL injuries than their male counterparts.

Previous assumptions that methods of training, risks of participation, and effects of exercise are the same for men and women are being challenged. Scientists are working to understand the gender differences in sports injuries.

Although poor conditioning has not been related to an increased incidence of ACL injuries specifically, it has been associated with an increase in injuries in general. For most American women, the basic level of conditioning is much lower than that of men. Studies at the U.S. Naval Academy revealed that overuse injuries were more frequent in women; however, as women became used to the rigors of training, the injury rates for men and women became similar.

Aside from conditioning level, other possible factors in women's sports injuries include structural difference of the knee and thigh muscles, fluctuating estrogen levels caused by menstruation, the fit of athletic shoes, and the way players jump, land, and twist. Also,

Table 54.2. Injuries in Adults, by Sport

Adults age 25 and over sustained an estimated 2.29 million sports and recreational injuries annually from 1997 through 1999. By sport, this number includes the following:

Recreational sports	370,000 injuries
Exercising	331,000 injuries
Basketball	276,000 injuries
Pedal cycling	231,000 injuries
Baseball/softball	205,000 injuries

Note: Recreational sports include racquet sports, golf, bowling, hiking, and other leisure sports. *Source:* National Health Interview Survey.

"the female triad," a combination of disordered eating, curtailed menstruation (amenorrhea), and loss of bone mass (osteoporosis), is increasingly more common in female athletes in some sports. Its true prevalence is unknown, but it appears to be greater in athletes, adolescents, and young adults, especially in people who are perfectionists and overachievers.

What Can Groups at High Risk Do to Prevent Sports Injuries?

Anyone who exercises is potentially at risk for a sports injury and should follow the injury prevention tips. But additional measures can be taken by groups at higher risk of injury.

General Tips for Preventing Injury

Whether you've never had a sports injury and you're trying to keep it that way or you've had an injury and don't want another, the following tips can help.

- Avoid bending knees past 90 degrees when doing half knee bends.

- Avoid twisting knees by keeping feet as flat as possible during stretches.

- When jumping, land with your knees bent.

- Do warmup exercises not just before vigorous activities like running, but also before less vigorous ones such as golf.

- Don't overdo.

- Do warmup stretches before activity. Stretch the Achilles tendon, hamstring, and quadriceps areas and hold the positions. Don't bounce.

- Cool down following vigorous sports. For example, after a race, walk or walk/jog for five minutes so your pulse comes down gradually.

- Wear properly fitting shoes that provide shock absorption and stability.

- Use the softest exercise surface available, and avoid running on hard surfaces like asphalt and concrete. Run on flat surfaces. Running uphill may increase the stress on the Achilles tendon and the leg itself.

Children

Preventing injuries in children is a team effort, requiring the support of parents, coaches, and the kids themselves. Here's what each should do to reduce injury risk.

What Parents and Coaches Can Do

- Try to group youngsters according to skill level and size, not by chronological age, particularly during contact sports. If this is not practical, modify the sport to accommodate the needs of children with varying skill levels.

- Match the child to the sport, and don't push the child too hard into an activity that she or he may not like or be physically capable of doing.

- Try to find sports programs where certified athletic trainers are present. These people, in addition to health care professionals, are trained to prevent, recognize, and give immediate care to sports injuries.

- See that all children get a preseason physical exam.

- Don't let (or insist that) a child play when injured. No child (or adult) should ever be allowed to work through the pain.

- Get the child medical attention if needed. A child who develops any symptom that persists or that affects athletic performance should be examined by a health care professional. Other clues that a child needs to see a health professional include inability to play following a sudden injury, visible abnormality of the arms and legs, and severe pain that prevents the use of an arm or leg.

- Provide a safe environment for sports. A poor playing field, unsafe gym sets, unsecured soccer goals, etc., can cause serious injury to children.

What Children Can Do

- Be in proper condition to play the sport. Get a preseason physical exam.

- Follow the rules of the game.

- Wear appropriate protective gear.

- Know how to use athletic equipment.

- Avoid playing when very tired or in pain.

- Make warmups and cooldowns part of your routine. Warmup exercises, such as stretching or light jogging, can help minimize the chances of muscle strain or other soft tissue injury. They also make the body's tissues warmer and more flexible. Cooldown exercises loosen the muscles that have tightened during exercise.

Adult Athletes

To prevent injuries, adult athletes should take the following precautions:

- Don't be a "weekend warrior," packing a week's worth of activity into a day or two. Try to maintain a moderate level of activity throughout the week.

- Learn to do your sport right. Using proper form can reduce your risk of "overuse" injuries such as tendonitis and stress fractures.

- Remember safety gear. Depending on the sport, this may mean knee or wrist pads or a helmet.

- Accept your body's limits. You may not be able to perform at the same level you did 10 or 20 years ago. Modify activities as necessary.

- Increase your exercise level gradually.

- Strive for a total body workout of cardiovascular, strength training, and flexibility exercises. Cross-training reduces injury while promoting total fitness.

Women

Increased emphasis on muscle strength and conditioning should be a priority for all women. Women should also be encouraged to maintain a normal body weight and avoid excessive exercise that affects the menstrual cycle. In addition, women should follow precautions listed above for other groups.

What Are Some Recent Advances in Treating Sports Injuries?

Today, the outlook for an injured athlete is far more optimistic than in the past. Sports medicine has developed some near-miraculous ways to help athletes heal and, in most cases, return to sports. Following are some procedures that have greatly advanced the treatment of sports injuries.

Arthroscopy

Most doctors agree that the single most important advance in sports medicine has been the development of arthroscopic surgery, or arthroscopy. Arthroscopy uses a small fiberoptic scope inserted through a small incision in the skin to see inside a joint. It is primarily a diagnostic tool, allowing surgeons to view joint problems without major surgery. Depending on the problem found, surgeons may use small tools inserted through additional incisions to repair the damage, such as a torn meniscus or a torn ligament that fails to heal naturally. Using arthroscopy, for example, a surgeon may reattach the torn ends of a ligament or reconstruct the ligament by using a piece (graft) of healthy ligament from the patient or from a cadaver.

Because arthroscopy uses tiny incisions, it results in less trauma, swelling, and scar tissue than conventional surgery, which in turn decreases hospitalization and rehabilitation times. Problems can be diagnosed earlier and treated without serious health risks or more invasive procedures. Furthermore, because injuries are often addressed at an earlier stage, operations are more likely to be successful.

Tissue Engineering

When joint cartilage is damaged by an injury, it doesn't heal on its own the way other tissues do. In recent years, however, the field of sports medicine and orthopaedic surgery has begun to develop techniques such as transplantation of one's own healthy cartilage or cells to improve healing. At present, this technique is used for small cartilage defects. Questions remain about its usefulness and cost.

Targeted Pain Relief

For people with painful sports injuries, new pain-killing medicated patches can be applied directly to the injury site. The patch is an effective method of delivering pain relief, especially for many people who prefer to put their pain medication exactly where it's needed rather than throughout their entire system.

Chapter 55

Exercise-Related Aches and Pains

Chapter Contents

Section 55.1

Achilles Tendon Disorders

Definition

Achilles tendonitis is inflammation, irritation, and swelling of the Achilles tendon (the tendon that connects the muscles of the calf to the heel).

Causes, Incidence, and Risk Factors

There are two large muscles in the calf, the gastrocnemius and soleus. These muscles generate the power for pushing off with the foot or going up on the toes. The large Achilles tendon connects these muscles to the heel.

These are important muscles for walking. This tendon can become inflamed, most commonly as a result of overuse or arthritis, although inflammation can also be associated with trauma and infection.

Tendonitis due to overuse is most common in younger individuals and can occur in walkers, runners, or other athletes, especially in sports like basketball that involve jumping. Jumping places a large amount of stress on the Achilles tendon.

Tendonitis from arthritis is more common in the middle aged and elderly population. Arthritis often causes extra bony growths around joints, and if this occurs around the heel where the Achilles tendon attaches to the heel bone, the tendon can become inflamed and painful.

Symptoms

Symptoms usually include pain in the affected heel when walking or running. The tendon is usually painful to touch and the skin over the tendon may be swollen and warm.

Achilles tendonitis may predispose the patient to Achilles rupture. Patients who experience this usually describe the injury as a sharp pain, like someone hit them in the back of the heel with a stick.

Signs and Tests

On physical exam, a doctor will look for tenderness along the tendon and for pain in the area of the tendon when the patient stands on their toes.

Imaging studies can also be helpful. X-rays can help diagnose arthritis and an MRI will demonstrate inflammation in the tendon.

Treatment

The initial treatment for Achilles tendonitis is usually non-steroidal anti-inflammatory drugs (NSAIDs), like aspirin and ibuprofen, and physical therapy to stretch the muscle-tendon unit and strengthen the muscles of the calf. In addition, any activity that aggravates the symptoms needs to be limited.

Occasionally, casting is used to immobilize the heel and allow the inflammation to quiet down. Functional braces or boots have also been used to limit ankle motion and help with inflammation.

If conservative treatment fails to improve symptoms, surgery may become necessary to remove inflamed tissue from around the tendon and to remove any part of the tendon that has become abnormal.

Expectations (Prognosis)

Conservative therapy is usually successful in improving symptoms, although they may recur if the offending activity is not limited or if the strength and flexibility of the tendon is not maintained.

When necessary, surgery has been shown to be very effective in improving pain symptoms. However, if pain does not improve with treatment and vigorous activity is continued, the tendon is at risk of completely tearing.

Complications

The worst complication is tearing of the tendon. This occurs because the inflamed tendon is abnormal and weak and continued activity can cause it to rupture. In this case surgical repair is necessary, but made more difficult because the tendon is not normal.

Calling Your Health Care Provider

If you have pain in the heel around the Achilles tendon that is worse with activity, contact your health care provider for evaluation and possible treatment for tendonitis.

Prevention

Prevention is very important in this disease. Maintaining strength and flexibility in the muscles of the calf will help reduce the risk of tendonitis. Overusing a weak or tight Achilles tendon is a setup for tendonitis.

Section 55.2

Knee Problems That Can Occur during Exercise

Excerpted from "Questions and Answers About Knee Problems," by the National Institute of Arthritis and Musculoskeletal and Skin Diseases (NIAMS, www.niams.nih.gov), NIH Publication No. 01-4912, May 2001. Reviewed by David A. Cooke, MD, on June 12, 2006.

The knees provide stable support for the body and allow the legs to bend and straighten. Both flexibility and stability are needed for standing and for motions like walking, running, crouching, jumping, and turning.

Several kinds of supporting and moving parts, including bones, cartilage, muscles, ligaments, and tendons, help the knees do their job. Any of these parts can be involved in pain or dysfunction.

What causes knee problems?

There are two general kinds of knee problems: mechanical and inflammatory.

- **Mechanical Knee Problems:** Some knee problems result from injury, such as a direct blow or sudden movements that strain the knee beyond its normal range of movement. Other problems, such as osteoarthritis in the knee, result from wear and tear on its parts.

- **Inflammatory Knee Problems:** Inflammation that occurs in certain rheumatic diseases, such as rheumatoid arthritis and systemic lupus erythematosus, can damage the knee.

What are joints?

The point at which two or more bones are connected is called a joint. In all joints, the bones are kept from grinding against each other by padding called cartilage. Bones are joined to bones by strong, elastic bands of tissue called ligaments. Tendons are tough cords of tissue that connect muscle to bone. Muscles work in opposing pairs to bend and straighten joints. While muscles are not technically part of a joint, they're important because strong muscles help support and protect joints.

What are the parts of the knee?

Like any joint, the knee is composed of bones and cartilage, ligaments, tendons, and muscles.

Bones and Cartilage

The knee joint is the junction of three bones: the femur (thighbone or upper leg bone), the tibia (shinbone or larger bone of the lower leg), and the patella (kneecap). The patella is 2 to 3 inches wide and 3 to 4 inches long. It sits over the other bones at the front of the knee joint and slides when the leg moves. It protects the knee and gives leverage to muscles.

The ends of the three bones in the knee joint are covered with articular cartilage, a tough, elastic material that helps absorb shock and allows the knee joint to move smoothly. Separating the bones of the knee are pads of connective tissue. One pad is called a meniscus. The plural is menisci. The menisci are divided into two crescent-shaped discs positioned between the tibia and femur on the outer and inner sides of each knee. The two menisci in each knee act as shock absorbers, cushioning the lower part of the leg from the weight of the rest of the body as well as enhancing stability.

Muscles

There are two groups of muscles at the knee. The quadriceps muscle comprises four muscles on the front of the thigh that work to straighten the leg from a bent position. The hamstring muscles, which bend the leg at the knee, run along the back of the thigh from the hip to just below the knee. Keeping these muscles strong with exercises such as walking up stairs or riding a stationary bicycle helps support and protect the knee.

Tendons and Ligaments

The quadriceps tendon connects the quadriceps muscle to the patella and provides the power to extend the leg. Four ligaments connect the femur and tibia and give the joint strength and stability:

- The medial collateral ligament (MCL) provides stability to the inner (medial) part of the knee.

- The lateral collateral ligament (LCL) provides stability to the outer (lateral) part of the knee.

- The anterior cruciate ligament (ACL), in the center of the knee, limits rotation and the forward movement of the tibia.

- The posterior cruciate ligament (PCL), also in the center of the knee, limits backward movement of the tibia.

Other ligaments are part of the knee capsule, which is a protective, fiber-like structure that wraps around the knee joint. Inside the capsule, the joint is lined with a thin, soft tissue called synovium.

Cartilage Injuries and Disorders

What is chondromalacia?

Chondromalacia, also called chondromalacia patellae, refers to softening of the articular cartilage of the kneecap. This disorder occurs most often in young adults and can be caused by injury, overuse, parts out of alignment, or muscle weakness. Instead of gliding smoothly across the lower end of the thighbone, the kneecap rubs against it, thereby roughening the cartilage underneath the kneecap. The damage may range from a slightly abnormal surface of the cartilage to a surface that has been worn away to the bone. Chondromalacia related to injury occurs when a blow to the kneecap tears off either a small piece of cartilage or a large fragment containing a piece of bone (osteochondral fracture).

What are the symptoms and how is it diagnosed?

The most frequent symptom is a dull pain around or under the kneecap that worsens when walking down stairs or hills. A person may also feel pain when climbing stairs or when the knee bears weight as it straightens. The disorder is common in runners and is also seen in skiers, cyclists, and soccer players. A patient's description of symptoms and a followup x-ray usually help the doctor make a diagnosis. Although arthroscopy can confirm the diagnosis, it's not performed unless the condition requires extensive treatment.

What is the treatment?

Many doctors recommend that patients with chondromalacia perform low-impact exercises that strengthen muscles, particularly the inner part of the quadriceps, without injuring joints. Swimming, riding a stationary bicycle, and using a cross-country ski machine are acceptable as long as the knee doesn't bend more than 90 degrees. Electrical stimulation may also be used to strengthen the muscles. If these treatments don't improve the condition, the doctor may perform arthroscopic surgery to smooth the surface of the cartilage and "wash out" the cartilage fragments that cause the joint to catch during bending and straightening. In more severe cases, surgery may be necessary to correct the angle of the kneecap and relieve friction with the cartilage or to reposition parts that are out of alignment.

Injuries to the Meniscus

What causes injuries to the meniscus?

The meniscus is easily injured by the force of rotating the knee while bearing weight. A partial or total tear may occur when a person quickly twists or rotates the upper leg while the foot stays still (for example, when dribbling a basketball around an opponent or turning to hit a tennis ball). If the tear is tiny, the meniscus stays connected to the front and back of the knee; if the tear is large, the meniscus may be left hanging by a thread of cartilage. The seriousness of a tear depends on its location and extent.

What are the symptoms?

Generally, when people injure a meniscus, they feel some pain, particularly when the knee is straightened. If the pain is mild, the person may continue moving. Severe pain may occur if a fragment of the meniscus catches between the femur and the tibia. Swelling may occur soon after injury if blood vessels are disrupted, or swelling may occur several hours later if the joint fills with fluid produced by the joint lining (synovium) as a result of inflammation. If the synovium is injured, it may become inflamed and produce fluid to protect itself. This makes the knee swell. Sometimes, an injury that occurred in the past but was not treated becomes painful months or years later, particularly if the knee is injured a second time. After any injury, the knee may click, lock, or feel weak. Although symptoms of meniscal injury may disappear on their own, they frequently persist or return and require treatment.

How are these injuries diagnosed?

In addition to listening to the patient's description of the onset of pain and swelling, the doctor may perform a physical examination and take x-rays of the knee. The examination may include a test in which the doctor bends the leg, then rotates the leg outward and inward while extending it. Pain or an audible click suggests a meniscal tear. An MRI may be recommended to confirm the diagnosis. Occasionally, the doctor may use arthroscopy to help diagnose and treat a meniscal tear.

What is the treatment?

If the tear is minor and the pain and other symptoms go away, the doctor may recommend a muscle-strengthening program. Exercises for meniscal problems are best started with guidance from a doctor and physical therapist or exercise therapist. The therapist will make sure that the patient does the exercises properly and without risking new or repeat injury. The following exercises after injury to the meniscus are designed to build up the quadriceps and hamstring muscles and increase flexibility and strength.

- warming up the joint by riding a stationary bicycle, then straightening and raising the leg (but not straightening it too much)

- extending the leg while sitting (a weight may be worn on the ankle for this exercise)

- raising the leg while lying on the stomach

- exercising in a pool (walking as fast as possible in chest-deep water, performing small flutter kicks while holding onto the side of the pool, and raising each leg to 90 degrees in chest-deep water while pressing the back against the side of the pool)

If the tear is more extensive, the doctor may perform arthroscopic or open surgery to see the extent of injury and to repair the tear. The doctor can sew the meniscus back in place if the patient is relatively young, if the injury is in an area with a good blood supply, and if the ligaments are intact. Most young athletes are able to return to active sports after meniscus repair.

If the patient is elderly or the tear is in an area with a poor blood supply, the doctor may cut off a small portion of the meniscus to even the surface. In some cases, the doctor removes the entire meniscus. However, osteoarthritis is more likely to develop in the knee if the meniscus is removed. Medical researchers are investigating a procedure called an allograft, in which the surgeon replaces the meniscus with one from a cadaver. A grafted meniscus is fragile and will shrink and tear easily. Researchers have also attempted to replace a meniscus with an artificial one, but this procedure is even less successful than an allograft.

Recovery after surgical repair takes several weeks, and postoperative activity is slightly more restricted than when the meniscus is removed. Nevertheless, putting weight on the joint actually fosters recovery. Regardless of the form of surgery, rehabilitation usually includes walking, bending the legs, and doing exercises that stretch and build up leg muscles. The best results of treatment for meniscal injury are obtained in people who do not show articular cartilage changes and who have an intact ACL.

Ligament Injuries

What are the causes of anterior and posterior cruciate ligament injuries?

Injury to the cruciate ligaments is sometimes referred to as a sprain. The ACL is most often stretched or torn (or both) by a sudden twisting motion (for example, when the feet are planted one way and the knees are turned another).

The PCL is most often injured by a direct impact, such as in an automobile accident or football tackle.

What are the symptoms and how is it diagnosed?

Injury to a cruciate ligament may not cause pain. Rather, the person may hear a popping sound, and the leg may buckle when he or she tries to stand on it. The doctor may perform several tests to see whether the parts of the knee stay in proper position when pressure is applied in different directions. A thorough examination is essential. An MRI is very accurate in detecting a complete tear, but arthroscopy may be the only reliable means of detecting a partial one.

What is the treatment?

For an incomplete tear, the doctor may recommend that the patient begin an exercise program to strengthen surrounding muscles. The doctor may also prescribe a brace to protect the knee during activity. For a completely torn ACL in an active athlete and motivated person, the doctor is likely to recommend surgery. The surgeon may reattach the torn ends of the ligament or reconstruct the torn ligament by using a piece (graft) of healthy ligament from the patient (autograft) or from a cadaver (allograft). Although synthetic ligaments have been tried in experiments, the results have not been as good as with human tissue. One of the most important elements in a patient's successful recovery after cruciate ligament surgery is a 4- to 6-month exercise and rehabilitation program that may involve using special exercise equipment at a rehabilitation or sports center. Successful surgery and rehabilitation will allow the patient to return to a normal lifestyle.

What is the most common cause of medial and lateral collateral ligament injuries?

The MCL is more easily injured than the LCL. The cause is most often a blow to the outer side of the knee that stretches and tears the ligament on the inner side of the knee. Such blows frequently occur in contact sports like football or hockey.

What are the symptoms and how is it diagnosed?

When injury to the MCL occurs, a person may feel a pop and the knee may buckle sideways. Pain and swelling are common. A thorough examination is needed to determine the kind and extent of the injury. To diagnose a collateral ligament injury, the doctor exerts pressure on the side of the knee to determine the degree of pain and the looseness of the joint. An MRI is helpful in diagnosing injuries to these ligaments.

What is the treatment?

Most sprains of the collateral ligaments will heal if the patient follows a prescribed exercise program. In addition to exercise, the doctor may recommend ice packs to reduce pain and swelling and a small sleeve-type brace to protect and stabilize the knee. A sprain may take 2 to 4 weeks to heal. A severely sprained or torn collateral ligament may be accompanied by a torn ACL, which usually requires surgical repair.

Tendon Injuries and Disorders

What causes tendonitis and ruptured tendons?

Knee tendon injuries range from tendonitis (inflammation of a tendon) to a ruptured (torn) tendon. If a person overuses a tendon during certain activities such as dancing, cycling, or running, the tendon stretches like a worn-out rubber band and becomes inflamed. Also, trying to break a fall may cause the quadriceps muscles to contract and tear the quadriceps tendon above the patella or the patellar tendon below the patella. This type of injury is most likely to happen in older people whose tendons tend to be weaker. Tendonitis of the patellar tendon is sometimes called jumper's knee because in sports that require jumping, such as basketball, the muscle contraction and force of hitting the ground after a jump strain the tendon. After repeated stress, the tendon may become inflamed or tear.

What are the symptoms and how is it diagnosed?

People with tendonitis often have tenderness at the point where the patellar tendon meets the bone. In addition, they may feel pain during running, hurried walking, or jumping. A complete rupture of the quadriceps or patellar tendon is not only painful, but also makes it difficult for a person to bend, extend, or lift the leg against gravity.

If there is not much swelling, the doctor will be able to feel a defect in the tendon near the tear during a physical examination. An x-ray will show that the patella is lower than normal in a quadriceps tendon tear and higher than normal in a patellar tendon tear. The doctor may use an MRI to confirm a partial or total tear.

What is the treatment?

Initially, the doctor may ask a patient with tendonitis to rest, elevate, and apply ice to the knee and to take medicines such as aspirin or ibuprofen to relieve pain and decrease inflammation and swelling. If the quadriceps or patellar tendon is completely ruptured, a surgeon will reattach the ends. After surgery, the patient will wear a cast for

3 to 6 weeks and use crutches. For a partial tear, the doctor might apply a cast without performing surgery.

Rehabilitating a partial or complete tear of a tendon requires an exercise program that is similar to but less vigorous than that prescribed for ligament injuries. The goals of exercise are to restore the ability to bend and straighten the knee and to strengthen the leg to prevent repeat injury. A rehabilitation program may last 6 months, although the patient can return to many activities before then.

What causes Osgood-Schlatter disease?

Osgood-Schlatter disease is caused by repetitive stress or tension on part of the growth area of the upper tibia (the apophysis). It is characterized by inflammation of the patellar tendon and surrounding soft tissues at the point where the tendon attaches to the tibia. The disease may also be associated with an injury in which the tendon is stretched so much that it tears away from the tibia and takes a fragment of bone with it. The disease most commonly affects active young people, particularly boys between the ages of 10 and 15, who play games or sports that include frequent running and jumping.

What are the symptoms and how is it diagnosed?

People with this disease experience pain just below the knee joint that usually worsens with activity and is relieved by rest. A bony bump that is particularly painful when pressed may appear on the upper edge of the tibia (below the kneecap). Usually, the motion of the knee is not affected. Pain may last a few months and may recur until the child's growth is completed.

Osgood-Schlatter disease is most often diagnosed by the symptoms. An x-ray may be normal, or show an injury, or, more typically, show that the growth area is in fragments.

What is the treatment?

Usually, the disease resolves without treatment. Applying ice to the knee when pain begins helps relieve inflammation and is sometimes used along with stretching and strengthening exercises. The doctor may advise the patient to limit participation in vigorous sports. Children who wish to continue moderate or less stressful sports activities may need to wear kneepads for protection and apply ice to the knee after activity. If there is a great deal of pain, sports activities may be limited until discomfort becomes tolerable.

What causes iliotibial band syndrome?

This is an overuse condition in which inflammation results when a band of a tendon rubs over the outer bone (lateral condyle) of the knee. Although iliotibial band syndrome may be caused by direct injury to the knee, it is most often caused by the stress of long-term overuse, such as sometimes occurs in sports training.

What are the symptoms and how is it diagnosed?

A person with this syndrome feels an ache or burning sensation at the side of the knee during activity. Pain may be localized at the side of the knee or radiate up the side of the thigh. A person may also feel a snap when the knee is bent and then straightened. Swelling is usually absent and knee motion is normal. The diagnosis of this disorder is typically based on the symptoms, such as pain at the outer bone, and exclusion of other conditions with similar symptoms.

What is the treatment?

Usually, iliotibial band syndrome disappears if the person reduces activity and performs stretching exercises followed by muscle-strengthening exercises. In rare cases when the syndrome doesn't disappear, surgery may be necessary to split the tendon so it isn't stretched too tightly over the bone.

Other Knee Injuries

What is osteochondritis dissecans?

Osteochondritis dissecans results from a loss of the blood supply to an area of bone underneath a joint surface and usually involves the knee. The affected bone and its covering of cartilage gradually loosen and cause pain. This problem usually arises spontaneously in an active adolescent or young adult. It may be due to a slight blockage of a small artery or to an unrecognized injury or tiny fracture that damages the overlying cartilage. A person with this condition may eventually develop osteoarthritis.

Lack of a blood supply can cause bone to break down (avascular necrosis). The involvement of several joints or the appearance of osteochondritis dissecans in several family members may indicate that the disorder is inherited.

What are the symptoms and how is it diagnosed?

If normal healing doesn't occur, cartilage separates from the diseased bone and a fragment breaks loose into the knee joint, causing weakness, sharp pain, and locking of the joint. An x-ray, MRI, or arthroscopy can determine the condition of the cartilage and can be used to diagnose osteochondritis dissecans.

How is it treated?

If cartilage fragments have not broken loose, a surgeon may fix them in place with pins or screws that are sunk into the cartilage to stimulate a new blood supply.

If fragments are loose, the surgeon may scrape down the cavity to reach fresh bone and add a bone graft and fix the fragments in position. Fragments that cannot be mended are removed, and the cavity is drilled or scraped to stimulate new cartilage growth. Research is being done to assess the use of cartilage cell and other tissue transplants to treat this disorder.

Preventing Knee Problems

Some knee problems, such as those resulting from an accident, can't be foreseen or prevented. However, a person can prevent many knee problems by following these suggestions:

- Before exercising or participating in sports, warm up by walking or riding a stationary bicycle, then do stretches. Stretching the muscles in the front of the thigh (quadriceps) and back of the thigh (hamstrings) reduces tension on the tendons and relieves pressure on the knee during activity.

- Strengthen the leg muscles by doing specific exercises (for example, by walking up stairs or hills, or by riding a stationary bicycle). A supervised workout with weights is another way to strengthen the leg muscles that support the knee.

- Avoid sudden changes in the intensity of exercise. Increase the force or duration of activity gradually.

- Wear shoes that both fit properly and are in good condition to help maintain balance and leg alignment when walking or running. Knee problems can be caused by flat feet or overpronated feet (feet that roll inward). People can often reduce some of these problems by wearing special shoe inserts (orthotics). Maintain a healthy weight to reduce stress on the knee. Obesity increases the risk of degenerative (wearing) conditions such as osteoarthritis of the knee.

Section 55.3

Muscle Soreness: Tips for Alleviating the Ache

Delayed muscle soreness. It's the name of the stiff pain you feel as you roll over and reach to turn off the morning alarm after a day in which you trained unusually hard or tried a new exercise.

Some people feel there's no better reward; others cease to exercise. What everyone should know is that there is a way to prevent this muscle soreness.

What Causes Sore Muscles?

There are two types of exercise-related muscle soreness. Immediate muscle soreness quickly dissipates and is the pain you feel during, or immediately after, exercise.

Delayed muscle soreness signals a natural adaptive process that the body initiates following intense exercise. It manifests 24 to 48 hours after the exercise session and spontaneously decreases after 72 hours.

Numerous studies have been conducted to determine the cause of delayed muscle soreness, and the theories have been many and controversial. The most current research attributes it to microscopic tears in the muscle and surrounding connective tissue following eccentric exercise.

Those who experience delayed muscle soreness include conditioned individuals who increase the intensity, frequency, or duration of their workouts or participate in an activity that they are unfamiliar with. Beginning exercisers, or those who have undergone a significant lapse in training, frequently experience soreness when starting a new exercise program.

Studies on the best methods to alleviate delayed muscle soreness are almost as abundant as the number of studies conducted to determine its cause.

Cryotherapy (the topical application of ice), massage, stretching, and the use of nonsteroidal anti-inflammatory drugs (NSAIDs), among other less conventional approaches, have been tested to determine if they can prevent delayed muscle soreness or are effective treatments. To date, no therapy that hastens the decrease of delayed muscle soreness has been found, however some of the therapies previously mentioned may have a minor impact if initiated immediately after intense or unusual exercise.

The Good News

Once you induce delayed onset muscle soreness at a specific exercise intensity, you shouldn't experience that sensation again until intensity is increased.

This is because delayed muscle soreness has been shown to produce a rapid adaptation response, which means that the muscles adapt to an exercise intensity. Until it is changed, soreness won't occur.

This is the basis for the most widely recommended approach to preventing delayed muscle soreness: Gradual progression and conservative increases in intensity, frequency, or duration. Preliminary light exercise may prevent the onset of soreness following a heavy eccentric exercise workout. [See Feeling a Little Eccentric? below.]

Beginners should exercise with light weights, two to three times per week for one or two months, then gradually build. Already-conditioned exercisers who want to try a new workout or sport also should begin gradually, taking care not to be overzealous.

Feeling a Little Eccentric?

A muscle contracts eccentrically when it lengthens under tension during exercise. For example, during a biceps curl, the biceps muscle shortens during the concentric lifting phase and lengthens during the eccentric lowering phase.

Eccentric contractions also can occur during aerobic activity, such as downhill running, in which the quadriceps muscle repeatedly lengthens against gravity to lower the center of mass and aid in shock absorption.

Section 55.4

Rotator Cuff Injuries and Other Shoulder Problems

Excerpted from "Questions and Answers about Shoulder Problems," a booklet published by the National Institute of Arthritis and Musculoskeletal and Skin Diseases (NIAMS, www.niams.nih.gov), NIH Publication No. 01-4865, May 2001. Reviewed by David A. Cooke, MD, on June 12, 2006.

How common are shoulder problems?

According to the American Academy of Orthopaedic Surgeons, about 4 million people in the United States seek medical care each year for shoulder sprain, strain, dislocation, or other problems. Each year, shoulder problems account for about 1.5 million visits to orthopaedic surgeons—doctors who treat disorders of the bones, muscles, and related structures.

What are the structures of the shoulder and how does the shoulder function?

The shoulder joint is composed of three bones: the clavicle (collarbone), the scapula (shoulder blade), and the humerus (upper arm bone). Two joints facilitate shoulder movement. The acromioclavicular (AC) joint is located between the acromion (part of the scapula that forms the highest point of the shoulder) and the clavicle. The glenohumeral joint, commonly called the shoulder joint, is a ball-and-socket type joint that helps move the shoulder forward and backward and allows the arm to rotate in a circular fashion or hinge out and up away from the body. (The "ball" is the top, rounded portion of the upper arm bone or humerus; the "socket," or glenoid, is a dish-shaped part of the outer edge of the scapula into which the ball fits.) The capsule is a soft tissue envelope that encircles the glenohumeral joint. It is lined by a thin, smooth synovial membrane.

The bones of the shoulder are held in place by muscles, tendons, and ligaments. Tendons are tough cords of tissue that attach the shoulder muscles to bone and assist the muscles in moving the shoulder.

Ligaments attach shoulder bones to each other, providing stability. For example, the front of the joint capsule is anchored by three gleno-humeral ligaments.

The rotator cuff is a structure composed of tendons that, with associated muscles, holds the ball at the top of the humerus in the glenoid socket and provides mobility and strength to the shoulder joint.

Two filmy sac-like structures called bursae permit smooth gliding between bone, muscle, and tendon. They cushion and protect the rotator cuff from the bony arch of the acromion.

What are the origin and causes of shoulder problems?

The shoulder is the most movable joint in the body. However, it is an unstable joint because of the range of motion allowed. It is easily subject to injury because the ball of the upper arm is larger than the shoulder socket that holds it. To remain stable, the shoulder must be anchored by its muscles, tendons, and ligaments. Some shoulder problems arise from the disruption of these soft tissues as a result of injury

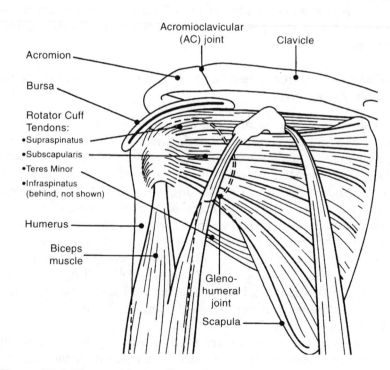

Figure 55.1. The structures of the shoulder.

or from overuse or underuse of the shoulder. Other problems arise from a degenerative process in which tissues break down and no longer function well.

Shoulder pain may be localized or may be referred to areas around the shoulder or down the arm. Disease within the body (such as gallbladder, liver, or heart disease, or disease of the cervical spine of the neck) also may generate pain that travels along nerves to the shoulder.

What is a shoulder dislocation?

The shoulder joint is the most frequently dislocated major joint of the body. In a typical case of a dislocated shoulder, a strong force that pulls the shoulder outward (abduction) or extreme rotation of the joint pops the ball of the humerus out of the shoulder socket. Dislocation commonly occurs when there is a backward pull on the arm that either catches the muscles unprepared to resist or overwhelms the muscles. When a shoulder dislocates frequently, the condition is referred to as shoulder instability. A partial dislocation where the upper arm bone is partially in and partially out of the socket is called a subluxation.

What are the signs of a dislocation and how is it diagnosed?

The shoulder can dislocate either forward, backward, or downward. Not only does the arm appear out of position when the shoulder dislocates, but the dislocation also produces pain. Muscle spasms may increase the intensity of pain. Swelling, numbness, weakness, and bruising are likely to develop. Problems seen with a dislocated shoulder are tearing of the ligaments or tendons reinforcing the joint capsule and, less commonly, nerve damage. Doctors usually diagnose a dislocation by a physical examination, and x-rays may be taken to confirm the diagnosis and to rule out a related fracture.

How is a dislocated shoulder treated?

Doctors treat a dislocation by putting the ball of the humerus back into the joint socket—a procedure called a reduction. The arm is then immobilized in a sling or a device called a shoulder immobilizer for several weeks. Usually the doctor recommends resting the shoulder and applying ice three or four times a day. After pain and swelling have been controlled, the patient enters a rehabilitation program that includes exercises to restore the range of motion of the shoulder and strengthen the muscles to prevent future dislocations. These exercises may progress from simple motion to the use of weights.

After treatment and recovery, a previously dislocated shoulder may remain more susceptible to reinjury, especially in young, active individuals. Ligaments may have been stretched or torn, and the shoulder may tend to dislocate again. A shoulder that dislocates severely or often, injuring surrounding tissues or nerves, usually requires surgical repair to tighten stretched ligaments or reattach torn ones.

Sometimes the doctor performs surgery through a tiny incision into which a small scope (arthroscope) is inserted to observe the inside of the joint. After this procedure, called arthroscopic surgery, the shoulder is generally immobilized for about 6 weeks and full recovery takes several months. Arthroscopic techniques involving the shoulder are relatively new and many surgeons prefer to repair a recurrent dislocating shoulder by the time-tested open surgery under direct vision. There are usually fewer repeat dislocations and improved movement following open surgery, but it may take a little longer to regain motion.

What is a shoulder separation?

A shoulder separation occurs where the collarbone (clavicle) meets the shoulder blade (scapula). When ligaments that hold the joint together are partially or completely torn, the outer end of the clavicle may slip out of place, preventing it from properly meeting the scapula. Most often the injury is caused by a blow to the shoulder or by falling on an outstretched hand.

What are the signs of a shoulder separation and how is it diagnosed?

Shoulder pain or tenderness and, occasionally, a bump in the middle of the top of the shoulder (over the AC joint) are signs that a separation may have occurred. Sometimes the severity of a separation can be detected by taking x-rays while the patient holds a light weight that pulls on the muscles, making a separation more pronounced.

How is a shoulder separation treated?

A shoulder separation is usually treated conservatively by rest and wearing a sling. Soon after injury, an ice bag may be applied to relieve pain and swelling. After a period of rest, a therapist helps the patient perform exercises that put the shoulder through its range of motion. Most shoulder separations heal within 2 or 3 months without further intervention. However, if ligaments are severely torn, surgical repair may be required to hold the clavicle in place. A doctor may wait to see if conservative treatment works before deciding whether surgery is required.

What are tendonitis, bursitis, and impingement syndrome of the shoulder?

These conditions are closely related and may occur alone or in combination. If the rotator cuff and bursa are irritated, inflamed, and swollen, they may become squeezed between the head of the humerus and the acromion. Repeated motion involving the arms, or the aging process involving shoulder motion over many years, may also irritate and wear down the tendons, muscles, and surrounding structures.

Tendonitis is inflammation (redness, soreness, and swelling) of a tendon. In tendonitis of the shoulder, the rotator cuff and/or biceps tendon become inflamed, usually as a result of being pinched by surrounding structures. The injury may vary from mild inflammation to involvement of most of the rotator cuff. When the rotator cuff tendon becomes inflamed and thickened, it may get trapped under the acromion. Squeezing of the rotator cuff is called impingement syndrome.

Tendonitis and impingement syndrome are often accompanied by inflammation of the bursa sacs that protect the shoulder. An inflamed bursa is called bursitis. Inflammation caused by a disease such as rheumatoid arthritis may cause rotator cuff tendonitis and bursitis. Sports involving overuse of the shoulder and occupations requiring frequent overhead reaching are other potential causes of irritation to the rotator cuff or bursa and may lead to inflammation and impingement.

What are the signs of tendonitis and bursitis?

Signs of these conditions include the slow onset of discomfort and pain in the upper shoulder or upper third of the arm and/or difficulty sleeping on the shoulder. Tendonitis and bursitis also cause pain when the arm is lifted away from the body or overhead. If tendonitis involves the biceps tendon (the tendon located in front of the shoulder that helps bend the elbow and turn the forearm), pain will occur in the front or side of the shoulder and may travel down to the elbow and forearm. Pain may also occur when the arm is forcefully pushed upward overhead.

How are these conditions diagnosed?

Diagnosis of tendonitis and bursitis begins with a medical history and physical examination. X-rays do not show tendons or the bursae but may be helpful in ruling out bony abnormalities or arthritis. The doctor may remove and test fluid from the inflamed area to rule out infection. Impingement syndrome may be confirmed when injection of a small amount of anesthetic (lidocaine hydrochloride) into the space under the acromion relieves pain.

How are tendonitis, bursitis, and impingement syndrome treated?

The first step in treating these conditions is to reduce pain and inflammation with rest, ice, and anti-inflammatory medicines such as aspirin, naproxen (Naprosyn), ibuprofen (Advil, Motrin, or Nuprin), or cox-2 inhibitors. In some cases the doctor or therapist will use ultrasound (gentle sound-wave vibrations) to warm deep tissues and improve blood flow. Gentle stretching and strengthening exercises are added gradually. These may be preceded or followed by use of an ice pack. If there is no improvement, the doctor may inject a corticosteroid medicine into the space under the acromion. While steroid injections are a common treatment, they must be used with caution because they may lead to tendon rupture. If there is still no improvement after 6 to 12 months, the doctor may perform either arthroscopic or open surgery to repair damage and relieve pressure on the tendons and bursae.

What is a torn rotator cuff?

One or more rotator cuff tendons may become inflamed from overuse, aging, a fall on an outstretched hand, or a collision. Sports requiring repeated overhead arm motion or occupations requiring heavy lifting also place a strain on rotator cuff tendons and muscles. Normally, tendons are strong, but a longstanding wearing down process may lead to a tear.

What are the signs of a torn rotator cuff?

Typically, a person with a rotator cuff injury feels pain over the deltoid muscle at the top and outer side of the shoulder, especially when the arm is raised or extended out from the side of the body. Motions like those involved in getting dressed can be painful. The shoulder may feel weak, especially when trying to lift the arm into a horizontal position. A person may also feel or hear a click or pop when the shoulder is moved.

How is a torn rotator cuff diagnosed?

Pain or weakness on outward or inward rotation of the arm may indicate a tear in a rotator cuff tendon. The patient also feels pain when lowering the arm to the side after the shoulder is moved backward and the arm is raised. A doctor may detect weakness but may not be able to determine from a physical examination where the tear is located. X-rays, if taken, may appear normal. An MRI [magnetic resonance imaging test] can help detect a full tendon tear, but does not detect partial tears. If the pain disappears after the doctor injects a small amount of anesthetic into the area, impingement is likely to be present. If there is no response to treatment, the doctor may use an arthrogram, rather than an MRI, to inspect the injured area and confirm the diagnosis.

How is a torn rotator cuff treated?

Doctors usually recommend that patients with a rotator cuff injury rest the shoulder, apply heat or cold to the sore area, and take medicine to relieve pain and inflammation. Other treatments might be added, such as electrical stimulation of muscles and nerves, ultrasound, or a cortisone injection near the inflamed area of the rotator cuff. The patient may need to wear a sling for a few days. If surgery is not an immediate consideration, exercises are added to the treatment program to build flexibility and strength and restore the shoulder's function. If there is no improvement with these conservative treatments and functional impairment persists, the doctor may perform arthroscopic or open surgical repair of the torn rotator cuff.

What is a frozen shoulder (adhesive capsulitis)?

As the name implies, movement of the shoulder is severely restricted in people with a "frozen shoulder." This condition, which doctors call adhesive capsulitis, is frequently caused by injury that leads to lack of use due to pain. Rheumatic disease progression and recent shoulder surgery can also cause frozen shoulder. Intermittent periods of use may cause inflammation. Adhesions (abnormal bands of tissue) grow between the joint surfaces, restricting motion. There is also a lack of synovial fluid, which normally lubricates the gap between the arm bone and socket to help the shoulder joint move. It is this restricted space between the capsule and ball of the humerus that distinguishes adhesive capsulitis from a less complicated painful, stiff shoulder. People with diabetes, stroke, lung disease, rheumatoid arthritis, and heart disease, or who have been in an accident, are at a higher risk for frozen shoulder. The condition rarely appears in people under 40 years old.

What are the signs of a frozen shoulder and how is it diagnosed?

With a frozen shoulder, the joint becomes so tight and stiff that it is nearly impossible to carry out simple movements, such as raising the arm. People complain that the stiffness and discomfort worsen at night. A doctor may suspect the patient has a frozen shoulder if a physical examination reveals limited shoulder movement. An arthrogram may confirm the diagnosis.

How is a frozen shoulder treated?

Treatment of this disorder focuses on restoring joint movement and reducing shoulder pain. Usually, treatment begins with nonsteroidal anti-inflammatory drugs and the application of heat, followed by gentle stretching exercises. These stretching exercises, which may be performed in the home with the help of a therapist, are the treatment of choice. In some cases, transcutaneous electrical nerve stimulation (TENS) with a small battery-operated unit may be used to reduce pain by blocking nerve impulses. If these measures are unsuccessful, the doctor may recommend manipulation of the shoulder under general anesthesia. Surgery to cut the adhesions is only necessary in some cases.

What happens when the shoulder is fractured?

A fracture involves a partial or total crack through a bone. The break in a bone usually occurs as a result of an impact injury, such as a fall or blow to the shoulder. A fracture usually involves the clavicle or the neck (area below the ball) of the humerus.

What are the signs of a shoulder fracture and how is it diagnosed?

A shoulder fracture that occurs after a major injury is usually accompanied by severe pain. Within a short time, there may be redness and bruising around the area. Sometimes a fracture is obvious because the bones appear out of position. Both diagnosis and severity can be confirmed by x-rays.

How is a shoulder fracture treated?

When a fracture occurs, the doctor tries to bring the bones into a position that will promote healing and restore arm movement. If the clavicle is fractured, the patient must at first wear a strap and sling around the chest to keep the clavicle in place. After removing the strap and sling, the doctor will prescribe exercises to strengthen the shoulder and restore movement. Surgery is occasionally needed for certain clavicle fractures.

Fracture of the neck of the humerus is usually treated with a sling or shoulder immobilizer. If the bones are out of position, surgery may be necessary to reset them. Exercises are also part of restoring shoulder strength and motion.

Section 55.5

Tennis Elbow (Lateral Epicondylitis)

Reproduced with permission from Tennis Elbow (Lateral Epicondylitis), in Johnson TR, (ed): *Your Orthopaedic Connection.* Rosemont, IL, American Academy of Orthopaedic Surgeons. Available at http://orthoinfo.aaos.org.

Description

Tennis elbow is a degenerative condition of the tendon fibers that attach on the bony prominence (epicondyle) on the outside (lateral side) of the elbow. The tendons involved are responsible for anchoring the muscles that extend or lift the wrist and hand.

Risk Factors/Prevention

Tennis elbow happens mostly in patients between the ages of 30 years to 50 years. It can occur in any age group. Tennis elbow can affect as many as half of athletes in racquet sports. However, most patients with tennis elbow are not active in racquet sports. Most of the time, there is not a specific traumatic injury before symptoms start. Many individuals with tennis elbow are involved in work or recreational activities that require repetitive and vigorous use of the forearm muscles. Some patients develop tennis elbow without any specific recognizable activity leading to symptoms.

Symptoms

Patients often complain of severe, burning pain on the outside part of the elbow. In most cases, the pain starts in a mild and slow fashion. It gradually worsens over weeks or months. The pain can be made worse by pressing on the outside part of the elbow or by gripping or lifting objects. Lifting even very light objects (such as a small book or a cup of coffee) can lead to significant discomfort. In more severe cases, pain can occur with simple motion of the elbow joint. Pain can radiate to the forearm.

To diagnose tennis elbow, tell the doctor your complete medical history. He or she will perform a physical examination.

- The doctor may press directly on the bony prominence on the outside part of the elbow to see if it causes pain.

- The doctor may also ask you to lift the wrist or fingers against pressure to see if that causes pain.

X-rays are not necessary. Rarely, MRI (magnetic resonance imaging) scans may be used to show changes in the tendon at the site of attachment onto the bone.

Treatment Options

In most cases, nonoperative treatment should be tried before surgery. Pain relief is the main goal in the first phase of treatment. The doctor may tell you to stop any activities that cause symptoms. You may need to apply ice to the outside part of the elbow. You may need to take acetaminophen or an anti-inflammatory medication for pain relief.

Orthotics can help diminish symptoms of tennis elbow. The doctor may want you to use counterforce braces and wrist splints. These can reduce symptoms by resting the muscles and tendons.

Symptoms should improve significantly within four weeks to six weeks. If not, the next step is a corticosteroid injection around the outside of the elbow. This can be very helpful in reducing pain. Corticosteroids are relatively safe medications. Most of their side effects (i.e., further degeneration of the tendon and wasting of the fatty tissue below the skin) occur after multiple injections. Avoid repeated injections (more than two or three in a specific site).

After pain is relieved, the next phase of treatment starts. Modifying activities can help make sure that symptoms do not come back. The doctor may want you to do physical therapy. This may include stretching and range of motion exercises and gradual strengthening of the affected muscles and tendons. Physical therapy can help complete recovery and give you back a painless and normally functioning elbow. Nonoperative treatment is successful in approximately 85 percent to 90 percent of patients with tennis elbow.

Treatment Options: Surgical

Surgery is considered only in patients who have incapacitating pain that does not get better after at least six months of nonoperative treatment.

The surgical procedure involves removing diseased tendon tissue and reattaching normal tendon tissue to bone. The procedure is an outpatient surgery; you do not need to stay in the hospital overnight. It can be performed under regional or general anesthesia.

- Most commonly, the surgery is performed through a small incision over the bony prominence on the outside of the elbow.

- Recently, an arthroscopic surgery method has been developed.

So far, no significant benefits have been found to using the arthroscopic method over the more traditional open incision.

After surgery, the elbow is placed in a small brace and the patient is sent home. About one week later, the sutures and splint are removed. Then exercises are started to stretch the elbow and restore range of motion. Light, gradual strengthening exercises are started two months after surgery. The doctor will tell you when you can return to athletic activity. This is usually approximately four months to six months after surgery. Tennis elbow surgery is considered successful in approximately 90 percent of patients.

Section 55.6

Shin Splints

Shin splints are pains in the front of the lower legs caused by exercise, usually after a period of relative inactivity.

Considerations

Shin splints can be caused by any of four types of problems, none of which is serious. All types of shin splints can be treated with rest.

Common Causes

Tibial shin splints are very common and affect both recreational and trained athletes. Runners are often affected.

Tibial periostitis occurs further toward the front of the leg than posterior tibial shin splints, and the bone itself is tender.

Anterior compartment syndrome affects the outer side of the front of the leg.

Stress fractures usually produce localized, sharp pain with tenderness 1 or 2 inches below the knee. A stress fracture is likely to occur 2 or 3 weeks into a new training program or after beginning a more strenuous training regimen.

Home Care

For posterior tibial and tibial periostitis shin splints, the healing process usually takes a week of rest with ice treatment for 20 minutes twice a day. Over-the-counter pain medications will also help. Do not resume running for another 2 to 4 weeks.

For anterior compartment syndrome, pain will usually subside as the muscles gradually accustom themselves to the vigorous exercise. Complete rest is probably not necessary.

For a stress fracture, rest for at least 1 month is required. Complete healing requires 4 to 6 weeks. Crutches can be used but typically are not necessary.

Call Your Health Care Provider

Although shin splints are seldom serious, you may need to call your health care provider:

- if the pain is prolonged and persistent, even with rest;
- if you are not sure your pain is caused by shin splints; or
- if there is no progress with home treatment after several weeks.

Section 55.7

Strains and Sprains: What They Are and What to Do

Reprinted with permission of the American College of Sports Medicine, Sprains & Strains: What They Are, What to Do About Them, written by Lynn Millar, Ph.D., PT, FACSM. This document was published in 2001 and reviewed by David A. Cooke, MD, on September 10, 2006.

We have all twisted an ankle or pulled a muscle at some time. But many of us are not sure what to do when this happens. This text discusses these basic types of injury and information regarding injury first aid and rehabilitation.

Sprains

A sprain is an injury to a joint ligament. Ligaments are the strong bands of tissue that connect one bone to another at a joint. The severity of the injury can be classified by the amount of tissue tearing, joint stability, pain, and swelling. The mildest sprain (first-degree) has little tearing, pain, or swelling and joint stability is good. The second-degree sprain has the broadest range of damage, with moderate instability, and moderate to severe pain and swelling. The most serious sprain is a third-degree sprain. The ligament is completely ruptured and the joint is unstable. There may be severe pain at first, but afterward there may be no pain. There will be a lot of swelling with this type of sprain, and often other tissues are damaged.

Strains

A strain is damage to muscle fibers and to the fibers that attach the muscle to the bone. Other names for a strain include "torn muscle," "muscle pulls," and "ruptured tendon." Muscle injuries are classified from first- (least severe) to third- (most severe) degree strains. A first-degree strain has little tissue tearing, mild tenderness, and pain with full range of motion. As with the sprains, the second-degree strain has a wide variability.

Muscle or tendon tissues have been torn, resulting in very painful, limited motion. There may be some observable swelling or a depression at the spot of the injury with a second-degree strain. The third-degree strain involves complete rupture of a part of the muscle unit. Motion will be severely decreased or absent. Pain will be severe at first, but the muscle may be painless after the initial injury.

Acute Treatment

There are several decisions that you must make when you injure yourself. Among the first of these is how serious the injury is and whether you should go to a health care provider. Look for deformities, swelling, and changes in skin color. If there are deformities, significant swelling, or pain, you should immobilize the area and seek medical help. Many fractures will not cause a deformity, thus if there is any doubt or concern you should get medical attention.

Stage One

Management of both sprains and strains follows the "PRICE" principle.

P—Protect from further injury

R—Restrict activity

I—Apply ice

C—Apply compression

E—Elevate the injured area

This principle limits the amount of swelling at the injury and improves the healing process. Splints, pads, and crutches will protect a joint or muscle from further injury when appropriately used (usually for more severe sprains or strains). Activity restriction (usually for 48 to 72 hours) will allow the healing process to begin. During the activity restriction, gentle movement of the muscle or joint should be started. Ice should be applied for 15 to 20 minutes every hour to hour and a half. Compression, such as an elastic bandage, should be kept on between icing; you may want to remove the bandage while sleeping, though keeping it compressed even during the night is best. Elevating the limb will also keep the swelling to a minimum. Acute treatment is the first stage of rehabilitation.

Important: If you suspect more than a mild injury, cannot put weight on the limb, or it gives way, you should consult with a health care provider.

Rehabilitation

Following the first 48 to 72 hours, it is important to start the next stage of rehabilitation. The second stage of rehabilitation focuses on gentle movement of the muscle or joint, mild resistive exercise, joint position training, and continued icing. When you are able to move without pain you can progress to the next stage of rehabilitation. During this stage you may gradually return to more strenuous activities, such as strengthening. A simple guide to how much you can do is pain. Pain should remain low during rehabilitation; if pain increases it usually means you have attempted to do too much.

Throughout your recovery you can still maintain an aerobic training program. Options for training include stationary bicycling, swimming, walking, or running in the water. If the injury is more than a mild sprain or strain it is best to consult your health care provider.

Here's an example of ankle rehabilitation.

Stage Two

After initial 48 to 72 hours swelling has stopped increasing and pain decreases

Range of Motion

- Towel pull with toes
- Draw the alphabet with ankle

Mild Resistive Exercises

- Foot press—up, down, and each side, against a solid object (no motion of the ankle)
- Tubing exercises in all motions (pain free)

Joint Position

- Standing with eyes closed—partial squats and shifts from side to side

Stage Three

Pain free; can walk without a limp

Range of Motion

- Stretching with towel

Strengthening

- Toe raises
- Hops—start forward and back, short hops
- Weights—Heavy tubing or cuff weights

Joint Position

- One-legged stand with eyes closed

Chapter 56

Foot Problems
That Plague Exercisers

Chapter Contents

Section 56.1

Fitness and Your Feet: Overcoming Blisters, Corns, Calluses, and Other Foot Problems

Fitness Planning

Striving for physical fitness is not to be taken lightly. The President's Council on Physical Fitness and Sports cautions that unless you are convinced of the benefits of fitness and the risks of unfitness, you will not succeed. Patience is essential. Don't try to do too much too soon; give yourself a chance to improve.

As you exercise, pay attention to what your body, including your feet, tells you. If you feel discomfort, you may be trying to do too much too fast. Ease up a bit or take a break and start again at another time. Drink fluids on hot days or during very strenuous activities to avoid heatstroke and heat exhaustion.

First Step—See Your Doctor

Before you start a fitness program, you should consult a physician for a complete physical and a podiatric physician for a foot exam. This is especially so if you are over 60, haven't had a physical checkup in the last year, have a disease or disability, or are taking medication. It is recommended that if you are 35 to 60, substantially overweight, easily fatigued, smoke excessively, have been physically inactive, or have a family history of heart disease, you should consult a physician.

Once you have been cleared to begin exercise, your first goal is to make physical activity a habit. The goals for your activity program, at whatever level of fitness you presently have, are (a) 30 minutes of exercise, (b) four times a week, and (c) at a comfortable pace. Stay true to these goals, and you will become fit.

Wear the Right Clothes and the Proper Shoes

For your fitness success, you should wear the right clothes and the proper shoes. Wear loose-fitting, light-colored and loosely woven clothing in hot weather and several layers of warm clothing in cold weather.

In planning for your equipment needs, don't ignore the part of your body that takes the biggest beating—your feet. Podiatric physicians recommend sturdy, properly fitted athletic shoes of proper width, with leather or canvas uppers, soles that are flexible (but only at the ball of the foot), cushioning, arch supports, and room for your toes. They also suggest a well-cushioned sock for reinforcement, preferably one with an acrylic fiber content so that some perspiration moisture is wicked away.

Because of the many athletic shoe brands, and styles within those brands, you may want to ask a podiatrist to help you select the shoe you need. Generally speaking, athletic shoes are available in sport-specific styles or cross-training models.

Foot Care for Fitness

The importance of foot care in exercising is stressed by the American Podiatric Medical Association. According to the American Academy of Podiatric Sports Medicine, an APMA affiliate, people don't realize the tremendous pressure that is put on their feet while exercising. For example, when a 150-pound jogger runs three miles, the cumulative impact on each foot is more than 150 tons.

Even without exercising, foot problems contribute to pain in knees, hips, and lower back, and also diminish work efficiency and leisure enjoyment. It is clear, however, that healthy feet are critical to a successful fitness program.

Further evidence for the necessity of proper foot care is the fact that there are more than 300 foot ailments. Although some are hereditary, many stem from the cumulative impact of a lifetime of abuse and neglect and, if left untreated, these foot ailments can prevent the successful establishment of fitness programs.

The Human Foot—A Biological Masterpiece

The human foot is a biological masterpiece. Like a finely tuned race car or a space shuttle, it is complex, containing within its relatively small size 26 bones (the two feet contain a quarter of all the bones in the body), 33 joints, and a network of more than 100 tendons, muscles, and ligaments, to say nothing of blood vessels and nerves.

Foot problems are among the most common health ills. Studies show that at least three quarters of the American population experience foot problems of some degree of seriousness at some time in their lives; only a small percentage of them seek medical treatment, apparently because most mistakenly believe that discomfort and pain are normal.

To keep your feet healthy for daily pursuits or for fitness, you should be familiar with the most common ills that affect them. Remember, though, that self-treatment can often turn a minor problem into a major one and is generally not advisable. If the conditions persist, you should see a podiatrist.

These conditions may also occur because of the impact of exercise on your feet:

Athlete's Foot

Athlete's foot is a skin disease, frequently starts between the toes, and can spread to other parts of the foot and body. It is caused by a fungus that commonly attacks the feet because the warm, dark, climate of shoes and such places as public locker rooms foster fungus growth. You can prevent infection by washing your feet daily in soap and water; drying carefully, especially between the toes; changing shoes and hose regularly to decrease moisture; and using foot powder on your feet and in your shoes on a daily basis.

Blisters

Blisters are caused by skin friction and moisture, often from active exercising in poorly fitting shoes. There are different schools of thought about whether to pop them. If the blister isn't large, apply an antiseptic and cover with a bandage, and leave it on until it falls off naturally in the bath or shower. If it is large, it may be appropriate to pop the blister with a sterile needle, by piercing it several times at its roof, then to drain the fluid as thoroughly as possible before applying an antiseptic and bandage. If the area appears infected or excessively inflamed, see your podiatrist. Keep your feet dry and wear socks as a cushion.

Corns and Calluses

Corns and calluses are protective layers of compacted, dead skin cells. They are caused by repeated friction and pressure from skin rubbing against bony areas or against an irregularity in a shoe (another reason to have your shoes properly fitted). Corns ordinarily form on the toes and calluses on the soles of the feet, but both can occur on either surface. Never cut corns or calluses with any instrument, and never apply home remedies, except under a podiatrist's instructions.

Heel Pain

Heel pain is generally traced to faulty biomechanics that place too much stress on the heel bone. Stress also can result from a bruise incurred while walking or jumping on hard surfaces or from poorly made or excessively worn footwear. Inserts designed to take the pressure off the heel are generally successful. Heel spurs are bony growths on the underside, forepart of the heel bone. Pain may result when inflammation develops at the point where the spur forms. Spurs can also occur without pain. Both heel pain and heel spurs are often associated with plantar fasciitis, an inflammation of the long band of supportive connective tissue running from the heel to the ball of the foot. There are many excellent treatments for heel pain and heel spurs. However, some general health conditions—arthritis and gout, for example—also cause heel pain.

Fitness and Your Podiatrist

A doctor of podiatric medicine can make an important contribution to your total health and to the success of your fitness program. Although podiatrists focus on foot care, they are aware of total health needs and should be seen as part of your annual medical checkup. If your foot ailments are related to a more generalized health problem, your podiatrist will consult with your primary physician or refer you to an appropriate specialist.

Section 56.2

Athlete's Foot

Athlete's foot is a skin disease caused by a fungus, usually occurring between the toes.

The fungus most commonly attacks the feet because shoes create a warm, dark, and humid environment, which encourages fungus growth.

The warmth and dampness of areas around swimming pools, showers, and locker rooms are also breeding grounds for fungi. Because the infection was common among athletes who used these facilities frequently, the term "athlete's foot" became popular.

Not all fungus conditions are athlete's foot. Other conditions, such as disturbances of the sweat mechanism, reaction to dyes or adhesives in shoes, eczema, and psoriasis, may mimic athlete's foot.

Symptoms

The signs of athlete's foot, singly or combined, are dry skin, itching, scaling, inflammation, and blisters. Blisters often lead to cracking of the skin. When blisters break, small raw areas of tissue are exposed, causing pain and swelling. Itching and burning may increase as the infection spreads.

Athlete's foot may spread to the soles of the feet and to the toenails. It can be spread to other parts of the body, notably the groin and underarms, by those who scratch the infection and then touch themselves elsewhere. The organisms causing athlete's foot may persist for long periods. Consequently, the infection may be spread by contaminated bed sheets or clothing to other parts of the body.

Prevention

It is not easy to prevent athlete's foot because it is usually contracted in dressing rooms, showers, and swimming pool locker rooms where bare feet come in contact with the fungus. However, you can do much to prevent infection by practicing good foot hygiene. Daily washing of the feet with soap and water; drying carefully, especially between the toes; and changing shoes and hose regularly to decrease moisture, help prevent the fungus from infecting the feet. Also helpful is daily use of a quality foot powder.

Tips

- Avoid walking barefoot; use shower shoes.
- Reduce perspiration by using talcum powder.
- Wear light and airy shoes.
- Wear socks that keep your feet dry, and change them frequently if you perspire heavily.

Treatment

Fungicidal and fungistatic chemicals, used for athlete's foot treatment, frequently fail to contact the fungi in the horny layers of the skin. Topical or oral antifungal drugs are prescribed with growing frequency. In mild cases of the infection it is important to keep the feet dry by dusting foot powder in shoes and hose. The feet should be bathed frequently and all areas around the toes dried thoroughly.

Consult Your Podiatrist

If an apparent fungus condition does not respond to proper foot hygiene and self-care, and there is no improvement within two weeks, consult your podiatrist. The podiatrist will determine if a fungus is the cause of the problem. If it is, a specific treatment plan, including the prescription of antifungal medication, applied topically or taken by mouth, will usually be suggested. Such a treatment appears to provide better resolution of the problem when the patient observes the course of treatment prescribed by the podiatrist; if it's shortened, failure of the treatment is common.

If the infection is caused by bacteria, antibiotics such as penicillin, which are effective against a broad spectrum of bacteria, may be prescribed.

Your podiatric physician/surgeon has been trained specifically and extensively in the diagnosis and treatment of all manner of foot conditions. This training encompasses all of the intricately related systems and structures of the foot and lower leg, including the neurological, circulatory, skin, and musculoskeletal systems (the musculoskeletal system includes the bones, joints, ligaments, tendons, muscles, and nerves).

Section 56.3

Morton's Neuroma

Overview

Morton's neuroma is an enlarged nerve that usually occurs in the third interspace, which is between the third and fourth toes.

Problems often develop in this area because part of the lateral plantar nerve combines with part of the medial plantar nerve here. When the two nerves combine, they are typically larger in diameter than those going to the other toes. Also, the nerve lies in subcutaneous tissue, just above the fat pad of the foot, close to an artery and vein. Above the nerve is a structure called the deep transverse metatarsal ligament. This ligament is very strong, holds the metatarsal bones together, and creates the ceiling of the nerve compartment. With each step, the ground pushes up on the enlarged nerve and the deep transverse metatarsal ligament pushes down. This causes compression in a confined space.

The reason the nerve enlarges has not been determined. Flat feet can cause the nerve to be pulled toward the middle (medially) more than normal, which can cause irritation and possibly enlargement of the nerve. The syndrome is more common in women than men, possibly because women wear confining shoes more often. High heels cause more weight to be transferred to the front of the foot and tight toe boxes create lateral compression. As a result, there is more force being applied in the area and the nerve compartment is squeezed on all sides. Under such conditions, even a minimal enlargement in the nerve can elicit pain.

Signs and Symptoms

The most common symptom of Morton's neuroma is localized pain in the interspace between the third and fourth toes. It can be sharp or dull, and is worsened by wearing shoes and by walking. Pain usually is less severe when the foot is not bearing weight.

Diagnosis

To diagnose Morton's neuroma the podiatrist commonly palpates the area to elicit pain, squeezing the toes from the side. Next he or she may try to feel the neuroma by pressing a thumb into the third interspace. The podiatrist then tries to elicit Mulder's sign, holding the patient's first, second, and third metatarsal heads with one hand and the fourth and fifth metatarsal heads in the other and pushing half the foot up and half the foot down slightly. In many cases of Morton's neuroma, this causes an audible click, known as Mulder's sign.

An x-ray should be taken to ensure that there is not a fracture. X-rays also can be used to examine the joints and bone density, ruling out arthritis (particularly rheumatoid arthritis and osteoarthritis).

An MRI scan (magnetic resonance imaging) is used to ensure that the compression is not caused by a tumor in the foot. An MRI also determines the size of the neuroma and whether the syndrome should be treated conservatively or aggressively. If surgery is indicated, the podiatrist can determine how much of the nerve must be resected. This is important, because different surgical techniques can be used, depending on the size and the position of the neuroma. Because MRIs are expensive, some insurance companies are reluctant to pay for them. If the podiatrist believes an MRI is necessary, he or she can persuade the insurance company to pay for it by presenting data to support the recommendation.

Treatment

In most cases, initial treatment consists of padding and taping to disperse weight away from the neuroma. If the patient has flat feet, an arch support is incorporated. The patient is instructed to wear shoes with wide toe boxes and avoid shoes with high heels. An injection of local anesthetic to relieve pain and a corticosteroid to reduce inflammation may be administered. The patient is advised to return in a week or two to monitor progress. If the pain has been relieved, the neuroma is probably small and caused by the structure of the patient's foot and the type of shoes the patient wears. It can be relieved by a custom-fitted orthotic that helps maintain the foot in a better position.

Conservative treatment does not work for most patients and minor surgery usually is necessary. Two surgical procedures are available. The dorsal approach involves making an incision on the top of the foot. This approach permits the patient to walk soon after surgery because the stitches are not on the weight-bearing side of the foot. The podiatrist maneuvers the instruments carefully through many structures and cuts the deep transverse metatarsal ligament, which typically causes most of the nerve compression. This procedure can lead to instability in the forefoot that may require attention in the future.

The second procedure involves a plantar approach, in which the incision is made on the sole of the foot. The patient must use crutches for about 3 weeks and the scar that forms can make walking uncomfortable. The advantage of the plantar approach is that the neuroma can be reached easily and resected without cutting any structures.

Surgical Complications

The surgical area contains very small blood vessels, nerves, and muscles and complications can occur. Once the neuroma is removed, the empty space may fill with blood, resulting in a painful hematoma. There is a risk for infection, necessitating careful monitoring by the podiatrist and patient. If the incision site becomes warm or red within a day or two after surgery, or if the patient runs a fever, the surgeon must be contacted immediately.

Recurrence is another possibility. The stump of nerve remaining after resection can begin to grow again. If this occurs, the nerve grows in width and length, creating a burning pain that can be treated by injection or further surgery.

Section 56.4

Plantar Fasciitis

Definition

Plantar fasciitis is an inflammation (irritation and swelling with presence of extra immune cells) of the thick tissue on the bottom of the foot that causes heel pain and disability.

Causes, Incidence, and Risk Factors

The plantar fascia is a very thick band of tissue that covers the bones on the bottom of the foot. This fascia can become inflamed and painful in some people, making walking more difficult.

Risk factors for plantar fasciitis include foot arch problems (both flat foot and high arches), obesity, sudden weight gain, running, and a tight Achilles tendon (the tendon connecting the calf muscles to the heel). A typical patient is an active man aged 40 to 70.

This condition is one of the most common orthopedic complaints relating to the foot.

Plantar fasciitis is commonly thought of as being caused by a heel spur, but research has found that this is not the case. On x-ray, heel spurs are seen commonly both in people with and without plantar fasciitis.

Symptoms

The most common complaint is pain in the bottom of the heel, usually worst in the morning and improving throughout the day. By the end of the day the pain may be replaced by a dull aching that improves with rest.

Treatment

Conservative treatment is almost always successful, given enough time. Duration of treatment can be anywhere from several months to 2 years before symptoms resolve, although about 90% of patients will be better in 9 months.

Initial treatment usually consists of heel stretching exercises, shoe inserts, night splints, and anti-inflammatory medications. If these fail, casting the affected foot in a short leg cast (a cast up to but not above the knee) for 3 to 6 weeks is very often successful in reducing pain and inflammation. Alternatively, a cast boot (which looks like a ski boot) may be used. It is still worn full time, but can be removed for bathing.

Some physicians will offer steroid injections, which provide lasting relief in about 50% of people. However, this injection is very painful and not for everyone.

In a few patients, non-surgical treatment fails and surgery to release the tight, inflamed fascia becomes necessary.

Expectations (Prognosis)

Nearly all patients will improve within 1 year of beginning non-surgical therapy, with no long-term problems. In the few patients requiring surgery, over 95% have relief of their heel pain.

Complications

A complication of non-operative therapy is continued pain. In surgical therapy, there is a risk of nerve injury, infection, rupture of the plantar fascia, and failure of the pain to improve.

Calling Your Health Care Provider

Contact your health care provider if you have symptoms of plantar fasciitis.

Prevention

Maintaining good flexibility around the ankle is probably the best way to prevent plantar fasciitis.

Chapter 57

Taking Care of Your Skin While You Sweat

Sports—the very activities we do for fun and fitness—can hurt skin if proper precautions aren't taken. Dermatologists say simple steps can keep sports and fitness enthusiasts out of harm's way.

Don't Sweat the Sweating

Joel E. Holloway, M.D., a board certified dermatologist who practices in Norman, Oklahoma, explained that perspiration is a necessary bodily function that cleanses the skin and keeps the body from becoming overheated. Problems resulting from perspiration can occur when restrictive clothing is worn, which prevents air from reaching the skin and evaporating perspiration.

"Occluding the skin can cause miliaria rubra, a type of heat rash," explained Dr. Holloway. "When the skin becomes too hydrated, the clothing occludes the little hole that the sweat tries to come out of, and causes big red bumps on the skin. This practice can also cause an elevated body temperature, which could lead to heat stroke or heat exhaustion."

Dr. Holloway suggests wearing loose clothing that allows sweat to soak through the fabric and run off.

Rubbed the Wrong Way

Chafing occurs when athletes wear clothing made of synthetic materials or clothing that does not fit well. Wearing athletic equipment, such as athletic supporters and cups, as well as staying in a wet bathing suit for hours after swimming, are other common causes of chafing. Rubbing against equipment can exacerbate folliculitis, which is an infection of the hair follicles. If chafing does not get better on its own, Dr. Holloway recommends the topical use of petrolatum jelly.

Sports and Acne

Acne mechanica is a form of acne that results from heat, pressure, occlusion, and friction, often caused by protective gear. To avoid this type of acne, dermatologists recommend that athletes wear clean, cotton clothing that doesn't fit too close to the skin. They should also wash the affected areas immediately following athletic activity and apply a keratolytic solution, such as one containing salicylic acid and resorcinol, directly to the rash. Dr. Holloway also cautioned that wearing makeup during sports activities could irritate acne.

Foot Fit

Alexa Boer Kimball, M.D., a board certified dermatologist and assistant professor at Stanford University Medical Center, Stanford, California, said blisters are a big problem for endurance athletes. "People have dropped out of races because of them," she related.

Dr. Kimball said athletes should make sure that their shoes fit well, and that their socks help to keep their feet dry because the wetter the feet, the greater the likelihood of friction and blisters. "It's a good idea for athletes to wear wool socks because wool keeps their feet warm but manages to keep moisture away. Polypropylene is usually pretty good. Cotton is horrible for socks," she said. "Wearing more than one pair of socks is helpful because then the friction is between the socks and not between your foot and the shoe."

Another tip: Don't break in a new pair of shoes during a long-distance race. Rather, train with a new pair of shoes until you are sure they fit well.

If it becomes necessary to pop a painful blister during an event, Dr. Kimball advises making a small incision of about ¼ inch at the base of the blister and applying a dressing to the wound. "My favorite dressings are healing strips (available at most drugstores). These are soft pads applied to the blister or scrape. They also promote wound healing and can be worn for days without rubbing off the feet," she said.

Athletes, especially runners, hikers, and others who depend on their feet, should buy shoes that fit correctly and replace shoes once they start to wear out. According to Dr. Holloway, shoes need to fit so that "toe box" is adequate and athletes don't slam their toes into the end of their shoes when they stop quickly. Shoes should also be laced tightly so that the toes don't slide around inside the shoe.

Athlete's foot is another common problem among athletes. The bothersome fungal infection can be avoided by keeping feet as dry and clean as possible. Antifungal powders and creams, purchased over the counter, can help, too.

Sun Safe

Athletes who compete and train outdoors must protect their skin from ultraviolet rays by applying sunscreens with a sun protection factor (SPF) of 15 or higher. Dr. Kimball suggests that endurance athletes consider gel-based sunscreens because they go on easily over sweaty or hair-bearing areas. Those who sweat a lot or swim should reapply sunscreens at least every two hours . Some experts suggest athletes wear clothing that offers SPF protection, however, Dr. Holloway suggested that regular clothing offers adequate protection. Drs. Holloway and Kimball agree that athletes should wear hats with extra material hanging down to cover the neck and ears.

Out in the Cold

According to Dr. Holloway, one of the biggest problems experienced by those who participate in cold weather sports or exercise is frostbite, a condition where feet, toes, hands, or fingers freeze, causing inadequate circulation. Frostbite can be avoided by wearing protective clothing, such as face masks, hats, gloves, and boots. Anyone who suspects they have frostbite should seek medical attention immediately.

Contact Sports

Dr. Holloway warned that athletes who compete in judo, wrestling, and other skin-to-skin contact sports must not compete if they have cold sores, molluscum, or other transmittable skin diseases. "We've got good medicines [to treat these athletes] now," he said. "Affected athletes ought to see a dermatologist right away so that they can get back to their sports as soon as possible."

Water Sports

The wrinkled skin that results from spending extended periods immersed in water is more prone to injury, rashes, and chafing. In general, skin will dehydrate after being in the water unless moisturizers are used.

Another problem, encountered by fair-haired swimmers, is "green hair." Too much chlorine is usually the culprit. "Problems also occur if the chemicals in the pool are too acidic and leach copper ions from the copper piping in the system; thus, dumping copper into the pool," Dr. Holloway said. According to Dr. Kimball, there are shampoos on the market that remove chlorine and copper from hair.

Ocean swimming presents other skin hazards, such as jellyfish stings and other bites. Swimmers who are bitten should see a dermatologist for treatment. Wet suits can protect athletes engaging in ocean-related sports.

Sweetness and Light

Some people react to exposure to ultraviolet light in combination with chemicals (such as perfumes or colognes). Those who wear fragrances and sweat in the sun could end up with a photoallergic or phototoxic reaction. Many perfumes and colognes contain oil of bergamot, an extract of the peel of a specific orange grown in the South of France and the Calabria district of Italy. When this oil comes in contact with the skin and the skin is exposed to sunlight, the oil of bergamot can cause the skin to discolor, a condition called berloque dermatitis. With repeated exposures to sunlight, the discoloration may become permanent. Sensitivities can also occur when people wear a deodorant-antiperspirant combination. The antiperspirants contain aluminum chloride, which when mixed with water can become hydrochloric acid and can cause burns under the arms, according to Dr. Holloway.

Lip Service

"Some lip balm use can result in a cycle—if you don't put it on, your lips become cracked and hurt, and if you do, they become irritated and shiny," Dr. Holloway said. "I see it every day with teenage kids who come to my office." When it comes to protecting the lips indoors, some dermatologists believe the best thing is petrolatum jelly or bees' wax—not a commercial lip balm. When out in the sun, however, lips need the same protection as any other exposed part of the body, therefore a lip protection balm with SPF 15 protection or greater is recommended.

Tips for Sun Safe Sports Activities

Athletes who participate in outdoor sports, as well as outdoor sports spectators, are at risk for high sun exposure and should take proper precautions to protect their skin. Bruce Robinson, M.D., a board-certified dermatologist who practices in Manhattan and is a clinical professor at Lenox Hill Hospital, New York City, offers these tips for sun-safe sporting.

- **After water sports, apply a moisturizer to avoid skin dehydration.** If you can, pick a time for your sports other than the hours of 10 a.m. to 4 p.m. Those are the peak times when you get the most ultraviolet exposure.

- **Use a proper SPF sunscreen—at least a number 15, but preferably a 30.** It's not necessary that you choose a sunscreen that claims to be waterproof. Instead, Dr. Robinson urges sports enthusiasts to find a sunscreen that is less irritating to the eyes, so that when you sweat the sunscreen won't be a concern. Micro-sized zinc oxide and titanium dioxide sunscreens are now available that work right away. Unlike other chemical sunscreens, you don't have to apply them 20 to 30 minutes before doing sports.

- **Reapply, reapply, reapply.** Apply sunscreen frequently—especially if you're sweating a lot. If you're a swimmer, you should apply it every time you get out of the pool. Apply a good amount of sunscreen (one palm full for each body area) in a thin layer.

- **Protective clothing is key.** Today, you can purchase clothing made with tighter weaves, specifically designed to offer sun protection. There are even new fabric treatment products that add UPF (ultraviolet protection factors) to clothing when added to the laundry.

- **Don't forget the hat.** Baseball caps shouldn't be your first choice. Rather, wear hats with a four-inch brim to protect your cheeks, ears, and nose from the sun. "We see quite a number of skin cancers on the ears," Dr. Robinson said.

- **Protect the whole body.** "If you look statistically at young women, the majority of melanomas occur on the lower legs. Apply sunscreen and wear proper clothing to protect all body parts," Dr. Robinson said. "Wear long sleeves to cover the arms if you can, and don't forget sunglasses with UVB and UVA protection. If you're a spectator, consider an umbrella."

- **Don't be fooled by winter sports.** Whether you're ascending a ski slope, or scaling Mount Everest, your sun resistance is going downhill. Because of the reduced atmosphere, you get more ultraviolet light as you increase in elevation. And while you might feel cooler skiing on the slopes, the truth is that the ultraviolet light bouncing off snow results in additional strong sun exposure for your skin. Some of what people deem windburn is really sunburn. Wear sunscreen as you would during summer sports.

- **Beware of skin changes.** Make it a point to check brown spots on your body for changes. Look for the warning signs of skin cancer.

We Can Work It out: Stay Skin Safe While Exercising in Health Clubs

Working out in a health club might protect an exerciser from the outdoor elements, such as sun exposure; nevertheless, the indoor environment presents skin hazards of its own.

Experts agree that people should look for gyms and health clubs that appear clean and encourage cleanliness. Exercisers also can take simple steps to protect themselves from fungal, bacterial and viral diseases that can be transmitted at health clubs, spas, and gyms.

"Exercisers need to approach the health club environment or any gym or workout facility as a significant source of possible infectious or contagious diseases," said John E. Wolf, Jr., M.D., a board-certified dermatologist and professor and chairman of the department of dermatology at Baylor College of Medicine in Houston.

Fungal Transmissions

Health clubs, pools, and spas do not pose an increased risk of fungal infection. Fungal transmissions can occur in any setting—and are as common in everyday life as they are in the locker room. Infected people walking barefoot in locker rooms, shower stalls, and in and around hot tubs and saunas can spread these fungi, however. Dr. Wolf suggests that people protect themselves by wearing sandals or slippers and keep their feet as dry and clean as possible to avoid athlete's foot and toenail fungi.

While the same fungus, *T. rubrum*, usually causes athlete's foot and toenail fungus, treatments for the two are different. Athlete's foot can be treated with various over-the-counter antifungal remedies. Toenail fungus, which leads to thickening and deformity of the toenail, is generally treated with oral or topical medications prescribed by a dermatologist. Proper treatment is important because toenail fungus can lead to other infections, open cuts, or sores. "This is particularly a problem in patients who have diabetes. Diabetics who have toenail fungus or athlete's foot fungus are more likely to develop secondary bacterial infections and ulcers of the skin," Dr. Wolf said. "Athlete's foot medications are not effective against toenail fungus. Toenail fungus is very hard to treat. Oral medications are often used to treat toenail fungus."

Exercisers should watch for fungi of the groin and other body areas. These tend to be caused by heat and humidity, as well as contact with infected equipment or skin. Make sure machines and mats are clean, and use a towel and protective clothing when working out.

Many of these fungal infections show up as rashes on the body. Dr. Wolf recommends seeing a dermatologist rather than trying to self-treat these rashes. Dermatologists can distinguish between fungal infections and other types of skin irritations with simple in-office tests and better target treatment.

Bacterial Infections

Exercise equipment can harbor the organisms that cause bacterial infections, such as impetigo, a mixed infection of streptococcus and staphylococcus bacteria. Impetigo, described as weeping, oozing and crusting of the skin in localized, honey-colored patches, often requires treatment with prescription antibiotics. Occasionally, it may appear as a blister or group of blisters.

A possible source for bacterial infection is the hot tub, according to K. William Kitzmiller, M.D., a board certified dermatologist who practices in Cincinnati, Ohio, and a volunteer clinical professor of dermatology at the University of Cincinnati Medical Center. "If the club's management doesn't keep the balance of chemicals right and doesn't clean the tubs, you can get into difficulty with hot tub folliculitis. It's a bacterium that gets lodged in the hair follicles and produces a superficial skin infection—like heat rash," he explained.

Dr. Kitzmiller recommends using an antibiotic soap to wash the body after exposure to a hot tub. Sometimes, exercisers who get folliculitis can treat it with a topical antibiotic ointment (such as over-the-counter medications like Polysporin or bacitracin). "If that doesn't produce prompt resolution, you should see your dermatologist," Dr. Kitzmiller said.

"This is an environment where you have multiple people using the same hot tub so it's very difficult for the spa managers to keep those truly clean," Dr. Wolf added.

Viral Infections

Viral infections may be spread in health club facilities. For instance, infected people walking barefoot on health club facility floors may transmit plantar warts, a wart on the sole of the foot that, because of pressure, develops a callus. For the most part, however, the risk of most viral infections like warts and herpes is low if the health club is clean and well maintained. "I think people can work out comfortably in health clubs," Dr. Kitzmiller said. "You should use common sense: use your own towel to exercise on, shower after with an antibacterial soap, and if the facility doesn't look clean, don't exercise there."

Chapter 58

How Much Is Too Much? Overtraining and Exercise Addiction

Chapter Contents

Section 58.1

Addiction to Exercise

"Male and female athletes and obligatory exercise" is reprinted
with permission of ANRED: Anorexia Nervosa and Related Eating
Disorders, Inc. http://www.anred.com.

Lay people know it as compulsive exercising. The person seems
addicted to his or her sport, which is often running or another intense
aerobic regimen. Researchers are calling it obligatory exercise. The
person feels obliged to pursue an excessive routine in spite of injuries, damaged relationships, and too much time taken off work in service of the activity.

Exercise Used as a Drug

At some point the over-exerciser begins to look like a drug addict.
He or she reports that the activity is no longer an enjoyable part of
life. It has taken over life and become the top priority under which
everything else is subordinate. Exercising is no longer a free choice;
it is now necessary and compulsory. It provides temporary feelings of
well being and even euphoria. The person believes he or she must do
the activity, and more and more of it. If he or she does not, he or she
feels overwhelming guilt and anxiety, which are sometimes described
as withdrawal.

Eventually the obligatory exerciser becomes obsessive in thought
and compulsive in deed. He or she may keep detailed records, scrupulously observe a rigid diet, and constantly focus on improving his
or her personal best.

Researchers say that prolonged, strenuous exercise stimulates the
body to produce substances similar to the opiate morphine. Debate
continues whether compulsive exercisers become physiologically addicted to these substances. If they do, then obligatory exercise is a
vicious circle where the biochemical products of activity lead to a self-
induced high, which in turn demands more activity to generate more
biochemical products.

The Social Context of Exercise Addiction

Sociologists say we live in an age of narcissism and self-absorption. We are preoccupied with ourselves and our bodies. Both men and women are expected to achieve perfect or near-perfect bodies: slim, toned, strong, agile, and aesthetically appealing. The closer people get to the cultural ideal, the more they notice the flaws that remain.

A preoccupation with appearance may grow out of a preoccupation with health and unrealistic expectations. We want to live to a hundred, never be sick, keep all our hair, have unlined faces and flat bellies, be attractive forever to romantic partners, and be strong, quick, and admirably competent. Paradoxically, in the United States, as increasing affluence and improving health care following World War II enabled more and more people to be better nourished and healthier, our satisfaction with our health and appearance has decreased.

Recognizing the Obligatory Exerciser

Recognition is relatively easy. These people talk of nothing but their sport, their training schedules, and their injuries. When injured, they will not take time off to heal unless immobilized. Obligatory runners with stress fractures, torn ligaments, and joint injuries have been known to work out in their walking casts.

Exercise addicts misuse their athletic achievements. Instead of enjoying their abilities as one part of a multifaceted life, they make exercising their whole life. They try to boost self-esteem, meet deep needs, and solve complex problems through performance excellence. Or they hide from emotional pain in workout schedules. It doesn't work, but instead of trying more effective behaviors, they raise their goals and standards, hoping that the increased effort will get the job done. It doesn't.

Many obligatory exercisers repress anger, have low self-esteem, and struggle with depression in spite of significant victories and achievements.

Warning Signs of Exercise Addiction

There are two warning signs. First, is your sport or workout schedule fun? If so, you are probably OK. Watch out, though, when the activity ceases being fun and becomes a duty, a chore, an obligation that is definitely not fun, but that you must do if you don't want to suffer guilt and anxiety.

541

The second danger sign is hearing repeated comments from family members, friends, romantic partners, coworkers, boss, and especially your physician to the effect that you are hurting yourself and losing perspective. The person who still has control heeds these warnings and backs off. The person who has lost control to excessive exercise will ignore sound advice and continue the compulsive behavior.

Elite athletes may be at special risk in this regard. They believe their single-minded discipline and ability to endure pain and injury set them apart and mark them as special people, even heroes, in a world gone comfortable and soft. Elite athletes who have become addicted to exercise, and to the lifestyle that is admired in their sports milieu, cannot see that they have fallen far from the goal of a healthy mind in a healthy body. They have become obsessive, compulsive, and vulnerable to permanent physical damage from minor injuries that they do not allow to heal by resting.

How Much Is Too Much Exercise?

Cardiovascular health requires that 2,000 to 3,500 calories be burned each week in aerobic exercise: running, jogging, dancing, brisk walking, and so forth. That can be accomplished by thirty minutes of exercise a day, six days a week, or less strenuous efforts (gardening, tennis, etc.) for an hour a day five days a week. After 3,500 hundred calories per week are burned, health benefits decrease, and the risk of injury increases.

Building and maintaining muscle and bone mass requires weight-bearing exercise. Individual requirements vary depending on age and level of fitness. We recommend you follow the advice of a competent trainer. Overdoing weight-bearing exercise can tear down muscle tissue instead of building it. It can also damage bones, joints, cartilage, tendons, and ligaments

Problems Associated with Obligatory Exercise

Obsessive thoughts, compulsive behaviors, self-worth measured only in terms of performance, damaged or ruined relationships, damaged careers, lower grades in school, stress fractures, and injured bones, joints, and soft tissues. Depression, guilt, and anxiety become problems when exercise is impossible.

If the exercise addict abuses steroid drugs in an effort to increase muscle mass, he or she faces additional risks: blurred vision, hallucinations, rages and tantrums, depression, acne, other skin problems, increased blood pressure, muscle cramps, joint pain, loss of sex drive, and mood swings.

Summary

For most of us, exercise is a good thing. It relaxes us and dissipates stress. It recharges our batteries so we can be more productive on the job and more attentive in relationships. In some cases exercise will lengthen our lives and make our sexual relationships more enjoyable.

For some people, however, those benefits are neutralized when exercise pushes everything else to the periphery of life. The well-balanced person enjoys home, career, hobbies, friends, physical activity, spiritual interests, and intellectual and cultural pursuits. Such a life is rich and satisfying. However, when one of these elements squeezes out the rest, the person becomes unbalanced. If you are concerned about yourself, talk to a coach, trainer, physician, or counselor about how you can regain a healthier perspective.

Section 58.2

Girls and Women at Risk: The Female Athlete Triad

Excerpted from the eMedicine article "Female Athlete Triad," by
Laura M. Gottschlich, D.O., Craig C. Young, M.D., and Boone Barrow, M.D.,
June 29, 2006. Used with permission from eMedicine.com, Inc., 2006.

The History of the Female Athlete Triad

Athletic activity by women and girls has dramatically increased in the last 30 years. Much of this increase can be attributed to Title IX legislation, which mandated that equal money and opportunities be made available to females at publicly funded institutions, particularly public schools, ranging from elementary schools to the universities. For the most part, this legislation has led to many health benefits, as generations of young women were given the chance to compete in a variety of sports. Women's athletics has grown to the point that, today, women's basketball has become a professional sport in the United States. The number of girls participating in youth baseball or tee-ball has risen from almost a rarity 20 years ago to rates nearly matching those of their male counterparts. Participation in high school sports has risen from 3.7% in 1972 to 40% in 2002, and participation in college spots has risen from 2% in 1972 to 43% in 2002.

With the increase in female participation in sports, the incidence of a triad of disorders particular to women has also increased. This triad, the female athlete triad, while more common in the athletic population, can also occur in the nonathletic population. Though first described at the 40th Annual American College of Sports Medicine Meeting in 1993, observations about bone mineral densities, stress fractures, eating disorders, and female athletics have been described for decades before the syndrome was named.

Often difficult to recognize, the female athlete triad can have a significant impact on morbidity and even mortality in a relatively young segment of the population. Indeed, the full impact of this syndrome may not be realized until these women reach menopause, when bone loss is accelerated.

Components of the Triad

The components of the triad are amenorrhea, disordered eating, and osteoporosis. Not all patients have all three components of the triad, and new data are beginning to emerge that even having only one or two elements of the triad greatly increases females' long-term morbidity.

Amenorrhea usually refers to secondary amenorrhea, although delayed menarche (primary amenorrhea) can occur in young athletes. By consensus, three to six consecutive missed menses is the requirement for diagnosis, although the continuum of normal menstruation may range from oligomenorrhea to amenorrhea.

Disordered eating includes anorexia nervosa and bulimia nervosa but is not limited to these diagnoses. The term disordered eating was coined to include pathologic eating behaviors that do not meet the strict *Diagnostic and Statistical Manual of Mental Disorders, Fourth Edition* (DSM-IV) requirements for anorexia or bulimia. This includes a spectrum of behaviors from as simple as the athlete not taking in enough food to offset the energy expended to preoccupation with eating and a fear of becoming fat by instituting measures such as food restrictions and/or the use of diet pills, laxatives, and/or diuretics.

In the young athletic population, osteoporosis refers to premature bone loss or inadequate bone formation leading to increased skeletal fragility, microarchitectural deterioration, and low bone mass. This can be manifested as multiple stress fractures or frank fractures. A high degree of suspicion is warranted in cases of unusual stress fractures (e.g., femoral neck, vertebral fractures) or in cases in which an athlete sustains stress fractures on a regular basis during her athletic career.

Frequency

United States

Although all female athletes are at risk for the female athlete triad or any of its components, sports that have an aesthetic component (e.g., ballet, figure skating, gymnastics) or sports tied to a weight class (e.g., tae kwon do, judo, wrestling) have a higher prevalence. Obtaining exact epidemiologic data is difficult because of the lack of reporting and/or gathering of data from athletes. Similar to individuals with anorexia or bulimia, many athletes with the triad try to hide their symptoms or behavior from friends, family, trainers, or coaches. This is the primary reason why diagnosis is so difficult. In fact, the vast majority of cases are diagnosed only after advanced symptoms become apparent. Milder cases may be extremely difficult to diagnose if the physician does not already have a high degree of suspicion.

The prevalence of disordered eating in the female athletic population has been estimated to be as high as 62%, with the incidence of anorexia nervosa and bulimia (as defined in the DSM-IV) estimated at 4% to 39%. The use of questionnaires, surveys, or similar modalities may not be accurate in assessing conditions such as the female athlete triad, in which the very nature of the disease leads the patient to hide her symptoms or abnormal behavior.

In the near future, epidemiologic data regarding the female athlete triad may become available. Many preparticipation physical questionnaires now include questions about whether the athlete is satisfied with her current weight and about how much weight she would like to gain or lose. These simple inquiries may reveal the first warning signs of the triad.

Functional Anatomy

Stress fractures and lower-extremity, pelvic, and vertebral fractures are most typical in the osteoporotic bone observed in those with the female athlete triad. These fractures are most likely due the increased stress sustained by these bones in the course of physical activity. In this respect, athletes with the triad are not unlike their healthy counterparts. However, those who have the triad or portions of it are more susceptible to multiple fractures, and they are more likely to sustain fractures in larger, less commonly affected bones (e.g., femoral neck, pelvis, vertebra).

Causes of Female Athlete Triad

The current theory is that the female athlete triad is caused by an energy drain/caloric deficit (i.e., athlete's energy expenditure exceeds her dietary energy intake). This disordered eating, whether subconscious or conscious, causes disruption of the hypothalamic-pituitary-ovarian axis, which results in decreased gonadotropin-releasing hormone (GnRH) pulsatility and low luteinizing hormone (LH) and follicle-stimulating hormone (FSH) levels. This, in turn, leads to decreased estrogen production, causing amenorrhea, and the decreased estrogen levels affect calcium resorption and bone accretion, causing osteoporosis.

A hormone called leptin has also garnered increased interest. Secreted by the adipocyte, it appears to influence the metabolic rate, and levels are proportional to a person's BMI. Leptin may be a significant mediator of reproductive function, and many studies have demonstrated that low levels of leptin correlate positively with amenorrhea and infertility. Furthermore, leptin receptors have been found on hypothalamic neurons involved in the control of GnRH pulsatility and in bone, which may also affect osteoblastic function.

As discussed previously, athletes in some sports linked to an aesthetic component or a weight class are more likely to have the triad. These athletes often attempt to reach unrealistic weight and body fat goals dictated by their sport, to the detriment of their health. Emotional stressors also can often be identified as inciting factors in athletes with the triad. Death of a coach or family member, growth spurts, illness that prevents training, and other events that an athlete cannot control often lead to disordered eating and excessive training—a portion of their life that they can control.

For many, moving to a university setting initiates the triad cascade. Some young women may move long distances away from their family and friends, and they have the added increase in responsibility and academic workload that most freshmen experience. Collegiate athletes have the additional pressure of performing up to the more difficult standards of collegiate competition, with a new coach and trainer and alongside athletes who may have had the benefit of 2 to 3 years of additional experience. Not surprisingly, the prevalence of the triad suddenly increases in college freshman.

Return to Play

In mild-to-moderate cases of the female athlete triad, many athletes continue to participate in their activity even while in treatment. Activity modifications should be in place, however, and the time that the patient spends exercising should be closely monitored. When inquiring about exercise times, the physician should ask about formal practice sessions and exercise away from the structured environment. Often, this extra activity is burning much of the athlete's caloric intake.

When the physician discusses exercise restrictions, the athlete often finds it easier to accept a restriction of her private workouts rather than her practice time with a team or coach. As with anorexia and bulimia, the triad is a secretive disorder. Just as the athlete may want to hide evidence of the disease, she may also try to hide evidence of the treatment. By allowing her to continue activity with her peers or coaches, she may not resist treatment.

Unless necessary, withdrawal from activity should not be used as a form of punishment for noncompliance or lack of objective improvement. This can often result of loss of the trust that has been built up and can lead to the athlete's resumption of self-directed exercise. Instead, the physician should work with the athlete to try to make her understand the necessity of the restrictions that are being set. This should minimize the likelihood of the athlete stopping therapy or being lost to follow-up.

If the athlete has been restricted from athletics because of poor compliance with the proscribed regimen or physical limitation (e.g., stress fracture), a slow resumption of exercise should be attempted. In advanced or difficult cases, resumption of activity should not be allowed until the athlete is within 10% to 15% of the suggested body weight. Even in cases in which the athlete meets the weight goal, only slow resumption should be attempted. If a physical limitation is required (e.g., to let a stress fracture heal), it may be needed for longer than usual to permit complete healing in the osteoporotic bone.

Complications

Continued bone loss leading to irreversible osteoporosis is the most worrisome complication of the triad. Some evidence suggests that bone mineral density can be regained to a small degree, but it is doubtful that significant loss can be completely corrected, even with years of therapy.

Multiple stress fractures or complete fractures can, of course, lead to increased incidence of osteoarthritis depending on the site of the fractures. Other fractures may heal without any long-term sequelae. Careful monitoring of these fractures should be provided, as they may take longer to heal than one would expect. The negative nutritional balance often leads to slowed or delayed healing of fractures.

End-stage eating disorders can result in more serious complications, such as prolonged hospitalization, cardiac arrhythmias, or even death. Anorexia nervosa has an estimated mortality rate of 15% once the diagnosis is made. Compared with others, athletes are less likely to meet the criteria for anorexia or bulimia, but significant morbidity and mortality can occur.

Prevention

Because of the difficulty in diagnosing the female athlete triad and in treating patients with the condition, prevention is fundamental in reducing morbidity and mortality rates. Early detection reduces symptoms and decreases the likelihood of serious long-term consequences.

Currently, there is substantial debate between physicians and the coaching community regarding the role of weigh-ins for sports. Some coaches or instructors have strict guidelines based on height or body type, and they set maximal weights for eligibility for competition. This regimented approach often places increased stress on the athlete and sends the wrong message about the importance of weight. It also does not account for how well the athlete has been performing in her sport (e.g., a situation in which the best athlete on the team is also 5 pounds over the weight limit).

The situation can be made worse when overweight athletes are "punished" with running or performing push-ups or when they are forced to weigh-in in front of the team. As a beginning step, the team physician should discourage such public weigh-ins and punishment and emphasize specific athletic achievement instead of weight.

The preparticipation physical examination presents an ideal opportunity to screen all female athletes for signs or symptoms of the triad. A high index of suspicion should be maintained for all female athletes because of the difficulty in diagnosing this disease. Many preparticipation questionnaires now include questions concerning the athlete's menstrual history and contentment with her current body weight. These questions often bring otherwise asymptomatic individuals to the attention of the medical and training staff. If these questions are not a part of the questionnaire, the physician should consider making them part of his or her routine examination. Most women will not volunteer this information unless asked; therefore, a proactive approach should be used in routine history taking.

Better education of team physicians, other health care providers, trainers, coaches, parents, and the athletes themselves should reduce the yearly incidence of the triad. Many young women consider oligomenorrhea or amenorrhea during the season or at times of peak activity a sign of hard work and dedication. Not long ago, the medical community considered athletic amenorrhea a benign condition and treated it as such. If both the athlete and physician are aware of the potential damage that can occur, they may be able to prevent this insidious disease.

Prognosis

For many athletes, the long-term prognosis is good. Few athletes with the female athlete triad are admitted to the hospital for inpatient treatment, and few die from their disease. However, significant long-term morbidity may affect these women later in life.

The diagnosis of the female athlete triad was established in the early 1990s, and this constellation of symptoms had been noted for years before a name was given to it. However, no long-term data about future problems are available. The first generation of athletes in whom this condition was diagnosed is still years away from menopause. Therefore, whether osteoporosis occurring at a younger age affects mortality or leads to more advanced osteoporosis later in life or an increased risk of significant fractures (e.g., hip fractures) is unknown.

For mild-to-moderate cases, some resolution of the osteoporosis is thought to occur. The lost bone mineral density is unlikely to be replaced in its entirety, and the bone mass that should have been accumulated during this important time in bone development may or may not be regained. However, many case reports show that bone density does not increase, and the losses may be permanent. Unfortunately, no long-term, double-blinded, controlled studies are available (and cannot be performed). As more information about the female athlete triad and its complications is gathered, everyone involved may better understand the significant morbidity that can occur years or decades after the disease is diagnosed and treated.

Education

Educating athletes may lead to earlier detection of the female athlete triad. If women know that amenorrhea is not a positive sign of hard work but a harbinger of disease, they may seek treatment sooner. Of course, the triad has a secretive nature, and once an athlete is showing signs of disordered eating, education may not be enough to help these women seek help. If the general athletic population is aware of the signs and symptoms of this disease, the disease might be caught in its early stages.

Physicians need to do better in educating trainers, coaches, and parents. These are the people who will have daily contact with the athlete, and they may be the persons who first raise concerns about a particular athlete. Taking the time to talk to the athletic staff about the warning signs may help in preventing the disease or catching it in its early stages.

Section 58.3

Fitness and Bone Health for Women: The Skeletal Risk of Overtraining

Excerpted from "Fitness and Bone Health for Women: The Skeletal Risk of Overtraining" by the National Institute of Arthritis and Musculoskeletal and Skin Diseases (NIAMS, www.niams.nih.gov), revised November 2005.

Are you exercising too much? Eating too little? Have your periods become irregular or stopped? If so, you may be putting yourself at high risk for several serious problems that could affect your health, your ability to remain active, and your risk for injuries. You also may be putting yourself at risk for developing osteoporosis, a disease in which bone density is decreased, leaving your bones vulnerable to fracture (breaking).

Why is missing my period such a big deal?

Some athletes see amenorrhea (the absence of menstrual periods) as a sign of successful training. Others see it as a great answer to a monthly inconvenience. And some young women accept it blindly, not stopping to think of the consequences. But missing your menstrual periods is often a sign of decreased estrogen levels. And lower estrogen levels can lead to osteoporosis, a disease in which your bones become brittle and more likely to break.

Usually, bones become brittle and break when women are much older, but some young women, especially those who exercise so much that their periods stop, develop brittle bones, and may start to have fractures at a very early age. Some 20-year-old female athletes have been said to have the bones of an 80-year-old woman. Even if bones don't break when you're young, low estrogen levels during the peak years of bone-building, the preteen and teen years, can affect bone density for the rest of your life. And studies show that bone growth lost during these years may not ever be regained.

Broken bones don't just hurt—they can cause lasting malformations. Have you noticed that some older women and men have a stooped posture? This is not a normal sign of aging. Fractures from osteoporosis have left their spines permanently altered.

Overtraining can cause other problems besides missed periods. If you don't take in enough calcium and vitamin D (among other nutrients) bone loss may result. This may lead to decreased athletic performance, decreased ability to exercise or train at desired levels of intensity or duration, and increased risk of injury.

Who is at risk for these problems?

Girls and women who may be trying to lose weight by restricting their eating and/or engaging in rigorous exercise regimes are at risk for these health problems. This may include serious athletes, "gym rats" (who spend considerable amounts of time and energy working out), and/or girls and women who believe "you can never be too thin."

How can I tell if someone I know, train with, or coach may be at risk for bone loss, fracture, and other health problems?

Here are some signs to look for:

- missed or irregular menstrual periods
- extreme and/or "unhealthy-looking" thinness
- extreme or rapid weight loss

- behaviors that reflect frequent dieting, such as: eating very little, not eating in front of others, trips to the bathroom following meals, preoccupation with thinness or weight, focus on low-calorie and diet foods, possible increase in the consumption of water and other no- and low-calorie foods and beverages, possible increase in gum chewing, limiting diet to one food group or eliminating a food group

- frequent intense bouts of exercise (e.g., taking an aerobics class, then running five miles, then swimming for an hour, followed by weightlifting, etc.)

- an "I can't miss a day of exercise/practice" attitude

- an overly anxious preoccupation with an injury

- exercising despite illness, inclement weather, injury, and other conditions that might lead someone else to take the day off

- an unusual amount of self-criticism and/or self-dissatisfaction

- indications of significant psychological or physical stress, including: depression, anxiety or nervousness, inability to concentrate, low levels of self-esteem, feeling cold all the time, problems sleeping, fatigue, injuries, talking about weight constantly.

How can I make needed changes to improve my bone health?

If you recognize some of these signs in yourself, the best thing you can do is to make your diet more healthful, and that includes consuming enough calories to support your activity level. It's best to check with a doctor to make sure your missed periods aren't a sign of some other problem and to get his or her help as you work toward a more healthy balance of food and exercise. Also, a doctor can help you take steps to protect your bones from further damage.

What can I do if I suspect a friend may have some of these signs?

First, be supportive. Approach your friend or teammate carefully and be sensitive. She probably won't appreciate a lecture about how she should be taking better care of herself. But maybe you could share this text with her or suggest that she talk to a trainer, coach, or doctor about the symptoms she's experiencing.

My friend drinks a lot of diet sodas. She says this helps keep her trim.

Often, girls and women who may be dieting will drink diet sodas rather than milk. Yet, milk and other dairy products are a good source of calcium, an essential ingredient for healthy bones. Drinking sodas instead of milk can be a problem, especially during the teen years when rapid bone growth occurs. If you (or your friend) find yourself addicted to sodas, try drinking half as many sodas each day, and gradually add more milk and dairy products to your diet. A frozen yogurt shake can be an occasional low-fat, tasty treat. Or try a fruit smoothie made with frozen yogurt, fruit, and/or calcium-enriched orange juice!

If you're a fitness instructor or trainer, it's important for you to be aware of problems associated with bone loss in today's active young women. As an instructor or trainer, you are the one who sees, leads, and perhaps even evaluates the training sessions and performances of your clients. You may know best when something seems to be amiss. You also may be the best person to help a zealous female exerciser recognize that she is putting herself at risk for bone loss and other health problems, and that she should establish new goals.

Trainers and instructors should also be aware of the implicit or explicit messages they send to their clients. An emphasis on health, strength, and fitness should be stressed, rather than an emphasis on thinness. Use caution when advising female clients to lose weight. And, if such a recommendation is deemed necessary, education and assistance regarding proper and safe weight management should be offered by knowledgeable personnel. As an instructor or trainer, it's best to maintain a professional rapport with your clients, so they can feel comfortable approaching you with concerns about their exercise training programs, appropriate exercise goals and time lines, body image and nutrition issues, as well as more personal problems regarding eating practices and menstruation.

My coach and I think I should lose just a little more weight. I want to be able to excel at my sport!

Years ago, it was not unusual for coaches to encourage athletes to be as thin as possible for many sports (dancing, gymnastics, figure skating, swimming, diving, running, etc.). However, many coaches are realizing that being too thin is unhealthy and can negatively affect performance. It is important to exercise and watch what you eat. However, it's also important to develop and maintain healthy bones and bodies. Without these, it will not matter how fast you can run, how thin you are, or how long you exercise each day. Balance is the key.

I'm still not convinced. If my bones become brittle, so what? What's the worst thing that could happen to me?

Brittle bones may not sound as scary as some other fatal or rare disease. The fact is that osteoporosis can lead to fractures. It can cause disability. Imagine having so many spine fractures that you've lost inches in height and walk bent over. Imagine looking down at the ground everywhere you go because you can't straighten your back. Imagine not being able to find clothes that fit you. Imagine having difficulty breathing and eating because your lungs and stomach are compressed into a smaller space. Imagine having difficulty walking, let alone exercising, because of pain and misshapen bones. Imagine constantly having to be aware of what you are doing and having to do things so slowly and carefully because of a very real fear and dread of a fracture—a fracture that could lead to a drastic change in your life, including pain, loss of independence, loss of mobility, loss of freedom, and more.

But osteoporosis isn't just an "older person's" disease. Young women also experience fractures. Imagine being sidelined because of a broken bone and not being able to get those good feelings you get from regular activity.

How can I eat for healthy bones?

How much calcium do I need? It is very important to your bone health that you receive adequate daily amounts of calcium, vitamin D, phosphorus, and magnesium. These are the vitamins and minerals that are most influential in building bones and teeth. This chart will help you decide how much calcium you need.

Table 58.1. Recommended Calcium Intakes (mg/day)

Ages	Amount
9 to 13	1,300
14 to 18	1,300
19 to 30	1,000

Source: National Academy of Sciences, 1997.

Part Seven

Maintaining Exercise Motivation

Chapter 59

Overcoming Barriers to Physical Fitness

Would you like to do more physical activity but do not know how to make it a part of your life? This chapter describes some common barriers to physical activity and ways to overcome them. After you read them, try writing down the top two or three barriers that you face. Then write down solutions that you think will work for you. You **can** make regular physical activity a part of your life.

Personal Barriers

Barrier: Between work, family, and other demands, I am too busy to exercise.

Solutions

- Make physical activity a priority. Carve out some time each week to be active and put it on your calendar. Try waking up a half-hour earlier to walk, scheduling lunchtime workouts, or taking an evening fitness class.

- Build physical activity into your routine chores. Rake the yard, wash the car, or do energetic housework. That way you do what needs to get done and move around, too.

From the brochure "Tips to Help You Get Active," by the Weight-control Information Network (win.niddk.nih.gov), part of the National Institute of Diabetes and Digestive and Kidney Diseases (NIDDK), NIH Publication No. 06-5578, January 2006.

- Make family time physically active. Plan a weekend hike through a park, family softball game, or an evening walk around the block.

Barrier: By the end of a long day, I am just too tired to work out.

Solutions

- Break your workout into three 10-minute segments each day. Taking three short walks during the day may seem easier and less tiring than one 30-minute workout, and is just as good for you.
- Find another time during the day to work out. If evening workouts are not for you, then try a bike ride before breakfast or a walk at lunchtime.
- Sneak physical activity into your days. Take stairs instead of elevators, park further away in parking lots, and walk in place while watching TV.

Barrier: I think my weight is fine, so I am not motivated to exercise.

Solutions

- Think about the other health benefits of physical activity. Regular physical activity may help lower cholesterol and blood pressure, and lower your odds of having heart disease, type 2 diabetes, or cancer. Research shows that people who are overweight, active, and fit live longer than people who are not overweight but are inactive and unfit. Also, physical activity may lift your mood and increase your energy level.
- Do it just for fun. Play a team sport, work in a garden, or learn a new dance and make getting fit something fun.
- Train for a charity event. You can work to help others while you work out.

Barrier: Getting on a treadmill or stationary bike is boring.

Solutions

- Meet a friend for workouts. If your buddy is on the next bike or treadmill, your workout will be less boring.

- Watch TV or listen to music or a book on tape while you walk or pedal indoors. Check out music or books on tape from your local library.

- Get outside. A change in scenery can relieve your boredom. If you are riding a bike outside, be sure to wear a helmet and learn safe rules of the road.

Barrier: I am afraid I will hurt myself.

Solutions

- Start slowly. If you are starting a new physical activity program, go slow at the start. Even if you are doing an activity that you once did well, start up again slowly to lower your risk of injury or burn-out.

- Choose moderate-intensity physical activities. You are not likely to hurt yourself by walking 30 minutes per day. Doing vigorous physical activities may increase your risk for injury, but moderate-intensity physical activity is low risk.

- Take a class. A knowledgeable group fitness instructor should be able to teach you how to move with proper form and lower risk for injury. The instructor can watch your actions during class and let you know if you are doing things right.

- Choose water workouts. Whether you swim laps or try water aerobics, working out in the water is easy on your joints and helps reduce sore muscles and injury.

- Work with a personal trainer. A certified personal trainer should be able to show you how to warm up, cool down, use fitness equipment like treadmills and weight-training machines, and use proper form to help lower your risk for injury. Personal training sessions may be cheap or costly, so find out about fees before making an appointment.

Barrier: I have never been into sports.

Solutions

- Find a physical activity that you enjoy. You do not have to be an athlete to benefit from physical activity. Try yoga, hiking, or planting a garden.

- Choose an activity that you can stick with, like walking. Just put one foot in front of the other. Use the time you spend walking to relax, talk with a friend or family member, or just enjoy the scenery.

Barrier: *I do not want to spend a lot of money to join a gym or buy workout gear.*

Solutions

- Choose free activities. Garden, take your children to the park to play, lift plastic milk jugs filled with water or sand, or take a walk.

- Find out if your job offers any discounts on memberships. Some companies get lower membership rates at fitness or community centers. Other companies will even pay for part of an employee's membership fee.

- Check out your local recreation or community center. These centers may cost less than other gyms, fitness centers, or health clubs.

- Choose physical activities that do not require any special gear. Walking requires only a pair of sturdy shoes. To dance, just turn on some music.

Barrier: *I do not have anyone to watch my kids while I work out.*

Solutions

- Do something physically active with your kids. Kids need physical activity, too. No matter what age your kids are, you can find an activity you can do together. Dance to music, take a walk, run around the park, or play basketball or soccer together.

- Take turns with another parent to watch the kids. One of you minds the kids while the other one works out.

- Hire a babysitter.

- Look for a fitness or community center that offers child care. Centers that have child care are becoming more popular. Cost and quality vary, so get all the information up front.

Barrier: *My family and friends are not physically active.*

Solutions

- Do not let that stop you. Do it for yourself. Enjoy the rewards—such as better sleep, a happier mood, more energy, and a stronger body—you get from working out.

- Join a class or sports league where people count on you to show up. If your basketball team or dance partner counts on you, you will not want to miss a workout, even if your family and friends are not involved.

Barrier: I would be embarrassed if my neighbors or friends saw me exercising.

Solutions

- Ask yourself if it really matters. You are doing something positive for your health and that is something to be proud of. You may even inspire others to get physically active, too.

- Invite a friend or neighbor to join you. You may feel less self-conscious if you are not alone.

- Go to a park, nature trail, or fitness or community center to be physically active.

Place Barriers

Barrier: My neighborhood does not have sidewalks.

Solutions

- Find a safe place to walk. Instead of walking in the street, walk in a friend or family member's neighborhood that has sidewalks. Walk during your lunch break at work. Find out if you can walk at a local school track.

- Work out in the yard. Do yard work or wash the car. These count as physical activity, too.

Barrier: The winter is too cold/summer is too hot to be active outdoors.

Solutions

- Walk around the mall.

- Join a fitness or community center. Find one that lets you pay only for the months or classes you want, instead of the whole year.

- Exercise at home. Work out to fitness videos or DVDs. Check a different one out from the library each week for variety.

Barrier: I do not feel safe exercising by myself.

Solutions

- Join or start a walking group. You can enjoy added safety and company as you walk.

- Take an exercise class at a nearby fitness or community center.

- Work out at home. You don't need a lot of space. Turn on the radio and dance or follow along with a fitness show on TV.

Health Barriers

Barrier: I have a health problem (diabetes, heart disease, asthma, arthritis) that I do not want to make worse.

Solutions

- Talk with your health care professional. Most health problems are helped by physical activity. Find out what physical activities you can safely do and follow advice about length and intensity of workouts.

- Start slowly. Take it easy at first and see how you feel before trying more challenging workouts. Stop if you feel out of breath, dizzy, faint, or nauseated, or if you have pain.

Barrier: I have an injury and do not know what physical activities, if any, I can do.

Solutions

- Talk with your health care professional. Ask your physician or physical therapist about what physical activities you can safely perform. Follow advice about length and intensity of workouts.

- Start slowly. Take it easy at first and see how you feel before trying more challenging workouts. Stop if you feel pain.

- Work with a personal trainer. A knowledgeable personal trainer should be able to help you design a fitness plan around your injury.

Moving Forward

What can I do to break through my roadblocks?

What are the top two or three roadblocks to physical activity that you face? What can you do to break through these barriers? Write down a list of the barriers you face and solutions you can use to overcome them.

What's next?

You have thought about ways to beat your roadblocks to physical activity. Now, create your road map for adding physical activity to your days in the following three steps.

#1. Know your goal.

Set up short-term goals, like walking 10 minutes a day, 3 days a week, and try to build up to at least 30 minutes of moderate-intensity physical activity on most days of the week—or preferably, every day of the week. Moderate-intensity physical activity makes you breathe harder, but you should still have enough breath to carry on a conversation. You may need to be physically active for more than 30 minutes a day to help you lose and keep off extra weight.

Track your progress by writing down your goals and what you have done each day, including the type of activity and how long you spent doing it. Seeing your progress in black and white can help keep you motivated.

#2. See your health care provider if necessary.

If you are a man and over age 40 or a woman and over age 50, or have a chronic health problem such as heart disease, high blood pressure, diabetes, osteoporosis, or obesity, talk to your health care provider before starting a vigorous physical activity program. You do not need to talk to your provider before starting an activity like walking.

#3. Answer questions about how physical activity will fit into your life.

Think about answers to the following four questions. You can write your answers down on a sheet of paper. Your answers will be your road map to your physical activity program.

- *What physical activities will you do?* List the activities you would like to do, such as walking, energetic yard work or house-work, joining a sports league, exercising with a video, dancing, swimming, bicycling, or taking a class at a fitness or community center. Think about sports or other activities that you enjoyed doing when you were younger. Could you enjoy one of these activities again?

- *When will you be physically active?* List the days and times you could do each activity on your list, such as first thing in the morning, during lunch break from work, after dinner, or on Saturday afternoon. Look at your calendar or planner to find the days and times that work best.

- *Who will remind you to get off the couch?* List the people—your spouse, sibling, parent, or friends—who can support your efforts to become physically active. Give them ideas about how they could be supportive, like offering encouraging words, watching your kids, or working out with you.

- *When will you start your physical activity program?* Set a date when you will start getting active. The date might be the first meeting of an exercise class you have signed up for, or a date you will meet a friend for a walk. Write the date on your calendar. Then stick to it. Before you know it, physical activity will become a regular part of your life.

Chapter 60

Staying Motivated to Exercise through Goal Setting

It's easy to sit back and think about all the reasons not to exercise (i.e., I'm tired, it hurts, I can't do much, or it's too hard). It is even easier not to contemplate the possibility of exercise. The hard part is making the conscious decision to make a change in your life and to write out or verbalize what that change will be. The hardest part is the first step, but the most gratifying experience is seeing the improvements you can make from that point forward. Remember that the most difficult step is merely getting out of bed and putting on your running shoes. After you walk out that door, the run is easy.

What is a goal?

A goal is an objective; something to strive for. Goals are said to direct an individual's attention to relevant activities and increase motivation to achieve a certain result. These goals can be both long- and short-term, and may reflect both outcome and process. The long-term or outcome goals represent the ultimate destination, the "big dream." Process or short-term goals are daily actions or behaviors that direct you to that final result. For example, a long-term goal may be, "I want

"Motivation through Goal Setting" by Jamie E. Robbins, Michigan State University, is reproduced from the National Center on Physical Activity and Disability at www.ncpad.org. It may be freely distributed in its entirety as long as it includes this notice but cannot be edited, modified, or otherwise altered without the express written permission of NCPAD. Contact NCPAD at 1-800-900-8086 for additional details.

to fit in my clothes from last year" and the short-term goals may include working out three times per week and cutting back on junk food. A common long-term goal for athletic teams concerns making it to a tournament or winning a championship. The process or short-term goals would deal with the amount of work put forth in everyday practice, times on runs, and other specific goals that can be measured and assessed throughout the season.

What is goal-setting and why should I use it?

Goal-setting allows you to decide what you want to accomplish and to set the guidelines for how you plan to get there. Other people often tell us what we need to do or what is expected of us, but goal-setting comes from your personal desire to improve and it ends with your effort and willingness to work for the outcome of choice.

Goal-setting simplifies and makes possible the attainment of a seemingly impossible dream. For example, it may seem unrealistic to say, "I want to run a marathon." However, it is feasible to say, "Tomorrow I will run 3 miles and Tuesday I will run 5 miles, until eventually I build up to the 26.1 miles." Eventually you will reach your goal, but the in-between steps are less grandiose and overwhelming.

The process of setting a goal also makes the possibility for success real because you are not only telling yourself, "This is what I want to do," but you also are telling other people, thereby making it concrete. By setting a goal publicly, you may increase your willingness to work through the tough times.

Goal-setting also aids in improving your focus on the important details that you need to address before achieving a goal. We are so busy, and it is so easy to lose focus or become distracted and focus on other responsibilities, thus abandoning our goals. However, by setting a goal and writing out the steps needed, you make your goal a priority.

Therefore, goal-setting puts the power in your hands to achieve an outcome you desire by focusing your attention, simplifying a seemingly large feat and by transforming some abstract wish into specific, daily, conquerable behaviors.

What constitutes a good goal?

What have I done before? Is my goal realistic given my abilities?

Looking at previous accomplishments or performances, or at previous failures, can help gauge where to set a goal initially. For example, if you want to start swimming, but you have never swum before, your first goal may be to just get to the pool.

How easily can I assess whether or not I achieved my goal? Are my goals specific and measurable so I can document my progress?

Specific goals are most effective in changing behavior because they help people recognize if they are achieving their goals, and if the goals are too easy or too difficult. "I want to do well" does not provide any context. Who do you want to do well in relation and what is "well"? A more valuable goal would be, "I want to lift the 10-pound dumbbell two more times with each arm than I did yesterday." A measurable goal is something you can assess throughout the process and therefore note progress or decline. So, instead of creating a goal to work hard when I'm in the gym, I would want a goal that uses amounts of time spent on workouts, amount of time to do a certain activity, or number of repetitions of a certain skill. These goals can be measured, charted, documented, and changed to fit the individual's needs.

Do I have short and long-term goals?

Goal-setting is like climbing stairs; the ultimate goal is the top, but you must use the entire staircase to accomplish that feat. For example, a long-term goal would be to bike a 10K race in May. A novice biker would need to set goals concerning how many days a week he or she wants to practice, how long the mileage will be each day, and eventually build from a slow 10-minute bike ride up to the desired 10K race. Remember that changes do not happen overnight. Often, people get discouraged when they do not see huge advances immediately or when change or progress appears to level off. It is important to remember that as you start to reach your peak in a certain area, improvements get smaller and smaller. For example, it is easier for a person who is 50 pounds overweight to lose weight than it is for a person who only needs to lose 5 pounds. Similarly it is easier for a person who is just beginning to run to drop his time over several weeks than it is for a person who has been running all her life and is near her peak potential. Because of this, short-term goals are important for maintaining motivation and by helping you to recognize where you began, where you are and where you are going.

It is beneficial to publicly acknowledge your goal.

This encourages other people to serve as a support system that can boost your motivation if it starts to wane. You can display signs in your house or office, or merely tell people what your goals are and how you plan to achieve them. A support system may consist of your best friends, your family, or your partners at work. The role they play is in understanding your goals and then pushing you in a positive way to stay on course to reach the outcome.

Finally, record your goals.

Keep track of what you have accomplished and where you have failed. A chart can help you assess your goals realistically and shift them according to your needs. If your goal is to exercise for 30 minutes a day, three days per week, and you accomplish this goal three weeks in a row, it may be time to increase your time spent exercising, or the number of days per week you choose to workout. It is easy to stay with a goal that is comfortable and a goal you can easily achieve, but the pride comes with setting a goal that pushes your limits.

Usefulness of Goal-Setting

Goal-setting can be used to start a workout program, plan for a test, or aid in planning a strategy to achieve any goal. This method provides the answers to both "What do I want?" and "How will I get there?" Having desires, hopes, and dreams is important. Doing something proactive to make those goals a reality is crucial.

How to Begin the Goal-Setting Process

List Your Goals

Make a list of general goals you have in a variety of areas, for example:

- do well in school or work,
- begin an exercise program,
- have fun, and
- visit my family more.

After listing your general goals, create a hierarchical list with (a) being most important to (d) being least important.

Assess Your Needs

After choosing the goal you most want to achieve, brainstorm all necessary factors that can influence your ability to achieve that goal.

For example, if you want to start an exercise program, what is the specific long-term goal? (i.e., work out for 30 minutes per day for three days per week). This is where you would look to see that the goal is realistic, specific, and measurable.

Plan a Route to Success

Next, write down the long-term goal and list the steps, or short-term goals, needed to achieve success. The progression would look something like the following example:

- Step one: Assess general fitness level by making an appointment to see a physician.
- Step two: Find a place to work out.
- Step three: Start workouts at an easy pace, two days per week for 20 minutes.
- Step four: Increase time of workout as comfort level increases.
- Step five: Increase days of week and length of workout.
- Final goal: Work out three times per week for 30 minutes.

It also is helpful to chart your progress. Create a calendar and document what you intend to do on a given day, and after the workout, document your actual achievements. You want to challenge yourself to work hard, but not push so hard that you never achieve the goal. If a goal is too difficult or too easy, you may be less inclined to try to achieve it and therefore it is important to assess the level correctly and change the goal as needed.

"The journey is the reward" (unknown); therefore, enjoy the process you take in achieving your goal. Setting a goal and trying to reach it is difficult and taxing at times, but the rewards are boundless. Goal-setting allows you to test your limits and demand more from yourself than you previously knew you had. It allows you to feel pride in accomplishing feats that once appeared to be out of reach. You can increase your self-concept by recognizing that you set a goal and you reached that goal because of your own effort, desire, and motivation to succeed.

Note

The information provided here is offered as a service only. The National Center on Physical Activity and Disability, University of Illinois at Chicago, the National Center on Accessibility, and the Rehabilitation Institute of Chicago do not formally recommend or endorse the equipment listed. As with any products or services, consumers should investigate and determine on their own which equipment best fits their needs and budget.

National Center on Physical Activity and Disability
Toll-Free: 800-900-8086
Fax: 312-355-4058
Website: http://www.ncpad.org
E-mail: ncpad@uic.edu

Books

1. Weinberg, R. S., and D. Gould, D. (1995). *Foundations of Sport and Exercise Psychology*. Champaign, IL: Human Kinetics.

2. Orlick, T. (1990). In *Pursuit of Excellence: How to Win in Sport and Life through Mental Training*. Champaign, IL: Human Kinetics Pub.

3. Gould, D. (2001). *Applied Sport Psychology: Goal Setting for Peak Performance*. Mountain View, CA: Mayfield Publishing Company.

4. Burton, D. (1992). In *Advances in Sport Psychology: The Jekyll / Hyde Nature of Goals: Reconceptualizing Goal-Setting in Sport*. Champaign, IL: Human Kinetics.

Journals

1. Wanlin, C. M., D.W. Hrycaiko, G.L. Martin, and M. Mahon. (1997). The Effects of Goal-Setting Package on the Performance of Speed Skaters. *Journal of Applied Sport Psychology,* 9(2), 212–228.

Chapter 61

Ten Tips for Sticking to Your Exercise Program

Now you're exercising again, and it feels great. Of course, it felt great last year, too, when you went to the gym every morning for almost the entire winter! If it feels so great, why do you keep quitting? You may be able to make your physical activity more consistent by using some of these tricks.

1. Start looking at exercise differently.

This is the big one, from my perspective, says James Gavin, PhD, sport psychologist and professor at Concordia University in Montreal, Quebec. All movement is exercise. People need to give themselves more options. Take the dog for a walk, bike to the store, take five-minute stretch breaks. If you don't count something as exercise unless it happens in the gym, goes on for 40 minutes, or requires a shower afterward, you're missing some of your best opportunities to stay active.

2. Think small.

This advice can be hardest for people who expect the most from themselves. Why bother walking around the block when you should be running your usual four miles? Because when you don't have time to do all four miles, a brisk hike can keep you from feeling that you've failed.

3. Set an agenda.

It helps to challenge yourself with a learning or performance agenda, says Gavin. Set a goal, such as increasing the speed, frequency, or duration of your activity. Maybe it's time to train for a marathon—or take a walk up the hill in the backyard without getting winded. (It's perfectly fine to think small for your performance agenda, too). Your trainer can help you determine appropriate goals.

4. Get off the beaten path.

Have you ever tried snowboarding? Bowling? Swing dancing? Body surfing? Chi kung? How about reversing your power walk route? Exercising at a different time of day? Physical activity isn't boring, but how you participate in it can be.

5. Use your brain.

The active mind needs to be engaged, says Gavin. If you're new to exercise, dissociate tactics, such as listening to music, watching TV, or playing computer games may help you stick with it—but stay aware of sensations that could signal injury or overdoing it. As you become more experienced, associative strategies, such as focusing on your breath or concentrating on the movement of your body, can help you enjoy exercise more.

6. Get an accountability partner.

Minneapolis lifestyle coach Kate Larsen suggests finding a friend, mentor, or coach to keep you honest. You can either exercise with your partner, or simply check in with him or her to report your progress.

7. Plan to stay active.

Don't decide in the moment if you can make the choice beforehand, says Larsen. Plan to park farther from the office and put your walking shoes in the car the night before. Plan to take that new yoga class next week, and call the babysitter now.

8. Face your fitness foes.

Does vacation throw your exercising schedule out of whack? Do projects at work overtake your activity time? Do injuries sideline you?

Boredom? Fear of success? Fitness foes can be beaten once they've been identified. You can change your vacation style, set work limits, get guidance for injury-free activity, find new challenges, or face your fears with counseling and support.

9. Go tribal.

Even if you are introverted, the presence of others in your exercise environment can be motivating. We pick up on other people's energy, Gavin points out. We get into the tribal rhythms of being fully alive. Choose places and times to exercise where there will be other people who are actively involved in exercise.

10. Use a script.

We tell ourselves things like, Skipping this one little walk won't matter all that much, according to Larsen. Next time, be prepared with an answer for this excuse. Use images of past successful experiences to remind yourself of how good exercise makes you feel. Or repeat a simple phrase to yourself, such as, Every little bit makes a big difference. If you use planning, flexibility, and imagination, you won't ever need to feel like a dropout again.

Chapter 62

Working out with Friends and Family

Chapter Contents

Section 62.1

Finding an Exercise Buddy or Joining a Club

From "Find a Buddy/Join a Club," a publication of the Office on Women's Health (www.womenshealth.gov) within the U.S. Department of Health and Human Services, 2004.

Let's face it. Exercise is one of the biggest challenges women face. The health benefits of staying physically active are well known, and women truly want to exercise for better health. So, why is it so hard to find motivation?

To find the motivation you need to get in shape, look for an exercise partner or even join a club. You will have fun communicating with others and improve your health at the same time.

Find a Buddy

"Being able to call someone for encouragement to keep on going is important," says Mary E. Clark, Program Chairperson of the Board of Directors for the Black Women's Agenda, a non-profit education and advocacy organization in Washington, D.C.

Finding a buddy does not have to be difficult. "Keep it simple," recommends Clark. "Pick someone who you would have to spend time with anyway, look for a family member or someone who's nearby, or tie it to something you have to do."

Consider these ideas to help you get moving.

- Look for someone who shares the same long-term physical fitness goals.

- Find someone with a similar fitness level so you can grow together.

- Make a plan that both you and your partner find enjoyable.

- Seek a variety of activities if doing the same thing bores you. Or stick to the one or two activities that you truly enjoy.

- Ask a coworker to join you for a walk around the block at lunchtime everyday.

- Find a virtual buddy and keep a fitness journal online.

Join a Club

If the social aspect of exercising with a group motivates you, then joining or starting a club may be your best path to fitness. Although the cost of joining a health club may be high, it may be a worthwhile investment. Here are specific tips on joining a club:

- Ask your local health club for pay-as-you-go options.

- Start or join a workplace walking or aerobic group.

- Look for more affordable community fitness centers that are sponsored by local counties.

- Start or join an exercise program at your neighborhood school, park and recreation service, or community college.

- Pursue group personal training. Get together with friends and hire a personal trainer for a more affordable way to get professional help.

- Look for walk-a-thons in the fall and in the spring. "It's a great way to join with a group for a worthy cause," says Clark.

- Start a fitness club at your church or join an existing one.

See your doctor to discuss your plan before starting an exercise program. He or she can address any health considerations and help you determine if the program you are considering is right for you.

Ask for specifics on such things as your cholesterol level, blood pressure, and how to take you heart rate.

Begin exercising at your current fitness level, and work up slowly. If you try to do too much at the beginning, you may face early burnout. Finding motivation to make exercise part of your regimen is a lifelong process that will bring many benefits and will put you on a path to better health.

Section 62.2

Staying Fit with Your Family

From "Play Sports with Your Kids," a publication of the Office on
Women's Health (www.womenshealth.gov) within the U.S. Department
of Health and Human Services, 2004.

Playing sports with your kids is an ideal way to keep the entire
family active. If you're trying to fit exercise into your schedule and
also spend more time with the family, staying active together will help
improve everyone's health and overall quality of life.

Modeling a healthy lifestyle is important, especially because "one
in four children are obese," says Verna Simpkins, Director of Membership and Program Initiatives for the Girl Scouts.

The Surgeon General's report on *Physical Activity and Health* finds
that:

- More than 60 percent of U.S. adults do not engage in the recommended amount of activity.

- Approximately 25 percent of U.S. adults are not at all active.

- Physical inactivity is more common among:

  - women than men;

  - African American and Hispanic adults than white adults; and

  - less affluent than more affluent populations.

Your children may be at risk of leading sedentary lives as well. The
Surgeon General's report finds that:

- Nearly half of American youths, aged 12 to 21 years, are not vigorously active on a regular basis.

- Inactivity among youths is more common among females than
males and more common among black females than among white
females.

- Participation in all types of physical activity declines strikingly
as age or grade in school increases.

But consider this. According to the Surgeon General's report, "Social support from family and friends has been consistently and positively related to regular physical activity."

So working out together is the inspiration everyone in your family needs. Begin by choosing activities that you can do together and that interest both you and your children. If your children are skeptical at first, motivate them. "Give the child some say in selecting the activities," recommends Simpkins. "Stress the fun and not necessarily the health benefits. It's not gym class. It's fun."

"Many adults had negative experiences in gym classrooms so we have to motivate the adults as well," continues Simpkins. Supporting each other to remain active is your secret formula for better health.

Begin right away by limiting sedentary activities such as watching television and playing video games. You don't have to engage in strenuous exercise to stay healthy. Simple activities that everyone enjoys are the key. Go for a walk in your neighborhood, or go to a school track or park if you prefer. "Walking is the number one recommended sport for endurance," says Simpkins. If your children are too young to walk, they will enjoy the fresh air while riding in the stroller.

Other possibilities to keep you moving:

- Shoot a round of basketball, play tag or touch football, or dance to your favorite music. If you or your children don't especially like team sports, modify the game to make it less competitive.

- Rake leaves, shovel snow, mow the grass, wash the car, or do any other chore that would be more fun if you had some company.

- Consult your local community center for free family services, such as swimming and dance classes.

- Take advantage of any natural resources in your surrounding area.

- Go bike riding on bike paths through the city, fly a kite in open spaces, or go hiking and bring a picnic basket.

It is well documented that staying physically active improves your health and helps prevent disease. According to the Surgeon General's report, physical activity reduces the risk of dying from coronary heart disease and of developing high blood pressure, colon cancer, and diabetes. Furthermore, it helps maintain healthy bones, muscles, and joints, and helps control weight, build lean muscle, and reduce body fat.

Even if your children participate in sports at school, it is important to provide encouragement and opportunities for physical activity at home. Staying active together will lead you and your family down a path to better health.

Part Eight

Additional Help and Information

Chapter 63

Glossary of Fitness Terms

Achilles tendonitis: A stretch, tear, or irritation to the tendon connecting the calf muscle to the back of the heel, Achilles tendon injuries can be sudden and agonizing. The most common cause of Achilles tendon tears is a problem called tendonitis, a degenerative condition caused by aging or overuse. When a tendon is weakened, trauma can cause it to rupture.

Acute fractures: Acute fractures can be simple (a clean break with little damage to the surrounding tissue) or compound (a break in which the bone pierces the skin with little damage to the surrounding tissue). Most acute fractures are emergencies.

Adipose tissue: Fat tissue in the body.

Aerobic: Conditions or processes that occur in the presence of, or requiring, oxygen.

This glossary contains terms excerpted from glossaries and documents produced by the following government agencies: Centers for Disease Control and Prevention (CDC); National Cancer Institute (NCI); National Heart, Lung, and Blood Institute (NHLBI); National Institute of Arthritis and Musculoskeletal and Skin Diseases (NIAMS); National Institute of Diabetes and Digestive and Kidney Diseases (NIDDK); National Institute on Aging (NIA); National Institute on Drug Abuse (NIDA); National Women's Health Information Center (NWHIC); the President's Council on Physical Fitness and Sports; and the U.S. Food and Drug Administration (FDA).

Aerobic exercise: An activity that uses the large muscles and involves increased breathing and heart rate over an extended period of time, usually a minimum of 20 minutes.

Agility: Ability to start, stop, and move the body quickly and in different directions.

Anabolic steroids: Human-made substances related to male sex hormones. Some athletes abuse anabolic steroids to enhance performance. Abuse of anabolic steroids can lead to serious health problems, some of which are irreversible. Major side effects can include liver tumors and cancer, jaundice, high blood pressure, kidney tumors, severe acne, and trembling. In males, side effects may include shrinking of the testicles and breast development. In females, side effects may include growth of facial hair, menstrual changes, and deepened voice. In teenagers, growth may be halted prematurely and permanently.

Androstenedione (andro): This product acts like a steroid once it is metabolized by the body and therefore can pose similar kinds of health risks as steroids.

Atherosclerosis: Atherosclerosis is the hardening and narrowing of the arteries. It is caused by the slow buildup of plaque on the inside of walls of the arteries. Arteries are blood vessels that carry oxygen-rich blood from the heart to other parts of the body.

Athlete's foot: A skin disease that can spread from the feet to other parts of the body and is caused by fungus. Signs are dry, scaly skin; itching; inflammation; and blisters.

Basal metabolic rate (BMR): A measure of the energy necessary for maintaining basic functions, such as breathing, heart rate, and digestion.

Blood pressure: The force of circulating blood on the walls of the arteries. Blood pressure is taken using two measurements: systolic (measured when the heart beats, when blood pressure is at its highest) and diastolic (measured between heart beats, when blood pressure is at its lowest). Blood pressure is written with the systolic blood pressure first, followed by the diastolic blood pressure (for example 120/80).

Body composition: The relative amount of body weight that is fat and nonfat.

Body mass index (BMI): Body mass index (BMI) is a number calculated from a person's weight and height. BMI is a reliable indicator of body fatness for people.

Bone mineral density (BMD) test: BMD tests can identify osteoporosis, determine the risk for fractures (broken bones), and measure response to osteoporosis treatment. The most widely recognized bone mineral density test is called a dual-energy x-ray absorptiometry or DXA test.

Bursitis: This condition involves inflammation of the bursae, small, fluid-filled sacs that help reduce friction between bones and other moving structures in the joints. The inflammation may result from arthritis in the joint or injury or infection of the bursae. Bursitis produces pain and tenderness and may limit the movement of nearby joints.

Caloric intake: Refers to the number of calories (energy content) consumed.

Calorie: Calories are a measure of how much energy a person gets from a serving of this food.

Carbohydrate loading: Carbohydrate loading is a technique used to increase the amount of glycogen in muscles. For five to seven days before an event, the athlete eats 10 to 12 grams of carbohydrate per kilogram body weight and gradually reduces the intensity of the workouts. The day before the event, the athlete rests and eats the same high-carbohydrate diet.

Carbohydrate: A sugar molecule. Carbohydrates can be small and simple (for example, glucose) or they can be large and complex (for example, polysaccharides such as starch, chitin or cellulose).

Cardiorespiratory function: A health-related component of physical fitness that relates to the ability of the circulatory and respiratory systems to supply oxygen during physical activity.

Cardiovascular: Having to do with the heart and blood vessels.

Cholesterol: A fat-like substance that is made by the body and is found naturally in animal foods such as meat, fish, poultry, eggs, and dairy products. Foods high in cholesterol include liver and organ meats, egg yolks, and dairy fats. Cholesterol is carried in the blood. When cholesterol levels are too high, some of the cholesterol is deposited on the walls of the blood vessels. Over time, the deposits can build up causing the blood vessels to narrow and blood flow to decrease.

Cooldown: A gradual decrease in the intensity of activity to restore a normal heart rate.

Coordination: Ability to do a task integrating movements of the body and different parts of the body.

Cryotherapy: The topical application of ice.

Cycling: Taking multiple doses of steroids over a specific period of time, stopping for a period, and starting again.

Dehydration: A deficit in body fluids.

Diabetes: A disease in which the body does not properly control the amount of sugar in the blood. As a result, the level of sugar in the blood is too high. This disease occurs when the body does not produce enough insulin or does not use it properly.

Electrolytes: Electrolytes are nutrients that affect fluid balance in the body and are necessary for nerves and muscles to function. Sodium and potassium are the two electrolytes most often added to sports drinks.

Endorphin: A morphine-like chemical that is made naturally in the brain and relieves pain.

Energy expenditure: The energy cost to the body of physical activity, usually measured in kilocalories.

Exercise (exercise training): Planned, structured, and repetitive bodily movement done to improve or maintain one or more components of physical fitness.

Exercise-induced asthma: Exercise-induced asthma (EIA) is a common form of asthma. It occurs only when a person exercises.

Fat: A major source of energy in the diet. All food fats have 9 calories per gram. Some kinds of fats, especially saturated fats, may cause blood cholesterol to increase and increase the risk for heart disease. Other fats, such as unsaturated fats do not increase blood cholesterol.

Female athlete triad: Disordered eating, absence of menstruation, and loss of bone mass, which may occur in female athletes.

Flexibility: Ability to move a joint through the full range of motion without discomfort or pain.

Folliculitis: An infection of the hair follicles.

Glucagon: A hormone produced by the pancreas that increases the level of glucose (sugar) in the blood.

Glucose: A type of sugar; the chief source of energy for living organisms.

Growth plate: A growth plate is the area of developing tissues at the end of the long bones in growing children and adolescents. When growth is complete, some time during adolescence, the growth plate is replaced by solid bone.

Healthy weight: Compared to overweight or obese, a body weight that is less likely to be linked with any weight-related health problems such as type 2 diabetes, heart disease, high blood pressure, high blood cholesterol, or others. A body mass index (BMI) of 18.5 up to 25 refers to a healthy weight, though not all individuals with a BMI in this range may be at a healthy level of body fat; they may have more body fat tissue and less muscle. A BMI of 25 up to 30 refers to overweight and a BMI of 30 or higher refers to obese.

Heat exhaustion: A heat-related injury that causes symptoms such as nausea, dizziness, weakness, headache, pale and moist skin, heavy perspiration, normal or low body temperature, weak pulse, dilated pupils, disorientation, fainting spells.

Heat stroke: A heat-related injury that causes headache, dizziness, confusion, and hot dry skin, possibly leading to vascular collapse, coma, and death.

Heel spurs (plantar fasciitis): Stretching or tearing of the plantar fascia, which runs along the bottom of the foot and supports the arch of the foot.

Hyperglycemia: Abnormally high levels of blood sugar.

Hypertension: A blood pressure of 140/90 or higher. Hypertension usually has no symptoms. It can harm the arteries and cause an increase in the risk of stroke, heart attack, kidney failure, and blindness. Also called high blood pressure.

Hypoglycemia: Abnormally low blood sugar.

Hypotension: Abnormally low blood pressure.

Kegel exercises: Exercises to strengthen the muscles that hold urine in the bladder.

Lactic acid: Lactic acid is a chemical byproduct of energy production in cells. The muscles produce lactic acid and lactate during exercise.

Lateral epicondylitis (tennis elbow): Injury to the tendons and muscles on the outside of the elbow, due to overuse or repetitive motion.

Ligament: A ligament is a band of tough, fibrous tissue that connects two or more bones at a joint and prevents excessive movement of the joint.

Maximal heart rate: Age-related maximal heart rate is determined by subtracting the person's age from 220. For example, for a 50-year-old person, the estimated maximum age-related heart rate would be calculated as 220 - 50 years = 170 beats per minute (bpm).

Metabolic equivalent (MET): The standard metabolic equivalent, or MET, level. This unit is used to estimate the amount of oxygen used by the body during physical activity. 1 MET = the energy (oxygen) used by the body as a person sits quietly, perhaps while talking on the phone or reading a book. The harder a person's body works during the activity, the higher the MET. Any activity that burns 3 to 6 METs is considered moderate-intensity physical activity. Any activity that burns > 6 METs is considered vigorous-intensity physical activity.

Metabolic: Having to do with metabolism.

Metabolism: The total of all chemical changes that take place in a cell or an organism. These changes produce energy and basic materials needed for important life processes.

Moderate physical activity: Activities that use large muscle groups and are at least equivalent to brisk walking.

Multiple-joint exercises: Multiple-joint exercises stress more than one joint or major muscle group. Examples include the bench press or squat.

Muscle group split routines: In strength training, performance of exercises for specific muscle groups during a workout.

Muscle: A muscle is a tissue composed of bundles of specialized cells that, when stimulated by nerve impulses, contract and produce movement.

Muscular endurance: Ability of the muscle to perform repetitive contractions over a prolonged period of time.

Muscular strength: Ability of the muscle to generate the maximum amount of force.

Negative energy balance: A condition in which energy output exceeds energy intake. This condition results in weight loss.

Non-weight-bearing activities: Activities that put less stress on the joints because a person does not have to lift or push his or her own weight.

Non-steroidal anti-inflammatory drugs (NSAID): These drugs temporarily relieve pain by blocking the body's production of chemicals known as prostaglandins, which are believed to be associated with the pain and inflammation of injuries and immune reactions.

Obese: Having an abnormally high, unhealthy amount of body fat. An adult who has a BMI of 30 or higher is considered obese.

Overweight: Being too heavy for one's height. It is defined as a body mass index (BMI) of 25 up to 30 kg per m^2. Body weight comes from fat, muscle, bone, and body water.

Pedometer: A device that measures the number of steps taken in a day.

Physical activity: Bodily movement that is produced by the contraction of skeletal muscle and that substantially increases energy expenditure.

Physical fitness: A set of attributes that persons have or achieve that relates to the ability to perform physical activity. Performance-related components of fitness include agility, balance, coordination, power, and speed. Health-related components of physical fitness include body composition, cardiorespiratory function, flexibility, and muscular strength/endurance.

Positive energy balance: A condition in which energy intake exceeds energy output for basal metabolic rate (BMR) and physical activities. Children, adolescents, and teenagers should be in positive energy balance. For these age groups, energy intake in excess of energy used for BMR and physical activities is used for growth or may be stored for use at a later time.

Power: Ability to exert muscular strength quickly.

Progressive overload: This process necessitates a gradual increase in the stress placed on the body during training. Without these additional demands, the human body has no reason to adapt any further than the current level of fitness.

Protein: A molecule made up of amino acids that are needed for the body to function properly. Proteins are the basis of body structures such as skin and hair and of substances such as enzymes, cytokines, and antibodies.

R.I.C.E.: Refers to rest, ice, compression, elevation, often used as a treatment for minor sprains and strains.

Resistance bands: These inexpensive latex bands often come in sets of three—light, medium, and heavy resistance. They provide resistance during both upper body and lower body strength exercises.

Rotator cuff: The rotator cuff is a structure composed of tendons that work along with associated muscles to hold the ball at the top of the humerus in the glenoid socket and provide mobility and strength to the shoulder joint.

Sedentary: Denotes a person who is relatively inactive and has a lifestyle characterized by a lot of sitting.

Shin splints: Pain along the tibia or shin bone, the large bone in the front of the lower leg. This pain can occur at the front outside part of the lower leg, including the foot and ankle (anterior shin splints) or at the inner edge of the bone where it meets the calf muscles (medial shin splints). Shin splints are primarily seen in runners, particularly those just starting a running program.

Single-joint exercises: Single-joint exercises stress one joint or major muscle group.

Specificity: The body's adaptations to training. The physiological adaptations to resistance training are specific to the muscle actions involved, velocity of movement, exercise range of motion, muscle groups trained, energy systems involved, and the intensity and volume of training.

Speed: Ability to move the whole body quickly.

Sprain: A sprain is an injury to a ligament—a stretching or a tearing. One or more ligaments can be injured during a sprain.

Stacking: When users often combine several different types of steroids to maximize their effectiveness while minimizing negative effects.

Strain: A strain is an injury to either a muscle or a tendon.

Strength training: Doing exercises with hand weights, elastic bands, or weight machines to build muscle mass.

Stress fracture: Where the ligament pulls off small pieces of bone.

Target heart rate: Target heart rate (THR) is a common way of judging how hard a person should exercise during endurance activities. It tells how fast the average person should try to make his or her heart beat during endurance sessions.

Tendonitis: This condition refers to inflammation of tendons (tough cords of tissue that connect muscle to bone) caused by overuse, injury, or a rheumatic condition. Tendonitis produces pain and tenderness and may restrict movement of nearby joints.

Tendon: A tendon is a tough, fibrous cord of tissue that connects muscle to bone.

Total-body workout: In strength training, performance of multiple exercises stressing all major muscle groups per session.

Training volume: The total number of sets and repetitions performed during a training session. Altering training volume can be accomplished by changing the number of exercises performed per session, the number of repetitions performed per set, or the number of sets per exercise.

Triglyceride: A form of fat in the blood. High triglyceride levels can raise heart disease risk.

Type 1 diabetes: Type 1 diabetes is a life-long condition in which the pancreas stops making insulin. Without insulin, the body is not able to use glucose (blood sugar) for energy. To treat the disease, a person must inject insulin, follow a diet plan, exercise daily, and test blood sugar several times a day. Type 1 diabetes usually begins before the age of 30.

Type 2 diabetes: Type 2 diabetes is the most common form of diabetes mellitus. People with type 2 diabetes produce insulin, but either do not make enough insulin or their bodies do not use the insulin they make. Most of the people who have this type of diabetes are overweight. Therefore, people with type 2 diabetes may be able to control their condition by losing weight through diet and exercise. They may also need to inject insulin or take medicine along with continuing to follow a healthy program of diet and exercise.

Upper/lower body split workouts: In strength training, performance of upper body exercises only during one workout and lower body exercises only during the next workout.

Variation: The systematic alteration of the resistance training program over time to allow for the training stimulus to remain optimal. It has been shown that systematic program variation is very effective for long-term progression.

Vigorous physical activity: Rhythmic, repetitive physical activities that use large muscle groups at 70 percent or more of maximum heart rate for age. An exercise heart rate of 70 percent of maximum heart rate for age is about 60 percent of maximal cardiorespiratory capacity and is sufficient for cardiorespiratory conditioning.

VO_2 max (maximal oxygen uptake): The maximum rate at which the body consumes oxygen during exhaustive exercise. VO_2 max is determined by the heart's ability to pump blood through the lungs to pick up oxygen, deliver oxygen to working muscles, and have muscles extract oxygen from the blood. VO_2 max reveals a person's level of aerobic capacity or fitness—the higher the better.

Warmup: Three to five minutes of low-level activity followed by a few minutes of stretching to prepare for exercise.

Weight control: Achieving and maintaining a healthy weight by eating well and getting regular physical activity.

Weight-bearing activities: These activities involve lifting or pushing a person's own body weight.

Weight cycle: Losing and gaining weight over and over again. Commonly called yo-yo dieting.

Yoga: Yoga is a system built on three main structures: exercise, breathing, and meditation. When yoga is practiced regularly, these systems are designed to work in unison and produce a clear mind and a strong body. There are four types or "paths" of yoga: Jnana, the path of knowledge; Bhakti, the path of devotion; Karma, the path of action; and Raja, the path of self-control. For each path, there are a number of different styles of yoga practiced. Hatha yoga (which is actually part of Raja yoga) is the form most popular in the West and focuses on postures and breathing.

Chapter 64

Directory of Fitness Resources

Government Agencies That Provide Information about Fitness and Exercise

Center for Nutrition Policy and Promotion
U.S. Department of Agriculture
3101 Park Center Drive, Rm. 1034
Alexandria, VA 22302-1594
Phone: 703-305-7600
Fax: 703-305-3400
Website: http://www.cnpp.usda.gov
E-mail: john.webster@cnpp.usda.gov

Centers for Disease Control and Prevention
1600 Clifton Road
Atlanta, GA 30333
Toll-Free: 800-311-3435
Phone: 404-639-3311
Website: http://www.cdc.gov
E-mail: cdcinfo@cdc.gov

Federal Trade Commission
CRC-240
Washington, DC 20580
Toll-Free: 877-FTC-HELP (382-4357)
Phone: 202-326-2222
Website: http://www.ftc.gov

Healthfinder®
U.S. Department of Health and Human Services
P.O. Box 1133
Washington, DC 20013-1133
Website: http://www.healthfinder.gov
E-mail: healthfinder@nhic.org

Resources in this chapter were compiled from several sources deemed reliable; all contact information was verified and updated in July 2006.

National Cancer Institute
Cancer Information Service
6116 Executive Boulevard
Room 3036A
Bethesda, MD 20892-8322
Toll-Free: 800-4-CANCER (422-6237)
TTY Toll-Free: 800-332-8615
Website: http://www.cancer.gov
E-mail: cancergovstaff@mail.nih.gov

National Center for Complementary and Alternative Medicine
NCCAM Clearinghouse
P.O. Box 7923
Gaithersburg, MD 20898-7923
Toll-Free: 888-644-6226
Phone: 301-519-3153
TTY: 866-464-3615
Fax: 866-464-3616
Website: http://nccam.nih.gov
E-mail: info@nccam.nih.gov

National Center for Health Statistics
3311 Toledo Road
Hyattsville, MD 20782
Toll-Free: 866-441-NCHS (441-6247)
Phone: 301-458-4000
Website: http://www.cdc.gov/nchs
E-mail: nchsquery@cdc.gov

National Diabetes Information Clearinghouse
1 Information Way
Bethesda, MD 20892-3560
Toll-Free: 800-860-8747
Fax: 703-738-4929
Website: http://diabetes.niddk.nih.gov
E-mail: ndic@info.niddk.nih.gov

National Digestive Diseases Information Clearinghouse
2 Information Way
Bethesda, MD 20892-3570
Toll-Free: 800-891-5389
Fax: 703-738-4929
Website: http://digestive.niddk.nih.gov
E-mail: nddic@info.niddk.nih.gov

National Heart, Lung, and Blood Institute Health Information Center
P.O. Box 30105
Bethesda, MD 20824-0105
Phone: 301-592-8573
TTY: 240-629-3255
Fax: 301-592-8563
Website: http://www.nhlbi.nih.gov
E-mail: nhlbiinfo@nhlbi.nih.gov

National Institute of Diabetes and Digestive and Kidney Diseases
Building 31, Room 9A04
31 Center Drive, MSC 2560
Bethesda, MD 20892-2560
NIDDK Information Clearinghouse Toll-Free: 800-891-5390
Website: http://www.niddk.nih.gov
E-mail: dkwebmaster@extra.niddk.nih.gov

National Institute of Arthritis and Musculoskeletal and Skin Diseases
1 AMS Circle
Bethesda, Maryland 20892-3675
Phone: 301-495-4484
Toll-Free: 877-22-NIAMS (226-4267)
Fax: 301-718-6366
TTY: 301-565-2966
Website: http://www.niams.nih.gov
E-mail: niamsinfo@mail.nih.gov

National Institute on Aging
P.O. Box 8057
Gaithersburg, MD 20892
Publications Toll-Free: 800-222-2225
Phone: 301-496-1752
TTY: 800-222-4225
Fax: 301-496-1072
Websites: http://www.nia.nih.gov, http://www.niapublications.org
E-mail: niainfo@nia.nih.gov

National Institute on Drug Abuse
6001 Executive Boulevard
Room 5213
Bethesda, MD 20892-9561
Phone: 301-443-1124
Website: http://www.drugabuse.gov
E-mail: information@nida.nih.gov

National Women's Health Information Center
8270 Willow Oaks Corporate Dr.
Fairfax, VA 22031
Toll-Free: 800-994-WOMAN (994-9662)
TTY: 888-220-5446
Website: http://www.4woman.gov

Office of Disease Prevention and Health Promotion
Office of Public Health and Science, Office of the Secretary
1101 Wootton Parkway
Suite LL100
Rockville, MD 20852
Phone: 240-453-8280
Fax: 240-453-8282
Website: http://odphp.osophs.dhhs.gov

Osteoporosis and Related Bone Diseases National Resource Center
2 AMS Circle
Bethesda, MD 20892-3676
Toll-Free: 800-624-BONE (624-2663)
Phone: 202-223-0344
Fax: 202-293-2356
TTY: 202-466-4315
Website: http://www.osteo.org
E-mail: NIAMSBONEINFO@mail.nih.gov

President's Council on Physical Fitness and Sports
Department W
200 Independence Ave., SW
Room 738-H
Washington, DC 20201-0004
Phone: 202-690-9000
Fax: 202-690-5211
Website: http://www.fitness.gov

U.S. Department of Health and Human Services
200 Independence Avenue, S.W.
Washington, DC 20201
Toll-Free: 877-696-6775
Phone: 202-619-0257
Website: http://www.hhs.gov

U.S. Food and Drug Administration
5600 Fishers Lane
Rockville, MD 20857-0001
Toll-Free: 888-463-6332
Website: http://www.fda.gov

U.S. National Library of Medicine
8600 Rockville Pike
Bethesda, MD 20894
Toll-Free: 888-346-3656
Phone: 301-594-5983
Website: http://www.nlm.nih.gov
E-mail: custserv@nlm.nih.gov

Weight-control Information Network (WIN)
1 WIN Way
Bethesda, MD 20892-3665
Toll-Free: 877-946-4627
Phone: 202-828-1025
Fax: 202-828-1028
Website: http://win.niddk.nih.gov
E-mail: win@info.niddk.nih.gov

Private Organizations That Provide Information about Fitness and Exercise

Action for Healthy Kids
4711 West Golf Road, Suite 625
Skokie, IL 60076
Toll-Free: 800-416-5136
Website: http://
www.actionforhealthykids.org
E-mail:
info@actionforhealthykids.org

Active Living by Design
400 Market Street, Suite 205
Chapel Hill, NC 27516
Phone: 919-843-ALBD (843-2523)
Fax: 919-843-3083
Website: http://
www.activelivingbydesign.org
E-mail:
info@activelivingbydesign.org

Aerobics and Fitness Association of America
15250 Ventura Boulevard
Suite 200
Sherman Oaks, CA 91403.
Toll-Free: 877-YOUR-BODY
(968-7263)
Fax: 818-990-5468
Website: http://www.afaa.com

Amateur Athletic Union
P.O. Box 22409
Lake Buena Vista, FL 32830
Phone: 407-934-7200
Fax: 407-934-7242
Website: http://
www.aausports.org

American Academy of Dermatology
P.O. Box 4014
Schaumburg, IL 60618-4014
Toll-Free: 866-503-SKIN (503-7546)
Fax: 847-240-1859
Website: http://www.aad.org
E-mail: MRC@aad.org

American Academy of Orthopaedic Surgeons
6300 North River Road
Rosemont, IL 60018-4262
Toll-Free: 800-346-AAOS (346-2267)
Phone: 847-823-7186
Fax: 847-823-8125
Website: http://www.aaos.org
E-mail: pemr@aaos.org

American Academy of Pediatrics
141 Northwest Point Boulevard
Elk Grove Village, IL, 60007
Phone: 847-434-4000
Fax: 847-434-8000
Website: http://www.aap.org
E-mail: kidsdocs@aap.org

American Academy of Physical Medicine and Rehabilitation
330 North Wabash Avenue
Suite 2500
Chicago, IL 60611-7617
Phone: 312-464-9700
Fax: 312-464-0227
Website: http://www.aapmr.org
E-mail: info@aapmr.org

American Alliance for Health, Physical Education, Recreation and Dance
1900 Association Drive
Reston, VA 20191
Toll-Free: 800-213-7193
Website: http://www.aahperd.org
E-mail: info@aahperd.org

American Association of Diabetes Educators
100 W. Monroe
Suite 400
Chicago, IL 60603
Toll-Free: 800-338-3633
Website: http://www.aadenet.org
E-mail: aade@aadenet.org

American College of Rheumatology
1800 Century Place
Suite 250
Atlanta, GA 30345-4300
Phone: 404-633-3777
Fax: 404-633-1870
Website: http://
www.rheumatology.org

American College of Sports Medicine
P.O. Box 1440
Indianapolis, IN 46206-1440
Phone: 317-637-9200
Fax: 317-634-7817
Website: http://www.acsm.org

American Council on Exercise
4851 Paramount Drive
San Diego, CA 92123
Toll-Free: 800-825-3636
Phone: 858-279-8227
Fax: 858-279-8064
Website: http://www.acefitness.org
E-mail: support@acefitness.org

American Diabetes Association
1701 North Beauregard Street
Alexandria, VA 22311
Toll-Free: 800-DIABETES (342-2383)
Website: http://www.diabetes.org
E-mail: AskADA@diabetes.org

American Dietetic Association
120 South Riverside Plaza
Suite 2000
Chicago, IL 60606-6995
Toll-Free: 800-877-1600
Website: http://www.eatright.org

American Fitness Professionals and Associates
P.O. Box 214
Ship Bottom, NJ 08008
Toll-Free: 800-494-7782
Phone: 609-978-7583
Website: http://www.afpafitness.com
E-mail: afpa@afpafitness.com

American Heart Association
7272 Greenville Avenue
Dallas, TX 75231
Toll-Free: 800-AHA-USA-1 (242-8721)
Website: http://www.americanheart.org

American Kinesiotherapy Association
Toll-Free: 800-296-2582
Website: http://www.akta.org
E-mail: ccbkt@aol.com

American Medical Association/Medem
649 Mission Street, 2nd Floor
San Francisco, CA 94105
Toll-Free: 877-926-3336
Phone: 415-644-3800
Fax: 415-644-3950
Website: http://www.medem.com
E-mail: info@medem.com

American Orthopaedic Society for Sports Medicine
6300 N. River Road, Suite 500
Rosemont, IL 60018
Phone: 847-292-4900
Fax: 847-292-4905
Website: http://www.sportsmed.org
E-mail: aossm@aossm.org

American Physical Therapy Association
1111 North Fairfax Street
Alexandria, VA 22314-1488
Toll-Free: 800-999-2782
Phone: 703-684-APTA (684-2782)
TDD: 703-683-6748
Fax: 703-684-7343
Website: http://www.apta.org

American Podiatric Medical Association
9312 Old Georgetown Road
Bethesda, MD 20814-1621
Toll-Free: 800-ASK-APMA (275-2672)
Phone: 301-571-9200
Fax: 301-530-2752
Website: http://www.apma.org
E-mail: askapma@apma.org

American Psychological Association
750 First Street, NE
Washington, DC 20002-4242
Toll-Free: 800-374-2721
Phone: 202-336-5500
TDD/TTY: 202-336-6123
Website: http://www.apa.org

American Public Health Association
800 I Street, NW
Washington, DC 20001
Phone: 202-777-2742
Fax: 202-777-2534
TTY: 202-777-2500
Website: http://www.apha.org
E-mail: comments@apha.org

American Red Cross
2025 E Street, NW
Washington, DC 20006
Toll-Free: 800-REDCROSS (733-2767)
Toll-Free: 800-257-7575 (Español)
Phone: 202-303-4498
Website: http://www.redcross.org

American Running Association
4405 East-West Highway
Suite 405
Bethesda, MD 20814
Toll-Free: 800-776-2732
Phone: 301-913-9517
Website: http://www.americanrunning.org
E-mail: run@americanrunning.org

American Tai Chi Association
2465 J-17 Centreville Road
Suite 150
Herndon, VA 20171
Website: http://www.americantaichi.org
E-mail: contact@americantaichi.net

American Medical Society for Sports Medicine
11639 Earnshaw
Overland Park, KS 66210
Phone: 913-327-1415
Fax: 913-327-1491
Website: http://
www.newamssm.org
E-mail: office@amssm.org

American Sports Medicine Institute
2660 10th Avenue South
Suite 505
Birmingham, AL 35205
Phone: 205-918-0000
Fax: 205-918-0800
Website: http://www.asmi.org

Anorexia Nervosa and Related Eating Disorders (ANRED)
Website: http://www.anred.com
E-mail: jarinor@rio.com

Aquatic Exercise Association
Toll-Free: 888-232-9283
Phone: 941-486-8600
Website: http://
www.aeawave.com
E-mail: info@aeawave.com

Arthritis Foundation
P.O. Box 7669
Atlanta, GA 30357-0669
Toll-Free: 800-568-4045
Phone: 404-872-7100
Website: http://www.arthritis.org

Center for the Study of Sport in Society
716 Columbus Avenue
Suite 161
Boston, MA 02120
Phone: 617-373-4025
Fax: 617-373-4566
Website: http://
www.sportinsociety.org
E-mail: sportinsociety@neu.edu

Cleveland Clinic
9500 Euclid Avenue
Cleveland, OH 44195
Toll-Free: 800-223-2273
Phone: 216-444-2200
TTY: 216-444-0261
Website: http://
www.clevelandclinic.org

Cooper Institute
12200 Preston Road
Dallas, TX 75230
Phone: 972-341-3200
Fax: 972-341-3224
Website: http://
www.cooperinst.org
E-mail: courses@cooperinst.org

Diabetes Exercise and Sports
8001 Montcastle Drive
Nashville, TN 37221
Toll-Free: 800-898-4322
Fax: 615-673-2077
Website: http://www.diabetes-exercise.org
E-mail: desa@diabetes-exercise.org

Disabled Sports USA
Website: http://www.dsusa.org
E-mail: information@dsusa.org

Exrx.net
http://www.exrx.net

Fifty Plus Lifelong Fitness
2483 E. Bayshore Road
Suite 202
Palo Alto, CA 94303
Phone: 650-843-1750
Fax: 650-843-1758
E-mail: info@50plus.org
Website: http://www.50plus.org

Gatorade Sports Science Institute
617 West Main Street
Barrington, Illinois 60010
Toll-Free: 800-616-GSSI (616-4774)
Website: http://www.gssiweb.org

Healthy Aging Campaign
P.O. Box 442
Unionville, PA 19375
Phone: 610-793-0979
Fax: 610-793-0978
Website: http://
www.healthyaging.net
E-mail: info@healthyaging.net

Human Kinetics
P.O. Box 5076
Champaign, IL 61825-5076
Toll-Free: 800-747-4457
Fax: 217-351-2674
Website: http://
www.humankinetics.com
E-mail: info@hkusa.com

IDEA Health & Fitness Association
10455 Pacific Center Court
San Diego, CA 92121-4339
Toll-Free: 800-999-4332, ext. 7
Fax: 858-535-8234
Website: http://www.ideafit.com
E-mail: contact@ideafit.com

Institute for Preventative Sports Medicine
P.O. Box 7032
Ann Arbor, MI 48107
Phone: 734-572-4577
Fax: 734-459-0814
Website: http://www.ipsm.org
E-mail: info@ipsm.org

International Fitness Association
12472 Lake Underhill Road, #341
Orlando, FL 32828
Toll-Free: 800-227-1976
Phone: 407-579-8610
Website: http://
www.ifafitness.com

International Food Information Council
1100 Connecticut Avenue, NW
Suite 430
Washington, DC 20036
Phone: 202-296-6540
Fax: 202-296-6547
Website: http://ific.org
E-mail: foodinfo@ific.org

International Health, Racquet and Sportsclub Association
263 Summer Street
Boston, MA 02210
Toll-Free: 800-228-4772
Phone: 617-951-0055
Fax: 617-951-0056
Website: http://cms.ihrsa.org
E-mail: info@ihrsa.org

International Sports Sciences Association
1015 Mark Avenue
Carpinteria, CA 93013
Toll-Free: 800-892-4772
Phone: 805-745-8111
Fax: 805-745-8119
Website: http://
www.issaonline.com
E-mail:
webmaster@issaonline.com

League of American Bicyclists
1612 K Street NW, Suite 800
Washington, DC 20006
Phone: 202-822-1333
Website: http://
www.bikeleague.org
E-mail:
bikeleague@bikeleague.org

Mature Fitness Awards USA
1850 West Winchester Road
Suite 213
Libertyville, IL 60048
Phone: 847-816-8660
Fax: 847-816-8662
Website: http://
www.fitnessday.com
E-mail: info@fitnessday.com

National Academy of Sports Medicine
26632 Agoura Road
Calabasas, CA 91302
Toll-Free: 800-460-NASM (460-6276)
Phone: 818-595-1200
Fax: 818-878-9511
Website: http://www.nasm.org

National Alliance for Youth Sports
2050 Vista Parkway
West Palm Beach, FL 33411
Toll-Free: 800-688-KIDS (688-5437)
Phone: 561-684-1141
Fax: 561-684-2546
Website: http://www.nays.org
E-mail: nays@nays.org

National Athletic Trainers' Association
2952 Stemmons Freeway
Dallas, TX 75247
Phone: 214-637-6282
Fax: 214-637-2206
Website: http://www.nata.org
E-mail: webmaster@nata.org

National Center on Physical Activity and Disability
1640 W. Roosevelt Road
Suite 711
Chicago, IL 60608-6904
Toll-Free: 800-900-8086
Fax: 312-355-4058
Website: http://www.ncpad.org
E-mail: ncpad@uic.edu

National Coalition for Promoting Physical Activity

1100 H Street NW
Suite 510
Washington, DC 20005
Fax: 202-454-7598
Website: http://www.ncppa.org
E-mail: info@ncppa.org

National Collegiate Athletic Association

700 W. Washington Street
P.O. Box 6222
Indianapolis, IN 46206-6222
Phone: 317-917-6222
Fax: 317-917-6888
Website: http://www.ncaa.org

National Disability Sports Alliance

25 West Independence Way
Kingston, RI 02881
Phone: 401-792-7130
Fax: 401-792-7132
Website: http://
www.ndsaonline.org
E-mail: info@ndsaonline.org

National Exercise Trainers Association

5955 Golden Valley Road
Suite 240
Minneapolis, MN 55422
Toll-Free: 800-AEROBIC (237-6242)
Phone: 763-545-2505
Fax: 763-545-2524
Website: http://www.ndeita.com
E-mail: neta@netafit.org

National Fibromyalgia Association

2200 N. Glassell Street, Suite A
Orange, CA 92865
Phone: 714-921-0150
Fax: 714-921-6920
Website: http://www.fmaware.org

National Fitness Therapy Association

P.O. Box 522
Winter Park, CO 80482
Website: http://www.nfta.org
E-mail: fitnesstherapy@nfta.org

National Jewish Medical and Research Center

1400 Jackson Street
Denver, CO 80206
Toll-Free: 800-222-LUNG (222-5864)
Phone: 303-388-4461
Website: http://
www.nationaljewish.org

National Osteoporosis Foundation

1232 22nd Street NW
Washington, DC 20037-1292
Phone: 202-223-2226
Website: http://www.nof.org
E-mail: webmaster@nof.org

National Recreation and Park Association

22377 Belmont Ridge Road
Ashburn, VA 20148-4150
Phone: 703-858-0784
Fax: 703-858-0794
Website: http://www.nrpa.org
E-mail: dvaira@nrpa.org

National Sports Center for the Disabled
P.O. Box 1290
Winter Park, CO 80482
Phone: 970-726-1540
Fax: 970-726-4112
Website: http://www.nscd.org

National Sporting Goods Association
1601 Feehanville Drive
Suite 300
Mt. Prospect, IL 60056
Toll-Free: 800-815-5422
Phone: 847-296-6742
Fax: 847-391-9827
Website: http://www.nsga.org
E-mail: info@nsga.org

National Strength and Conditioning Association
1885 Bob Johnson Drive
Colorado Springs, CO 80906
Toll-Free: 800-815-6826
Phone: 719-632-6722
Fax: 719-632-6367
Website: http://www.nsca-lift.org
E-mail: nsca@nsca-lift.org

National Stroke Association
9707 E. Easter Lane
Centennial, CO 80112
Toll-Free: 800-STROKES (787-6537)
Fax: 303-649-1328
Website: http://www.stroke.org
E-mail: info@stroke.org

Nemours Foundation Center for Children's Health Media
1600 Rockland Road
Wilmington, DE 19803
Phone: 302-651-4000
Fax: 302-651-4055
Website: http://www.kidshealth.org
E-mail: info@kidshealth.org

Nicholas Institute of Sports Medicine and Athletic Trauma
130 East 77th Street
10th Floor
New York, NY 10021
Phone: 212-434-2700
Website: http://www.nismat.org
E-mail: info@nismat.org

PE Central
P.O. Box 10262
Blacksburg, VA 24062
Phone: 540-953-1043
Fax: 800-783-8124
Website: http://www.pecentral.org
E-mail: pec@pecentral.org

PE4Life
810 Baltimore, Suite 100
Kansas City, MO 64105-1706
Phone: 816-472-PE4L (472-7345)
Fax: 816-474-7329
Website: http://www.pe4life.org

Pedestrian and Bicycle Information Center
730 Martin Luther Jr. Boulevard
Suite 300
Campus Box 3430
Chapel Hill, NC 27599-3430
Phone: 919-962-2203
Fax: 919-962-8710
Website: http://www.bicyclinginfo.org
E-mail: pbic@pedbikeinfo.org

Pilates Method Alliance
P.O. Box 370906
Miami, FL 33137-0906
Toll-Free: 866-573-4945
Phone: 305-573-4946
Fax: 305-573-4461
Website: http://www.pilatesmethodalliance.org
E-mail: info@pilatesmethodalliance.org

Road Runners Club of America
8965 Guilford Road, Suite 150
Columbia, MD 21046
Phone: 410-290-3890
Fax: 410-290-3893
Website: http://www.rrca.org
E-mail: office@rrca.org

Shape Up America
808 17th Street NW, Suite 600
Washington, DC 20006
Website: http://www.shapeup.org
E-mail: info@shapeup.org

SPARK
438 Camino Del Rio South
Suite 110
San Diego, CA 92108
Toll-Free: 800-SPARK PE (772-7573)
Phone: 619-293-7990
Fax: 619-293-7992
Website: http://www.sparkpe.org
E-mail: spark@sparkpe.org

Special Olympics International
1133 19th Street, NW
Washington, DC 20036
Phone: 202-628-3630
Fax: 202-824-0200
Website: http://www.specialolympics.org
E-mail: info@specialolympics.org

U.S. Deaf Sports Federation
102 North Krohn Place
Sioux Falls, SD 57103-1800
Phone: 605-367-5760
Fax: 605-367-5958
TTY: 605-367-5761
Website: http://www.usdeafsports.org
E-mail: HomeOffice@usdeafsports.org

United States Association of Blind Athletes
33 N. Institute Street
Colorado Springs, CO 80903
Phone: 719-630-0422
Fax: 719-630-0616
Website: http://www.usaba.org
E-mail: rortiz@usaba.org

United States Olympic Committee

1 Olympic Plaza
Colorado Springs, CO 80909
Phone: 719-632-5551
Website: http://www.olympic-usa.org
E-mail: media@usoc.org

United States Paralympics

1 Olympic Plaza
Colorado Springs, CO 80909
Phone: 719-866-2030
Fax: 719-866-2029
Website: http://www.usolympicteam.com/paralympics
E-mail: paralympicinfo@usoc.org

Wellness Councils of America

9802 Nicholas Street, Suite 315
Omaha, NE 68114
Phone: 402-827-3590
Fax: 402-827-3594
Website: http://www.welcoa.org
E-mail: wellworkplace@welcoa.org

Wheelchair Sports Revised

Website: http://www.wsusa.org
E-mail: wsusa@aol.com

Women's Sports Foundation

Eisenhower Park
East Meadow, NY 11554
Toll-Free: 800-227-3988
Phone: 516-542-4700
Fax: 516-542-4716
Website: http://www.womenssportsfoundation.org
E-mail: info@womenssportsfoundation.org

World Health Organization

Avenue Appia 20
1211 Geneva 27
Switzerland
Phone: + 41 22 791 21 11
Fax: + 41 22 791 3111
Website: http://www.who.int/en
E-mail: info@who.int

YMCA of the USA

101 North Wacker Drive
Chicago, IL 60606
Phone: 800-872-9622
Website: http://www.ymca.net
E-mail: fulfillment@ymca.net

Yoga Research and Education Center

P.O. Box 448
Ukiah, CA 95482
Website: http://www.yrec.org
E-mail: webmaster@yrec.org

YWCA

1015 18th Street NW, Suite 1100
Washington, DC 20036
Phone: 202-467-0801
Fax: 202-467-0802
Website: http://www.ywca.org
E-mail: info@ywca.org

Index

Index

Page numbers followed by 'n' indicate a footnote. Page numbers in *italics* indicate a table or illustration.

A

609

617

SCDS *see* sudden cardiac death
  syndrome
scleroderma 432
sedentary, defined 590
sedentary lifestyles
  calorie intake 28
  chronic diseases 12–13
  physical activity 8
  statistics 13
  students 331
self-esteem
  balance training 292
  cancer treatment 447
  exercise 33, 56
  physical activity 17
  tobacco use 402
seniors
  exercise recommendations 367–70
  exercise safety 369–70, 371–75
  see also age factor
Shape Up America, contact
  information 605
shin splints
  defined 590
  described 471–72, 514–15
shoulder blade *see* scapula
shoulder exercises 288, 307, 421–22,
  426–27
shoulder joint *see* glenohumeral joint
shoulder problems 503–11
shoulder rotation exercise 282, *283*
shoulder separation 506–7
side effects
  nonsteroidal anti-inflammatory
    drugs 477
  supplements 104–5
side reaches *195*
Simpkins, Verna 578–79
simple fracture, described 473, 583
single hip rotation exercise 282, *283*
single-joint exercises, defined 590
"Six-Pack Abs Electronically?"
  (FDA) 172n
ski machines 184–85
skin care 531–38
sleep apnea
  obesity 20
  weight management 8
sleep disorders, strength training 242

slings, sports injuries 477
snacks, childhood athletics 82
Snyder, Stephen 45–46
soccer, injury prevention 467
social well-being, physical activity 17
socioeconomic status, obesity 19
sodium
  dietary intake levels 96–97
  healthy diets 65
  hyponatremia 98–100
  sports drinks 586
softball
  injury prevention 467
  injury statistics *480*, *482*
sore muscles 501–2
space requirements, home gyms 150
SPARK, contact information 605
special needs
  health/fitness facilities 143–44
  personal trainers 137
Special Olympics International,
  contact information 605
specificity
  defined 590
  exercise programs 120
  resistance exercises 260
speed, defined 590
splints, sports injuries 477–78
sports
  alternatives 339–42
  aquatic exercise 209
  asthma 404–5
  childhood injury prevention 463–68
  disabilities 458–59
  energy expenditure *30*, 40
  exercise 57
  preparticipation evaluations
    343–47
  social well-being 17
  tobacco use 400–402
  see also individual sports
sports drinks
  athletes 97
  childhood athletics 81
  electrolytes 586
sports injuries, overview 469–86
sports nutrition 69–74, 83–94
  see also athletes; diet and nutrition
"Sports Supplements" (NWHIC) 101n

Health Reference Series
COMPLETE CATALOG
List price $87 per volume. **School and library price $78 per volume.**

Adolescent Health Sourcebook, 2nd Edition

Basic Consumer Health Information about the Physical, Mental, and Emotional Growth and Development of Adolescents, Including Medical Care, Nutritional and Physical Activity Requirements, Puberty, Sexual Activity, Acne, Tanning, Body Piercing, Common Physical Illnesses and Disorders, Eating Disorders, Attention Deficit Hyperactivity Disorder, Depression, Bullying, Hazing, and Adolescent Injuries Related to Sports, Driving, and Work

Along with Substance Abuse Information about Nicotine, Alcohol, and Drug Use, a Glossary, and Directory of Additional Resources

Edited by Joyce Brennfleck Shannon. 683 pages. 2006. 0-7808-0943-2.

"It is written in clear, nontechnical language aimed at general readers. . . . Recommended for public libraries, community colleges, and other agencies serving health care consumers."
— *American Reference Books Annual, 2003*

"Recommended for school and public libraries. Parents and professionals dealing with teens will appreciate the easy-to-follow format and the clearly written text. This could become a 'must have' for every high school teacher." — *E-Streams, Jan '03*

"A good starting point for information related to common medical, mental, and emotional concerns of adolescents." — *School Library Journal, Nov '02*

"This book provides accurate information in an easy to access format. It addresses topics that parents and caregivers might not be aware of and provides practical, useable information."
— *Doody's Health Sciences Book Review Journal, Sep-Oct '02*

"Recommended reference source."
— *Booklist, American Library Association, Sep '02*

AIDS Sourcebook, 3rd Edition

Basic Consumer Health Information about Acquired Immune Deficiency Syndrome (AIDS) and Human Immunodeficiency Virus (HIV) Infection, Including Facts about Transmission, Prevention, Diagnosis, Treatment, Opportunistic Infections, and Other Complications, with a Section for Women and Children, Including Details about Associated Gynecological Concerns, Pregnancy, and Pediatric Care

Along with Updated Statistical Information, Reports on Current Research Initiatives, a Glossary, and Directories of Internet, Hotline, and Other Resources

Edited by Dawn D. Matthews. 664 pages. 2003. 0-7808-0631-X.

"The 3rd edition of the *AIDS Sourcebook*, part of Omnigraphics' *Health Reference Series*, is a welcome update. . . . This resource is highly recommended for academic and public libraries."
— *American Reference Books Annual, 2004*

"Excellent sourcebook. This continues to be a highly recommended book. There is no other book that provides as much information as this book provides."
— *AIDS Book Review Journal, Dec-Jan '00*

"Recommended reference source."
— *Booklist, American Library Association, Dec '99*

Alcoholism Sourcebook, 2nd Edition

Basic Consumer Health Information about Alcohol Use, Abuse, and Dependence, Featuring Facts about the Physical, Mental, and Social Health Effects of Alcohol Addiction, Including Alcoholic Liver Disease, Pancreatic Disease, Cardiovascular Disease, Neurological Disorders, and the Effects of Drinking during Pregnancy

Along with Information about Alcohol Treatment, Medications, and Recovery Programs, in Addition to Tips for Reducing the Prevalence of Underage Drinking, Statistics about Alcohol Use, a Glossary of Related Terms, and Directories of Resources for More Help and Information

Edited by Amy L. Sutton. 653 pages. 2006. 0-7808-0942-4.

"This title is one of the few reference works on alcoholism for general readers. For some readers this will be a welcome complement to the many self-help books on the market. Recommended for collections serving general readers and consumer health collections."
— *E-Streams, Mar '01*

"This book is an excellent choice for public and academic libraries."
— *American Reference Books Annual, 2001*

"Recommended reference source."
— *Booklist, American Library Association, Dec '00*

"Presents a wealth of information on alcohol use and abuse and its effects on the body and mind, treatment, and prevention." — *SciTech Book News, Dec '00*

"Important new health guide which packs in the latest consumer information about the problems of alcoholism." — *Reviewer's Bookwatch, Nov '00*

SEE ALSO *Drug Abuse Sourcebook, Substance Abuse Sourcebook*

Allergies Sourcebook, 2nd Edition

Basic Consumer Health Information about Allergic Disorders, Triggers, Reactions, and Related Symptoms, Including Anaphylaxis, Rhinitis, Sinusitis, Asthma, Dermatitis, Conjunctivitis, and Multiple Chemical Sensitivity

Along with Tips on Diagnosis, Prevention, and Treatment, Statistical Data, a Glossary, and a Directory of Sources for Further Help and Information

Edited by Annemarie S. Muth. 598 pages. 2002. 0-7808-0376-0.

"This book brings a great deal of useful material together. . . . This is an excellent addition to public and consumer health library collections."
— *American Reference Books Annual, 2003*

"This second edition would be useful to laypersons with little or advanced knowledge of the subject matter. This book would also serve as a resource for nursing and other health care professions students. It would be useful in public, academic, and hospital libraries with consumer health collections."
— *E-Streams, Jul '02*

Alternative Medicine Sourcebook

SEE *Complementary & Alternative Medicine Sourcebook, 3rd Edition*

Alzheimer's Disease Sourcebook, 3rd Edition

Basic Consumer Health Information about Alzheimer's Disease, Other Dementias, and Related Disorders, Including Multi-Infarct Dementia, AIDS Dementia Complex, Dementia with Lewy Bodies, Huntington's Disease, Wernicke-Korsakoff Syndrome (Alcohol-Reated Dementia), Delirium, and Confusional States

Along with Information for People Newly Diagnosed with Alzheimer's Disease and Caregivers, Reports Detailing Current Research Efforts in Prevention, Diagnosis, and Treatment, Facts about Long-Term Care Issues, and Listings of Sources for Additional Information

Edited by Karen Bellenir. 645 pages. 2003. 0-7808-0666-2.

"This very informative and valuable tool will be a great addition to any library serving consumers, students and health care workers."
— *American Reference Books Annual, 2004*

"This is a valuable resource for people affected by dementias such as Alzheimer's. It is easy to navigate and includes important information and resources."
— *Doody's Review Service, Feb '04*

"Recommended reference source."
— *Booklist, American Library Association, Oct '99*

SEE ALSO *Brain Disorders Sourcebook*

Arthritis Sourcebook, 2nd Edition

Basic Consumer Health Information about Osteoarthritis, Rheumatoid Arthritis, Other Rheumatic Disorders, Infectious Forms of Arthritis, and Diseases with Symptoms Linked to Arthritis, Featuring Facts about Diagnosis, Pain Management, and Surgical Therapies

Along with Coping Strategies, Research Updates, a Glossary, and Resources for Additional Help and Information

Edited by Amy L. Sutton. 593 pages. 2004. 0-7808-0667-0.

"This easy-to-read volume is recommended for consumer health collections within public or academic libraries."
— *E-Streams, May '05*

"As expected, this updated edition continues the excellent reputation of this series in providing sound, usable health information. . . . Highly recommended."
— *American Reference Books Annual, 2005*

"Excellent reference."
— *The Bookwatch, Jan '05*

Asthma Sourcebook, 2nd Edition

Basic Consumer Health Information about the Causes, Symptoms, Diagnosis, and Treatment of Asthma in Infants, Children, Teenagers, and Adults, Including Facts about Different Types of Asthma, Common Co-Occurring Conditions, Asthma Management Plans, Triggers, Medications, and Medication Delivery Devices

Along with Asthma Statistics, Research Updates, a Glossary, a Directory of Asthma-Related Resources, and More

Edited by Karen Bellenir. 609 pages. 2006. 0-7808-0866-5.

"A worthwhile reference acquisition for public libraries and academic medical libraries whose readers desire a quick introduction to the wide range of asthma information."
— *Choice, Association of College & Research Libraries, Jun '01*

"Recommended reference source."
— *Booklist, American Library Association, Feb '01*

"Highly recommended."
— *The Bookwatch, Jan '01*

"There is much good information for patients and their families who deal with asthma daily."
— *American Medical Writers Association Journal, Winter '01*

"This informative text is recommended for consumer health collections in public, secondary school, and community college libraries and the libraries of universities with a large undergraduate population."
— *American Reference Books Annual, 2001*

Attention Deficit Disorder Sourcebook

Basic Consumer Health Information about Attention Deficit/Hyperactivity Disorder in Children and Adults, Including Facts about Causes, Symptoms, Diagnostic Criteria, and Treatment Options Such as Medications, Behavior Therapy, Coaching, and Homeopathy

Along with Reports on Current Research Initiatives, Legal Issues, and Government Regulations, and Featuring a Glossary of Related Terms, Internet Resources, and a List of Additional Reading Material

Edited by Dawn D. Matthews. 470 pages. 2002. 0-7808-0624-7.

"Recommended reference source."
—Booklist, American Library Association, Jan '03

"This book is recommended for all school libraries and the reference or consumer health sections of public libraries." —American Reference Books Annual, 2003

∎

Back & Neck Sourcebook, 2nd Edition

Basic Consumer Health Information about Spinal Pain, Spinal Cord Injuries, and Related Disorders, Such as Degenerative Disk Disease, Osteoarthritis, Scoliosis, Sciatica, Spina Bifida, and Spinal Stenosis, and Featuring Facts about Maintaining Spinal Health, Self-Care, Pain Management, Rehabilitative Care, Chiropractic Care, Spinal Surgeries, and Complementary Therapies

Along with Suggestions for Preventing Back and Neck Pain, a Glossary of Related Terms, and a Directory of Resources

Edited by Amy L. Sutton. 633 pages. 2004. 0-7808-0738-3.

"Recommended . . . an easy to use, comprehensive medical reference book." —E-Streams, Sep '05

"The strength of this work is its basic, easy-to-read format. Recommended." —Reference and User Services Quarterly, American Library Association, Winter '97

∎

Blood & Circulatory Disorders Sourcebook, 2nd Edition

Basic Consumer Health Information about the Blood and Circulatory System and Related Disorders, Such as Anemia and Other Hemoglobin Diseases, Cancer of the Blood and Associated Bone Marrow Disorders, Clotting and Bleeding Problems, and Conditions That Affect the Veins, Blood Vessels, and Arteries, Including Facts about the Donation and Transplantation of Bone Marrow, Stem Cells, and Blood and Tips for Keeping the Blood and Circulatory System Healthy

Along with a Glossary of Related Terms and Resources for Additional Help and Information

Edited by Amy L. Sutton. 659 pages. 2005. 0-7808-0746-4.

"Highly recommended pick for basic consumer health reference holdings at all levels."
—The Bookwatch, Aug '05

"Recommended reference source."
—Booklist, American Library Association, Feb '99

"An important reference sourcebook written in simple language for everyday, non-technical users. "
—Reviewer's Bookwatch, Jan '99

Brain Disorders Sourcebook, 2nd Edition

Basic Consumer Health Information about Acquired and Traumatic Brain Injuries, Infections of the Brain, Epilepsy and Seizure Disorders, Cerebral Palsy, and Degenerative Neurological Disorders, Including Amyotrophic Lateral Sclerosis (ALS), Dementias, Multiple Sclerosis, and More

Along with Information on the Brain's Structure and Function, Treatment and Rehabilitation Options, Reports on Current Research Initiatives, a Glossary of Terms Related to Brain Disorders and Injuries, and a Directory of Sources for Further Help and Information

Edited by Sandra J. Judd. 625 pages. 2005. 0-7808-0744-8.

"Highly recommended pick for basic consumer health reference holdings at all levels."
—The Bookwatch, Aug '05

"Belongs on the shelves of any library with a consumer health collection." —E-Streams, Mar '00

"Recommended reference source."
—Booklist, American Library Association, Oct '99

SEE ALSO Alzheimer's Disease Sourcebook

∎

Breast Cancer Sourcebook, 2nd Edition

Basic Consumer Health Information about Breast Cancer, Including Facts about Risk Factors, Prevention, Screening and Diagnostic Methods, Treatment Options, Complementary and Alternative Therapies, Post-Treatment Concerns, Clinical Trials, Special Risk Populations, and New Developments in Breast Cancer Research

Along with Breast Cancer Statistics, a Glossary of Related Terms, and a Directory of Resources for Additional Help and Information

Edited by Sandra J. Judd. 595 pages. 2004. 0-7808-0668-9.

"This book will be an excellent addition to public, community college, medical, and academic libraries."
—American Reference Books Annual, 2006

"It would be a useful reference book in a library or on loan to women in a support group."
—Cancer Forum, Mar '03

"Recommended reference source."
—Booklist, American Library Association, Jan '02

"This reference source is highly recommended. It is quite informative, comprehensive and detailed in nature, and yet it offers practical advice in easy-to-read language. It could be thought of as the 'bible' of breast cancer for the consumer." —E-Streams, Jan '02

"From the pros and cons of different screening methods and results to treatment options, Breast Cancer Sourcebook provides the latest information on the subject."
—Library Bookwatch, Dec '01

"This thoroughgoing, very readable reference covers all aspects of breast health and cancer. . . . Readers will find much to consider here. Recommended for all public and patient health collections."

— *Library Journal, Sep '01*

SEE ALSO Cancer Sourcebook for Women, Women's Health Concerns Sourcebook

■

Breastfeeding Sourcebook

Basic Consumer Health Information about the Benefits of Breastmilk, Preparing to Breastfeed, Breastfeeding as a Baby Grows, Nutrition, and More, Including Information on Special Situations and Concerns Such as Mastitis, Illness, Medications, Allergies, Multiple Births, Prematurity, Special Needs, and Adoption

Along with a Glossary and Resources for Additional Help and Information

Edited by Jenni Lynn Colson. 388 pages. 2002. 0-7808-0332-9.

"Particularly useful is the information about professional lactation services and chapters on breastfeeding when returning to work. . . . *Breastfeeding Sourcebook* will be useful for public libraries, consumer health libraries, and technical schools offering nurse assistant training, especially in areas where Internet access is problematic."
— *American Reference Books Annual, 2003*

SEE ALSO Pregnancy & Birth Sourcebook

■

Burns Sourcebook

Basic Consumer Health Information about Various Types of Burns and Scalds, Including Flame, Heat, Cold, Electrical, Chemical, and Sun Burns

Along with Information on Short-Term and Long-Term Treatments, Tissue Reconstruction, Plastic Surgery, Prevention Suggestions, and First Aid

Edited by Allan R. Cook. 604 pages. 1999. 0-7808-0204-7.

"This is an exceptional addition to the series and is highly recommended for all consumer health collections, hospital libraries, and academic medical centers."
— *E-Streams, Mar '00*

"This key reference guide is an invaluable addition to all health care and public libraries in confronting this ongoing health issue."
— *American Reference Books Annual, 2000*

"Recommended reference source."
— *Booklist, American Library Association, Dec '99*

SEE ALSO Dermatological Disorders Sourcebook

■

Cancer Sourcebook, 4th Edition

Basic Consumer Health Information about Major Forms and Stages of Cancer, Featuring Facts about Head and Neck Cancers, Lung Cancers, Gastrointestinal Cancers, Genitourinary Cancers, Lymphomas, Blood Cell Cancers, Endocrine Cancers, Skin Cancers, Bone Cancers, Sarcomas, and Others, and Including Information about Cancer Treatments and Therapies,

Identifying and Reducing Cancer Risks, and Strategies for Coping with Cancer and the Side Effects of Treatment

Along with a Cancer Glossary, Statistical and Demographic Data, and a Directory of Sources for Additional Help and Information

Edited by Karen Bellenir. 1,119 pages. 2003. 0-7808-0633-6.

"With cancer being the second leading cause of death for Americans, a prodigious work such as this one, which locates centrally so much cancer-related information, is clearly an asset to this nation's citizens and others."
— *Journal of the National Medical Association, 2004*

"This title is recommended for health sciences and public libraries with consumer health collections."
— *E-Streams, Feb '01*

". . . can be effectively used by cancer patients and their families who are looking for answers in a language they can understand. Public and hospital libraries should have it on their shelves."
— *American Reference Books Annual, 2001*

"Recommended reference source."
— *Booklist, American Library Association, Dec '00*

SEE ALSO Breast Cancer Sourcebook, Cancer Sourcebook for Women, Pediatric Cancer Sourcebook, Prostate Cancer Sourcebook

■

Cancer Sourcebook for Women, 3rd Edition

Basic Consumer Health Information about Leading Causes of Cancer in Women, Featuring Facts about Gynecologic Cancers and Related Concerns, Such as Breast Cancer, Cervical Cancer, Endometrial Cancer, Uterine Sarcoma, Vaginal Cancer, Vulvar Cancer, and Common Non-Cancerous Gynecologic Conditions, in Addition to Facts about Lung Cancer, Colorectal Cancer, and Thyroid Cancer in Women

Along with Information about Cancer Risk Factors, Screening and Prevention, Treatment Options, and Tips on Coping with Life after Cancer Treatment, a Glossary of Cancer Terms, and a Directory of Resources for Additional Help and Information

Edited by Amy L. Sutton. 715 pages. 2006. 0-7808-0867-3.

"An excellent addition to collections in public, consumer health, and women's health libraries."
— *American Reference Books Annual, 2003*

"Overall, the information is excellent, and complex topics are clearly explained. As a reference book for the consumer it is a valuable resource to assist them to make informed decisions about cancer and its treatments."
— *Cancer Forum, Nov '02*

"Highly recommended for academic and medical reference collections."
— *Library Bookwatch, Sep '02*

"This is a highly recommended book for any public or consumer library, being reader friendly and containing accurate and helpful information."
— *E-Streams, Aug '02*

Cardiovascular Diseases & Disorders Sourcebook, 3rd Edition

Basic Consumer Health Information about Heart and Vascular Diseases and Disorders, Such as Angina, Heart Attacks, Arrhythmias, Cardiomyopathy, Valve Disease, Atherosclerosis, and Aneurysms, with Information about Managing Cardiovascular Risk Factors and Maintaining Heart Health, Medications and Procedures Used to Treat Cardiovascular Disorders, and Concerns of Special Significance to Women

Along with Reports on Current Research Initiatives, a Glossary of Related Medical Terms, and a Directory of Sources for Further Help and Information

Edited by Sandra J. Judd. 713 pages. 2005. 0-7808-0739-1.

"This updated sourcebook is still the best first stop for comprehensive introductory information on cardiovascular diseases."
—*American Reference Books Annual, 2006*

"Recommended for public libraries and libraries supporting health care professionals."
—*E-Streams, Sep '05*

"This should be a standard health library reference."
—*The Bookwatch, Jun '05*

"Recommended reference source."
—*Booklist, American Library Association, Dec '00*

". . . comprehensive format provides an extensive overview on this subject."
—*Choice, Association of College & Research Libraries*

Caregiving Sourcebook

Basic Consumer Health Information for Caregivers, Including a Profile of Caregivers, Caregiving Responsibilities and Concerns, Tips for Specific Conditions, Care Environments, and the Effects of Caregiving

Along with Facts about Legal Issues, Financial Information, and Future Planning, a Glossary, and a Listing of Additional Resources

Edited by Joyce Brennfleck Shannon. 600 pages. 2001. 0-7808-0331-0.

"Essential for most collections."
—*Library Journal, Apr 1, 2002*

"An ideal addition to the reference collection of any public library. Health sciences information professionals may also want to acquire the *Caregiving Sourcebook* for their hospital or academic library for use as a ready reference tool by health care workers interested in aging and caregiving."
—*E-Streams, Jan '02*

"Recommended reference source."
—*Booklist, American Library Association, Oct '01*

Child Abuse Sourcebook

Basic Consumer Health Information about the Physical, Sexual, and Emotional Abuse of Children, with Additional Facts about Neglect, Munchausen Syndrome by Proxy (MSBP), Shaken Baby Syndrome, and Controversial Issues Related to Child Abuse, Such as Withholding Medical Care, Corporal Punishment, and Child Maltreatment in Youth Sports, and Featuring Facts about Child Protective Services, Foster Care, Adoption, Parenting Challenges, and Other Abuse Prevention Efforts

Along with a Glossary of Related Terms and Resources for Additional Help and Information

Edited by Dawn D. Matthews. 620 pages. 2004. 0-7808-0705-7.

"A valuable and highly recommended resource for school, academic and public libraries whether used on its own or as a starting point for more in-depth research."
—*E-Streams, Apr '05*

"Every week the news brings cases of child abuse or neglect, so it is useful to have a source that supplies so much helpful information. . . . Recommended. Public and academic libraries, and child welfare offices."
—*Choice, Association of College & Research Libraries, Mar '05*

"Packed with insights on all kinds of issues, from foster care and adoption to parenting and abuse prevention."
—*The Bookwatch, Nov '04*

SEE ALSO: *Domestic Violence Sourcebook, 2nd Edition*

Childhood Diseases & Disorders Sourcebook

Basic Consumer Health Information about Medical Problems Often Encountered in Pre-Adolescent Children, Including Respiratory Tract Ailments, Ear Infections, Sore Throats, Disorders of the Skin and Scalp, Digestive and Genitourinary Diseases, Infectious Diseases, Inflammatory Disorders, Chronic Physical and Developmental Disorders, Allergies, and More

Along with Information about Diagnostic Tests, Common Childhood Surgeries, and Frequently Used Medications, with a Glossary of Important Terms and Resource Directory

Edited by Chad T. Kimball. 662 pages. 2003. 0-7808-0458-9.

"This is an excellent book for new parents and should be included in all health care and public libraries."
—*American Reference Books Annual, 2004*

SEE ALSO: *Healthy Children Sourcebook*

Colds, Flu & Other Common Ailments Sourcebook

Basic Consumer Health Information about Common Ailments and Injuries, Including Colds, Coughs, the Flu, Sinus Problems, Headaches, Fever, Nausea and

Vomiting, Menstrual Cramps, Diarrhea, Constipation, Hemorrhoids, Back Pain, Dandruff, Dry and Itchy Skin, Cuts, Scrapes, Sprains, Bruises, and More

Along with Information about Prevention, Self-Care, Choosing a Doctor, Over-the-Counter Medications, Folk Remedies, and Alternative Therapies, and Including a Glossary of Important Terms and a Directory of Resources for Further Help and Information

Edited by Chad T. Kimball. 638 pages. 2001. 0-7808-0435-X.

"A good starting point for research on common illnesses. It will be a useful addition to public and consumer health library collections."
— American Reference Books Annual, 2002

"Will prove valuable to any library seeking to maintain a current, comprehensive reference collection of health resources. . . . Excellent reference."
— The Bookwatch, Aug '01

"Recommended reference source."
— Booklist, American Library Association, Jul '01

■

Communication Disorders Sourcebook

Basic Information about Deafness and Hearing Loss, Speech and Language Disorders, Voice Disorders, Balance and Vestibular Disorders, and Disorders of Smell, Taste, and Touch

Edited by Linda M. Ross. 533 pages. 1996. 0-7808-0077-X.

"This is skillfully edited and is a welcome resource for the layperson. It should be found in every public and medical library." — Booklist Health Sciences Supplement, American Library Association, Oct '97

■

Complementary & Alternative Medicine Sourcebook, 3rd Edition

Basic Consumer Health Information about Complementary and Alternative Medical Therapies, Including Acupuncture, Ayurveda, Traditional Chinese Medicine, Herbal Medicine, Homeopathy, Naturopathy, Biofeedback, Hypnotherapy, Yoga, Art Therapy, Aromatherapy, Clinical Nutrition, Vitamin and Mineral Supplements, Chiropractic, Massage, Reflexology, Crystal Therapy, Therapeutic Touch, and More

Along with Facts about Alternative and Complementary Treatments for Specific Conditions Such as Cancer, Diabetes, Osteoarthritis, Chronic Pain, Menopause, Gastrointestinal Disorders, Headaches, and Mental Illness, a Glossary, and a Resource List for Additional Help and Information

Edited by Sandra J. Judd. 657 pages. 2006. 0-7808-0864-9.

"Recommended for public, high school, and academic libraries that have consumer health collections. Hospital libraries that also serve the public will find this to be a useful resource." — E-Streams, Feb '03

"Recommended reference source."
—Booklist, American Library Association, Jan '03

"An important alternate health reference."
—MBR Bookwatch, Oct '02

"A great addition to the reference collection of every type of library." — American Reference Books Annual, 2000

■

Congenital Disorders Sourcebook, 2nd Edition

Basic Consumer Health Information about Nonhereditary Birth Defects and Disorders Related to Prematurity, Gestational Injuries, Congenital Infections, and Birth Complications, Including Heart Defects, Hydrocephalus, Spina Bifida, Cleft Lip and Palate, Cerebral Palsy, and More

Along with Facts about the Prevention of Birth Defects, Fetal Surgery and Other Treatment Options, Research Initiatives, a Glossary of Related Terms, and Resources for Additional Information and Support

Edited by Sandra J. Judd. 647 pages. 2006. 0-7808-0945-9.

"Recommended reference source."
— Booklist, American Library Association, Oct '97

SEE ALSO Pregnancy & Birth Sourcebook

■

Consumer Issues in Health Care Sourcebook

Basic Information about Health Care Fundamentals and Related Consumer Issues, Including Exams and Screening Tests, Physician Specialties, Choosing a Doctor, Using Prescription and Over-the-Counter Medications Safely, Avoiding Health Scams, Managing Common Health Risks in the Home, Care Options for Chronically or Terminally Ill Patients, and a List of Resources for Obtaining Help and Further Information

Edited by Karen Bellenir. 618 pages. 1998. 0-7808-0221-7.

"Both public and academic libraries will want to have a copy in their collection for readers who are interested in self-education on health issues."
—American Reference Books Annual, 2000

"The editor has researched the literature from government agencies and others, saving readers the time and effort of having to do the research themselves. Recommended for public libraries."
— Reference and User Services Quarterly, American Library Association, Spring '99

"Recommended reference source."
— Booklist, American Library Association, Dec '98

■

Contagious Diseases Sourcebook

Basic Consumer Health Information about Infectious Diseases Spread by Person-to-Person Contact through Direct Touch, Airborne Transmission, Sexual Contact, or Contact with Blood or Other Body Fluids, Including Hepatitis, Herpes, Influenza, Lice, Measles, Mumps, Pinworm, Ringworm, Severe Acute Respiratory Syndrome (SARS), Streptococcal Infections, Tuberculosis, and Others

Along with Facts about Disease Transmission, Anti-microbial Resistance, and Vaccines, with a Glossary and Directories of Resources for More Information

Edited by Karen Bellenir. 643 pages. 2004. 0-7808-0736-7.

"This easy-to-read volume is recommended for consumer health collections within public or academic libraries." — E-Streams, May '05

"This informative book is highly recommended for public libraries, consumer health collections, and secondary schools and undergraduate libraries." — American Reference Books Annual, 2005

"Excellent reference." — The Bookwatch, Jan '05

Contagious & Non-Contagious Infectious Diseases Sourcebook

Basic Information about Contagious Diseases like Measles, Polio, Hepatitis B, and Infectious Mononucleosis, and Non-Contagious Infectious Diseases like Tetanus and Toxic Shock Syndrome, and Diseases Occurring as Secondary Infections Such as Shingles and Reye Syndrome

Along with Vaccination, Prevention, and Treatment Information, and a Section Describing Emerging Infectious Disease Threats

Edited by Karen Bellenir and Peter D. Dresser. 566 pages. 1996. 0-7808-0075-3.

SEE ALSO Infectious Diseases Sourcebook

Death & Dying Sourcebook, 2nd Edition

Basic Consumer Health Information about End-of-Life Care and Related Perspectives and Ethical Issues, Including End-of-Life Symptoms and Treatments, Pain Management, Quality-of-Life Concerns, the Use of Life Support, Patients' Rights and Privacy Issues, Advance Directives, Physician-Assisted Suicide, Caregiving, Organ and Tissue Donation, Autopsies, Funeral Arrangements, and Grief

Along with Statistical Data, Information about the Leading Causes of Death, a Glossary, and Directories of Support Groups and Other Resources

Edited by Joyce Brennfleck Shannon. 653 pages. 2006. 0-7808-0871-1.

"Public libraries, medical libraries, and academic libraries will all find this sourcebook a useful addition to their collections." — American Reference Books Annual, 2001

"An extremely useful resource for those concerned with death and dying in the United States." — Respiratory Care, Nov '00

"Recommended reference source." — Booklist, American Library Association, Aug '00

"This book is a definite must for all those involved in end-of-life care." — Doody's Review Service, 2000

Dental Care & Oral Health Sourcebook, 2nd Edition

Basic Consumer Health Information about Dental Care, Including Oral Hygiene, Dental Visits, Pain Management, Cavities, Crowns, Bridges, Dental Implants, and Fillings, and Other Oral Health Concerns, Such as Gum Disease, Bad Breath, Dry Mouth, Genetic and Developmental Abnormalities, Oral Cancers, Orthodontics, and Temporomandibular Disorders

Along with Updates on Current Research in Oral Health, a Glossary, a Directory of Dental and Oral Health Organizations, and Resources for People with Dental and Oral Health Disorders

Edited by Amy L. Sutton. 609 pages. 2003. 0-7808-0634-4.

"This book could serve as a turning point in the battle to educate consumers in issues concerning oral health." — American Reference Books Annual, 2004

"Unique source which will fill a gap in dental sources for patients and the lay public. A valuable reference tool even in a library with thousands of books on dentistry. Comprehensive, clear, inexpensive, and easy to read and use. It fills an enormous gap in the health care literature." — Reference & User Services Quarterly, American Library Association, Summer '98

"Recommended reference source." — Booklist, American Library Association, Dec '97

Depression Sourcebook

Basic Consumer Health Information about Unipolar Depression, Bipolar Disorder, Postpartum Depression, Seasonal Affective Disorder, and Other Types of Depression in Children, Adolescents, Women, Men, the Elderly, and Other Selected Populations

Along with Facts about Causes, Risk Factors, Diagnostic Criteria, Treatment Options, Coping Strategies, Suicide Prevention, a Glossary, and a Directory of Sources for Additional Help and Information

Edited by Karen Belleni. 602 pages. 2002. 0-7808-0611-5.

"Depression Sourcebook is of a very high standard. Its purpose, which is to serve as a reference source to the lay reader, is very well served." — Journal of the National Medical Association, 2004

"Invaluable reference for public and school library collections alike." — Library Bookwatch, Apr '03

"Recommended for purchase." — American Reference Books Annual, 2003

Dermatological Disorders Sourcebook, 2nd Edition

Basic Consumer Health Information about Conditions and Disorders Affecting the Skin, Hair, and Nails, Such as Acne, Rosacea, Rashes, Dermatitis, Pigmentation Disorders, Birthmarks, Skin Cancer, Skin Injuries, Psoriasis, Scleroderma, and Hair Loss, Including Facts about Medications and Treatments for Dermatological

Disorders and Tips for Maintaining Healthy Skin, Hair, and Nails

Along with Information about How Aging Affects the Skin, a Glossary of Related Terms, and a Directory of Resources for Additional Help and Information

Edited by Amy L. Sutton. 645 pages. 2005. 0-7808-0795-2.

". . . comprehensive, easily read reference book."
—*Doody's Health Sciences Book Reviews, Oct '97*

SEE ALSO *Burns Sourcebook*

■

Diabetes Sourcebook, 3rd Edition

Basic Consumer Health Information about Type 1 Diabetes (Insulin-Dependent or Juvenile-Onset Diabetes), Type 2 Diabetes (Noninsulin-Dependent or Adult-Onset Diabetes), Gestational Diabetes, Impaired Glucose Tolerance (IGT), and Related Complications, Such as Amputation, Eye Disease, Gum Disease, Nerve Damage, and End-Stage Renal Disease, Including Facts about Insulin, Oral Diabetes Medications, Blood Sugar Testing, and the Role of Exercise and Nutrition in the Control of Diabetes

Along with a Glossary and Resources for Further Help and Information

Edited by Dawn D. Matthews. 622 pages. 2003. 0-7808-0629-8.

"This edition is even more helpful than earlier versions. . . . It is a truly valuable tool for anyone seeking readable and authoritative information on diabetes."
—*American Reference Books Annual, 2004*

"An invaluable reference." —*Library Journal, May '00*

Selected as one of the 250 "Best Health Sciences Books of 1999." —*Doody's Rating Service, Mar-Apr '00*

"Provides useful information for the general public."
—*Healthlines, University of Michigan Health Management Research Center, Sep/Oct '99*

". . . provides reliable mainstream medical information . . . belongs on the shelves of any library with a consumer health collection." —*E-Streams, Sep '99*

"Recommended reference source."
—*Booklist, American Library Association, Feb '99*

■

Diet & Nutrition Sourcebook, 3rd Edition

Basic Consumer Health Information about Dietary Guidelines and the Food Guidance System, Recommended Daily Nutrient Intakes, Serving Proportions, Weight Control, Vitamins and Supplements, Nutrition Issues for Different Life Stages and Lifestyles, and the Needs of People with Specific Medical Concerns, Including Cancer, Celiac Disease, Diabetes, Eating Disorders, Food Allergies, and Cardiovascular Disease

Along with Facts about Federal Nutrition Support Programs, a Glossary of Nutrition and Dietary Terms, and Directories of Additional Resources for More Information about Nutrition

Edited by Joyce Brennfleck Shannon. 633 pages. 2006. 0-7808-0800-2.

"This book is an excellent source of basic diet and nutrition information." —*Booklist Health Sciences Supplement, American Library Association, Dec '00*

"This reference document should be in any public library, but it would be a very good guide for beginning students in the health sciences. If the other books in this publisher's series are as good as this, they should all be in the health sciences collections."
—*American Reference Books Annual, 2000*

"This book is an excellent general nutrition reference for consumers who desire to take an active role in their health care for prevention. Consumers of all ages who select this book can feel confident they are receiving current and accurate information." —*Journal of Nutrition for the Elderly, Vol. 19, No. 4, 2000*

SEE ALSO *Digestive Diseases & Disorders Sourcebook, Eating Disorders Sourcebook, Gastrointestinal Diseases & Disorders Sourcebook, Vegetarian Sourcebook*

■

Digestive Diseases & Disorders Sourcebook

Basic Consumer Health Information about Diseases and Disorders that Impact the Upper and Lower Digestive System, Including Celiac Disease, Constipation, Crohn's Disease, Cyclic Vomiting Syndrome, Diarrhea, Diverticulosis and Diverticulitis, Gallstones, Heartburn, Hemorrhoids, Hernias, Indigestion (Dyspepsia), Irritable Bowel Syndrome, Lactose Intolerance, Ulcers, and More

Along with Information about Medications and Other Treatments, Tips for Maintaining a Healthy Digestive Tract, a Glossary, and Directory of Digestive Diseases Organizations

Edited by Karen Bellenir. 335 pages. 2000. 0-7808-0327-2.

"This title would be an excellent addition to all public or patient-research libraries."
—*American Reference Books Annual, 2001*

"This title is recommended for public, hospital, and health sciences libraries with consumer health collections." —*E-Streams, Jul-Aug '00*

"Recommended reference source."
—*Booklist, American Library Association, May '00*

SEE ALSO *Eating Disorders Sourcebook, Gastrointestinal Diseases & Disorders Sourcebook*

■

Disabilities Sourcebook

Basic Consumer Health Information about Physical and Psychiatric Disabilities, Including Descriptions of Major Causes of Disability, Assistive and Adaptive Aids, Workplace Issues, and Accessibility Concerns

Along with Information about the Americans with Disabilities Act, a Glossary, and Resources for Additional Help and Information

Edited by Dawn D. Matthews. 616 pages. 2000. 0-7808-0389-2.

"It is a must for libraries with a consumer health section." — *American Reference Books Annual, 2002*

"A much needed addition to the Omnigraphics Health Reference Series. A current reference work to provide people with disabilities, their families, caregivers or those who work with them, a broad range of information in one volume, has not been available until now. . . . It is recommended for all public and academic library reference collections." — *E-Streams, May '01*

"An excellent source book in easy-to-read format covering many current topics; highly recommended for all libraries." — *Choice, Association of College & Research Libraries, Jan '01*

"Recommended reference source." — *Booklist, American Library Association, Jul '00*

■

Domestic Violence Sourcebook, 2nd Edition

Basic Consumer Health Information about the Causes and Consequences of Abusive Relationships, Including Physical Violence, Sexual Assault, Battery, Stalking, and Emotional Abuse, and Facts about the Effects of Violence on Women, Men, Young Adults, and the Elderly, with Reports about Domestic Violence in Selected Populations, and Featuring Facts about Medical Care, Victim Assistance and Protection, Prevention Strategies, Mental Health Services, and Legal Issues

Along with a Glossary of Related Terms and Resources for Additional Help and Information

Edited by Dawn D. Matthews. 628 pages. 2004. 0-7808-0669-7.

"Educators, clergy, medical professionals, police, and victims and their families will benefit from this realistic and easy-to-understand resource." — *American Reference Books Annual, 2005*

"Recommended for all collections supporting consumer health information. It should also be considered for any collection needing general, readable information on domestic violence." — *E-Streams, Jan '05*

"This sourcebook complements other books in its field, providing a one-stop resource . . . Recommended." — *Choice, Association of College & Research Libraries, Jan '05*

"Interested lay persons should find the book extremely beneficial. . . . A copy of *Domestic Violence and Child Abuse Sourcebook* should be in every public library in the United States." — *Social Science & Medicine, No. 56, 2003*

"This is important information. The Web has many resources but this sourcebook fills an important societal need. I am not aware of any other resources of this type." — *Doody's Review Service, Sep '01*

"Recommended reference source." — *Booklist, American Library Association, Apr '01*

"Important pick for college-level health reference libraries." — *The Bookwatch, Mar '01*

"Because this problem is so widespread and because this book includes a lot of issues within one volume, this work is recommended for all public libraries." — *American Reference Books Annual, 2001*

SEE ALSO *Child Abuse Sourcebook*

■

Drug Abuse Sourcebook, 2nd Edition

Basic Consumer Health Information about Illicit Substances of Abuse and the Misuse of Prescription and Over-the-Counter Medications, Including Depressants, Hallucinogens, Inhalants, Marijuana, Stimulants, and Anabolic Steroids

Along with Facts about Related Health Risks, Treatment Programs, Prevention Programs, a Glossary of Abuse and Addiction Terms, a Glossary of Drug-Related Street Terms, and a Directory of Resources for More Information

Edited by Catherine Ginther. 607 pages. 2004. 0-7808-0740-5.

"Commendable for organizing useful, normally scattered government and association-produced data into a logical sequence." — *American Reference Books Annual, 2006*

"This easy-to-read volume is recommended for consumer health collections within public or academic libraries." — *E-Streams, Sep '05*

"An excellent library reference." — *The Bookwatch, May '05*

"Containing a wealth of information, this book will be useful to the college student just beginning to explore the topic of substance abuse. This resource belongs in libraries that serve a lower-division undergraduate or community college clientele as well as the general public." — *Choice, Association of College & Research Libraries, Jun '01*

"Recommended reference source." — *Booklist, American Library Association, Feb '01*

SEE ALSO *Alcoholism Sourcebook, Substance Abuse Sourcebook*

■

Ear, Nose & Throat Disorders Sourcebook, 2nd Edition

Basic Consumer Health Information about Disorders of the Ears, Hearing Loss, Vestibular Disorders, Nasal and Sinus Problems, Throat and Vocal Cord Disorders, and Otolaryngologic Cancers, Including Facts about Ear Infections and Injuries, Genetic and Congenital Deafness, Sensorineural Hearing Disorders, Tinnitus, Vertigo, Ménière Disease, Rhinitis, Sinusitis, Snoring, Sore Throats, Hoarseness, and More

Along with Reports on Current Research Initiatives, a Glossary of Related Medical Terms, and a Directory of Sources for Further Help and Information

Edited by Sandra J. Judd. 659 pages. 2006. 0-7808-0872-X.

"Overall, this sourcebook is helpful for the consumer seeking information on ENT issues. It is recommended for public libraries."
—American Reference Books Annual, 1999

"Recommended reference source."
—Booklist, American Library Association, Dec '98

■

Eating Disorders Sourcebook

Basic Consumer Health Information about Eating Disorders, Including Information about Anorexia Nervosa, Bulimia Nervosa, Binge Eating, Body Dysmorphic Disorder, Pica, Laxative Abuse, and Night Eating Syndrome

Along with Information about Causes, Adverse Effects, and Treatment and Prevention Issues, and Featuring a Section on Concerns Specific to Children and Adolescents, a Glossary, and Resources for Further Help and Information

Edited by Dawn D. Matthews. 322 pages. 2001. 0-7808-0335-3.

"Recommended for health science libraries that are open to the public, as well as hospital libraries. This book is a good resource for the consumer who is concerned about eating disorders." — E-Streams, Mar '02

"This volume is another convenient collection of excerpted articles. Recommended for school and public library patrons; lower-division undergraduates; and two-year technical program students."
—Choice, Association of College & Research Libraries, Jan '02

"Recommended reference source."
— Booklist, American Library Association, Oct '01

SEE ALSO Diet & Nutrition Sourcebook, Digestive Diseases & Disorders Sourcebook, Gastrointestinal Diseases & Disorders Sourcebook

■

Emergency Medical Services Sourcebook

Basic Consumer Health Information about Preventing, Preparing for, and Managing Emergency Situations, When and Who to Call for Help, What to Expect in the Emergency Room, the Emergency Medical Team, Patient Issues, and Current Topics in Emergency Medicine

Along with Statistical Data, a Glossary, and Sources of Additional Help and Information

Edited by Jenni Lynn Colson. 494 pages. 2002. 0-7808-0420-1.

"Handy and convenient for home, public, school, and college libraries. Recommended."
— Choice, Association of College & Research Libraries, Apr '03

"This reference can provide the consumer with answers to most questions about emergency care in the United States, or it will direct them to a resource where the answer can be found."
—American Reference Books Annual, 2003

"Recommended reference source."
— Booklist, American Library Association, Feb '03

■

Endocrine & Metabolic Disorders Sourcebook

Basic Information for the Layperson about Pancreatic and Insulin-Related Disorders Such as Pancreatitis, Diabetes, and Hypoglycemia; Adrenal Gland Disorders Such as Cushing's Syndrome, Addison's Disease, and Congenital Adrenal Hyperplasia; Pituitary Gland Disorders Such as Growth Hormone Deficiency, Acromegaly, and Pituitary Tumors; Thyroid Disorders Such as Hypothyroidism, Graves' Disease, Hashimoto's Disease, and Goiter; Hyperparathyroidism; and Other Diseases and Syndromes of Hormone Imbalance or Metabolic Dysfunction

Along with Reports on Current Research Initiatives

Edited by Linda M. Shin. 574 pages. 1998. 0-7808-0207-1.

"Omnigraphics has produced another needed resource for health information consumers."
—American Reference Books Annual, 2000

"Recommended reference source."
— Booklist, American Library Association, Dec '98

■

Environmental Health Sourcebook, 2nd Edition

Basic Consumer Health Information about the Environment and Its Effect on Human Health, Including the Effects of Air Pollution, Water Pollution, Hazardous Chemicals, Food Hazards, Radiation Hazards, Biological Agents, Household Hazards, Such as Radon, Asbestos, Carbon Monoxide, and Mold, and Information about Associated Diseases and Disorders, Including Cancer, Allergies, Respiratory Problems, and Skin Disorders

Along with Information about Environmental Concerns for Specific Populations, a Glossary of Related Terms, and Resources for Further Help and Information

Edited by Dawn D. Matthews. 673 pages. 2003. 0-7808-0632-8.

"This recently updated edition continues the level of quality and the reputation of the numerous other volumes in Omnigraphics' Health Reference Series."
—American Reference Books Annual, 2004

"An excellent updated edition."
—The Bookwatch, Oct '03

"Recommended reference source."
— Booklist, American Library Association, Sep '98

"This book will be a useful addition to anyone's library." — Choice Health Sciences Supplement, Association of College & Research Libraries, May '98

"... a good survey of numerous environmentally induced physical disorders ... a useful addition to anyone's library."
— *Doody's Health Sciences Book Reviews, Jan '98*

■

Environmentally Induced Disorders Sourcebook

SEE *Environmental Health Sourcebook, 2nd Edition*

■

Ethnic Diseases Sourcebook

Basic Consumer Health Information for Ethnic and Racial Minority Groups in the United States, Including General Health Indicators and Behaviors, Ethnic Diseases, Genetic Testing, the Impact of Chronic Diseases, Women's Health, Mental Health Issues, and Preventive Health Care Services

Along with a Glossary and a Listing of Additional Resources

Edited by Joyce Brennfleck Shannon. 664 pages. 2001. 0-7808-0336-1.

"Recommended for health sciences libraries where public health programs are a priority."
— *E-Streams, Jan '02*

"Not many books have been written on this topic to date, and the *Ethnic Diseases Sourcebook* is a strong addition to the list. It will be an important introductory resource for health consumers, students, health care personnel, and social scientists. It is recommended for public, academic, and large hospital libraries."
— *American Reference Books Annual, 2002*

"Recommended reference source."
— *Booklist, American Library Association, Oct '01*

"Will prove valuable to any library seeking to maintain a current, comprehensive reference collection of health resources.... An excellent source of health information about genetic disorders which affect particular ethnic and racial minorities in the U.S."
— *The Bookwatch, Aug '01*

■

Eye Care Sourcebook, 2nd Edition

Basic Consumer Health Information about Eye Care and Eye Disorders, Including Facts about the Diagnosis, Prevention, and Treatment of Common Refractive Problems Such as Myopia, Hyperopia, Astigmatism, and Presbyopia, and Eye Diseases, Including Glaucoma, Cataract, Age-Related Macular Degeneration, and Diabetic Retinopathy

Along with a Section on Vision Correction and Refractive Surgeries, Including LASIK and LASEK, a Glossary, and Directories of Resources for Additional Help and Information

Edited by Amy L. Sutton. 543 pages. 2003. 0-7808-0635-2.

"... a solid reference tool for eye care and a valuable addition to a collection."
— *American Reference Books Annual, 2004*

■

Family Planning Sourcebook

Basic Consumer Health Information about Planning for Pregnancy and Contraception, Including Traditional Methods, Barrier Methods, Hormonal Methods, Permanent Methods, Future Methods, Emergency Contraception, and Birth Control Choices for Women at Each Stage of Life

Along with Statistics, a Glossary, and Sources of Additional Information

Edited by Amy Marcaccio Keyzer. 520 pages. 2001. 0-7808-0379-5.

"Recommended for public, health, and undergraduate libraries as part of the circulating collection."
— *E-Streams, Mar '02*

"Information is presented in an unbiased, readable manner, and the sourcebook will certainly be a necessary addition to those public and high school libraries where Internet access is restricted or otherwise problematic." — *American Reference Books Annual, 2002*

"Recommended reference source."
— *Booklist, American Library Association, Oct '01*

"Will prove valuable to any library seeking to maintain a current, comprehensive reference collection of health resources.... Excellent reference."
— *The Bookwatch, Aug '01*

SEE ALSO *Pregnancy & Birth Sourcebook*

■

Fitness & Exercise Sourcebook, 3rd Edition

Basic Consumer Health Information about the Physical and Mental Benefits of Fitness, Including Cardiorespiratory Endurance, Muscular Strength, Muscular Endurance, and Flexibility, with Facts about Sports Nutrition and Exercise-Related Injuries and Tips about Physical Activity and Exercises for People of All Ages and for People with Health Concerns

Along with Advice on Selecting and Using Exercise Equipment, Maintaining Exercise Motivation, a Glossary of Related Terms, and a Directory of Resources for More Help and Information

Edited by Amy L. Sutton. 663 pages. 2007. 0-7808-0946-7.

"This work is recommended for all general reference collections."
— *American Reference Books Annual, 2002*

"Highly recommended for public, consumer, and school grades fourth through college." — *E-Streams, Nov '01*

"Recommended reference source."
— *Booklist, American Library Association, Oct '01*

"The information appears quite comprehensive and is considered reliable. . . . This second edition is a welcomed addition to the series."
— *Doody's Review Service, Sep '01*

Food & Animal Borne Diseases Sourcebook

Basic Information about Diseases That Can Be Spread to Humans through the Ingestion of Contaminated Food or Water or by Contact with Infected Animals and Insects, Such as Botulism, E. Coli, Hepatitis A, Trichinosis, Lyme Disease, and Rabies

Along with Information Regarding Prevention and Treatment Methods, and Including a Special Section for International Travelers Describing Diseases Such as Cholera, Malaria, Travelers' Diarrhea, and Yellow Fever, and Offering Recommendations for Avoiding Illness

Edited by Karen Bellenir and Peter D. Dresser. 535 pages. 1995. 0-7808-0033-8.

"Targeting general readers and providing them with a single, comprehensive source of information on selected topics, this book continues, with the excellent caliber of its predecessors, to catalog topical information on health matters of general interest. Readable and thorough, this valuable resource is highly recommended for all libraries."
— Academic Library Book Review, Summer '96

"A comprehensive collection of authoritative information." *— Emergency Medical Services, Oct '95*

■

Food Safety Sourcebook

Basic Consumer Health Information about the Safe Handling of Meat, Poultry, Seafood, Eggs, Fruit Juices, and Other Food Items, and Facts about Pesticides, Drinking Water, Food Safety Overseas, and the Onset, Duration, and Symptoms of Foodborne Illnesses, Including Types of Pathogenic Bacteria, Parasitic Protozoa, Worms, Viruses, and Natural Toxins

Along with the Role of the Consumer, the Food Handler, and the Government in Food Safety; a Glossary, and Resources for Additional Help and Information

Edited by Dawn D. Matthews. 339 pages. 1999. 0-7808-0326-4.

"This book is recommended for public libraries and universities with home economic and food science programs." *— E-Streams, Nov '00*

"Recommended reference source."
— Booklist, American Library Association, May '00

"This book takes the complex issues of food safety and foodborne pathogens and presents them in an easily understood manner. [It does] an excellent job of covering a large and often confusing topic."
— American Reference Books Annual, 2000

■

Forensic Medicine Sourcebook

Basic Consumer Information for the Layperson about Forensic Medicine, Including Crime Scene Investigation, Evidence Collection and Analysis, Expert Testimony, Computer-Aided Criminal Identification, Digital Imaging in the Courtroom, DNA Profiling, Accident Reconstruction, Autopsies, Ballistics, Drugs and Explosives Detection, Latent Fingerprints, Product Tampering, and Questioned Document Examination

Along with Statistical Data, a Glossary of Forensics Terminology, and Listings of Sources for Further Help and Information

Edited by Annemarie S. Muth. 574 pages. 1999. 0-7808-0232-2.

"Given the expected widespread interest in its content and its easy to read style, this book is recommended for most public and all college and university libraries."
— E-Streams, Feb '01

"Recommended for public libraries."
— Reference & User Services Quarterly, American Library Association, Spring 2000

"Recommended reference source."
— Booklist, American Library Association, Feb '00

"A wealth of information, useful statistics, references are up-to-date and extremely complete. This wonderful collection of data will help students who are interested in a career in any type of forensic field. It is a great resource for attorneys who need information about types of expert witnesses needed in a particular case. It also offers useful information for fiction and nonfiction writers whose work involves a crime. A fascinating compilation. All levels."
— Choice, Association of College & Research Libraries, Jan '00

"There are several items that make this book attractive to consumers who are seeking certain forensic data. . . . This is a useful current source for those seeking general forensic medical answers."
— American Reference Books Annual, 2000

■

Gastrointestinal Diseases & Disorders Sourcebook, 2nd Edition

Basic Consumer Health Information about the Upper and Lower Gastrointestinal (GI) Tract, Including the Esophagus, Stomach, Intestines, Rectum, Liver, and Pancreas, with Facts about Gastroesophageal Reflux Disease, Gastritis, Hernias, Ulcers, Celiac Disease, Diverticulitis, Irritable Bowel Syndrome, Hemorrhoids, Gastrointestinal Cancers, and Other Diseases and Disorders Related to the Digestive Process

Along with Information about Commonly Used Diagnostic and Surgical Procedures, Statistics, Reports on Current Research Initiatives and Clinical Trials, a Glossary, and Resources for Additional Help and Information

Edited by Sandra J. Judd. 681 pages. 2006. 0-7808-0798-7.

". . . very readable form. The successful editorial work that brought this material together into a useful and understandable reference makes accessible to all readers information that can help them more effectively understand and obtain help for digestive tract problems."
— Choice, Association of College & Research Libraries, Feb '97

Genetic Disorders Sourcebook, 3rd Edition

Basic Consumer Health Information about Hereditary Diseases and Disorders, Including Facts about the Human Genome, Genetic Inheritance Patterns, Disorders Associated with Specific Genes, Such as Sickle Cell Disease, Hemophilia, and Cystic Fibrosis, Chromosome Disorders, Such as Down Syndrome, Fragile X Syndrome, and Turner Syndrome, and Complex Diseases and Disorders Resulting from the Interaction of Environmental and Genetic Factors, Such as Allergies, Cancer, and Obesity

Along with Facts about Genetic Testing, Suggestions for Parents of Children with Special Needs, Reports on Current Research Initiatives, a Glossary of Genetic Terminology, and Resources for Additional Help and Information

Edited by Karen Bellenir. 777 pages. 2004. 0-7808-0742-1.

"This text is recommended for any library with an interest in providing consumer health resources."
— *E-Streams, Aug '05*

"This is a valuable resource for anyone wishing to have an understandable description of any of the topics or disorders included. The editor succeeds in making complex genetic issues understandable."
— *Doody's Book Review Service, May '05*

"A good acquisition for public libraries."
— *American Reference Books Annual, 2005*

"Excellent reference." — *The Bookwatch, Jan '05*

"Recommended reference source."
— *Booklist, American Library Association, Apr '01*

"Important pick for college-level health reference libraries." — *The Bookwatch, Mar '01*

Head Trauma Sourcebook

Basic Information for the Layperson about Open-Head and Closed-Head Injuries, Treatment Advances, Recovery, and Rehabilitation

Along with Reports on Current Research Initiatives

Edited by Karen Bellenir. 414 pages. 1997. 0-7808-0208-X.

Headache Sourcebook

Basic Consumer Health Information about Migraine, Tension, Cluster, Rebound and Other Types of Headaches, with Facts about the Cause and Prevention of Headaches, the Effects of Stress and the Environment, Headaches during Pregnancy and Menopause, and Childhood Headaches

Along with a Glossary and Other Resources for Additional Help and Information

Edited by Dawn D. Matthews. 362 pages. 2002. 0-7808-0337-X.

"Highly recommended for academic and medical reference collections." — *Library Bookwatch, Sep '02*

Health Insurance Sourcebook

Basic Information about Managed Care Organizations, Traditional Fee-for-Service Insurance, Insurance Portability and Pre-Existing Conditions Clauses, Medicare, Medicaid, Social Security, and Military Health Care

Along with Information about Insurance Fraud

Edited by Wendy Wilcox. 530 pages. 1997. 0-7808-0222-5.

"Particularly useful because it brings much of this information together in one volume. This book will be a handy reference source in the health sciences library, hospital library, college and university library, and medium to large public library."
— *Medical Reference Services Quarterly, Fall '98*

Awarded "Books of the Year Award"
— *American Journal of Nursing, 1997*

"The layout of the book is particularly helpful as it provides easy access to reference material. A most useful addition to the vast amount of information about health insurance. The use of data from U.S. government agencies is most commendable. Useful in a library or learning center for healthcare professional students."
— *Doody's Health Sciences Book Reviews, Nov '97*

Healthy Aging Sourcebook

Basic Consumer Health Information about Maintaining Health through the Aging Process, Including Advice on Nutrition, Exercise, and Sleep, Help in Making Decisions about Midlife Issues and Retirement, and Guidance Concerning Practical and Informed Choices in Health Consumerism

Along with Data Concerning the Theories of Aging, Different Experiences in Aging by Minority Groups, and Facts about Aging Now and Aging in the Future; and Featuring a Glossary, a Guide to Consumer Help, Additional Suggested Reading, and Practical Resource Directory

Edited by Jenifer Swanson. 536 pages. 1999. 0-7808-0390-6.

"Recommended reference source."
— *Booklist, American Library Association, Feb '00*

SEE ALSO *Physical & Mental Issues in Aging Sourcebook*

Healthy Children Sourcebook

Basic Consumer Health Information about the Physical and Mental Development of Children between the Ages of 3 and 12, Including Routine Health Care, Preventative Health Services, Safety and First Aid, Healthy Sleep, Dental Care, Nutrition, and Fitness, and Featuring Parenting Tips on Such Topics as Bed-

wetting, *Choosing Day Care, Monitoring TV and Other Media, and Establishing a Foundation for Substance Abuse Prevention*

Along with a Glossary of Commonly Used Pediatric Terms and Resources for Additional Help and Information.

Edited by Chad T. Kimball. 647 pages. 2003. 0-7808-0247-0.

"It is hard to imagine that any other single resource exists that would provide such a comprehensive guide of timely information on health promotion and disease prevention for children aged 3 to 12."

—*American Reference Books Annual, 2004*

"The strengths of this book are many. It is clearly written, presented and structured."

—*Journal of the National Medical Association, 2004*

SEE ALSO *Childhood Diseases & Disorders Sourcebook*

■

Healthy Heart Sourcebook for Women

Basic Consumer Health Information about Cardiac Issues Specific to Women, Including Facts about Major Risk Factors and Prevention, Treatment and Control Strategies, and Important Dietary Issues

Along with a Special Section Regarding the Pros and Cons of Hormone Replacement Therapy and Its Impact on Heart Health, and Additional Help, Including Recipes, a Glossary, and a Directory of Resources

Edited by Dawn D. Matthews. 336 pages. 2000. 0-7808-0329-9.

"A good reference source and recommended for all public, academic, medical, and hospital libraries."

—*Medical Reference Services Quarterly, Summer '01*

"Because of the lack of information specific to women on this topic, this book is recommended for public libraries and consumer libraries."

—*American Reference Books Annual, 2001*

"Contains very important information about coronary artery disease that all women should know. The information is current and presented in an easy-to-read format. The book will make a good addition to any library."

—*American Medical Writers Association Journal, Summer '00*

"Important, basic reference."

—*Reviewer's Bookwatch, Jul '00*

SEE ALSO *Cardiovascular Diseases & Disorders Sourcebook, Women's Health Concerns Sourcebook*

■

Heart Diseases & Disorders Sourcebook

SEE *Cardiovascular Diseases & Disorders Sourcebook, 3rd Edition*

Hepatitis Sourcebook

Basic Consumer Health Information about Hepatitis A, Hepatitis B, Hepatitis C, and Other Forms of Hepatitis, Including Autoimmune Hepatitis, Alcoholic Hepatitis, Nonalcoholic Steatohepatitis, and Toxic Hepatitis, with Facts about Risk Factors, Screening Methods, Diagnostic Tests, and Treatment Options

Along with Information on Liver Health, Tips for People Living with Chronic Hepatitis, Reports on Current Research Initiatives, a Glossary of Terms Related to Hepatitis, and a Directory of Sources for Further Help and Information

Edited by Sandra J. Judd. 597 pages. 2005. 0-7808-0749-9.

"Highly recommended."

—*American Reference Books Annual, 2006*

■

Household Safety Sourcebook

Basic Consumer Health Information about Household Safety, Including Information about Poisons, Chemicals, Fire, and Water Hazards in the Home

Along with Advice about the Safe Use of Home Maintenance Equipment, Choosing Toys and Nursery Furniture, Holiday and Recreation Safety, a Glossary, and Resources for Further Help and Information

Edited by Dawn D. Matthews. 606 pages. 2002. 0-7808-0338-8.

"This work will be useful in public libraries with large consumer health and wellness departments."

—*American Reference Books Annual, 2003*

"As a sourcebook on household safety this book meets its mark. It is encyclopedic in scope and covers a wide range of safety issues that are commonly seen in the home."

—*E-Streams, Jul '02*

■

Hypertension Sourcebook

Basic Consumer Health Information about the Causes, Diagnosis, and Treatment of High Blood Pressure, with Facts about Consequences, Complications, and Co-Occurring Disorders, Such as Coronary Heart Disease, Diabetes, Stroke, Kidney Disease, and Hypertensive Retinopathy, and Issues in Blood Pressure Control, Including Dietary Choices, Stress Management, and Medications

Along with Reports on Current Research Initiatives and Clinical Trials, a Glossary, and Resources for Additional Help and Information

Edited by Dawn D. Matthews and Karen Bellenir. 613 pages. 2004. 0-7808-0674-3.

"Academic, public, and medical libraries will want to add the *Hypertension Sourcebook* to their collections."

—*E-Streams, Aug '05*

"The strength of this source is the wide range of information given about hypertension."

—*American Reference Books Annual, 2005*

Immune System Disorders Sourcebook, 2nd Edition

Basic Consumer Health Information about Disorders of the Immune System, Including Immune System Function and Response, Diagnosis of Immune Disorders, Information about Inherited Immune Disease, Acquired Immune Disease, and Autoimmune Diseases, Including Primary Immune Deficiency, Acquired Immunodeficiency Syndrome (AIDS), Lupus, Multiple Sclerosis, Type 1 Diabetes, Rheumatoid Arthritis, and Graves' Disease

Along with Treatments, Tips for Coping with Immune Disorders, a Glossary, and a Directory of Additional Resources.

Edited by Joyce Brennfleck Shannon. 671 pages. 2005. 0-7808-0748-0

"Highly recommended for academic and public libraries." — *American Reference Books Annual, 2006*

"The updated second edition is a 'must' for any consumer health library seeking a solid resource covering the treatments, symptoms, and options for immune disorder sufferers. . . . An excellent guide."
— *MBR Bookwatch, Jan '06*

Infant & Toddler Health Sourcebook

Basic Consumer Health Information about the Physical and Mental Development of Newborns, Infants, and Toddlers, Including Neonatal Concerns, Nutrition Recommendations, Immunization Schedules, Common Pediatric Disorders, Assessments and Milestones, Safety Tips, and Advice for Parents and Other Caregivers

Along with a Glossary of Terms and Resource Listings for Additional Help

Edited by Jenifer Swanson. 585 pages. 2000. 0-7808-0246-2.

"As a reference for the general public, this would be useful in any library." — *E-Streams, May '01*

"Recommended reference source."
— *Booklist, American Library Association, Feb '01*

"This is a good source for general use."
— *American Reference Books Annual, 2001*

Infectious Diseases Sourcebook

Basic Consumer Health Information about Non-Contagious Bacterial, Viral, Prion, Fungal, and Parasitic Diseases Spread by Food and Water, Insects and Animals, or Environmental Contact, Including Botulism, E. Coli, Encephalitis, Legionnaires' Disease, Lyme Disease, Malaria, Plague, Rabies, Salmonella, Tetanus, and Others, and Facts about Newly Emerging Diseases, Such as Hantavirus, Mad Cow Disease, Monkeypox, and West Nile Virus

Along with Information about Preventing Disease Transmission, the Threat of Bioterrorism, and Current

Research Initiatives, with a Glossary and Directory of Resources for More Information

Edited by Karen Bellenir. 634 pages. 2004. 0-7808-0675-1.

"This reference continues the excellent tradition of the *Health Reference Series* in consolidating a wealth of information on a selected topic into a format that is easy to use and accessible to the general public."
— *American Reference Books Annual, 2005*

"Recommended for public and academic libraries."
— *E-Streams, Jan '05*

Injury & Trauma Sourcebook

Basic Consumer Health Information about the Impact of Injury, the Diagnosis and Treatment of Common and Traumatic Injuries, Emergency Care, and Specific Injuries Related to Home, Community, Workplace, Transportation, and Recreation

Along with Guidelines for Injury Prevention, a Glossary, and a Directory of Additional Resources

Edited by Joyce Brennfleck Shannon. 696 pages. 2002. 0-7808-0421-X.

"This publication is the most comprehensive work of its kind about injury and trauma."
— *American Reference Books Annual, 2003*

"This sourcebook provides concise, easily readable, basic health information about injuries. . . . This book is well organized and an easy to use reference resource suitable for hospital, health sciences and public libraries with consumer health collections."
— *E-Streams, Nov '02*

"Practitioners should be aware of guides such as this in order to facilitate their use by patients and their families." — *Doody's Health Sciences Book Review Journal, Sep-Oct '02*

"Recommended reference source."
— *Booklist, American Library Association, Sep '02*

"Highly recommended for academic and medical reference collections." — *Library Bookwatch, Sep '02*

Kidney & Urinary Tract Diseases & Disorders Sourcebook

SEE Urinary Tract & Kidney Diseases & Disorders Sourcebook, 2nd Edition

Learning Disabilities Sourcebook, 2nd Edition

Basic Consumer Health Information about Learning Disabilities, Including Dyslexia, Developmental Speech and Language Disabilities, Non-Verbal Learning Disorders, Developmental Arithmetic Disorder, Developmental Writing Disorder, and Other Conditions That Impede Learning Such as Attention Deficit/ Hyperac-

tivity Disorder, Brain Injury, Hearing Impairment, Kline-felter Syndrome, Dyspraxia, and Tourette's Syndrome

Along with Facts about Educational Issues and Assistive Technology, Coping Strategies, a Glossary of Related Terms, and Resources for Further Help and Information

Edited by Dawn D. Matthews. 621 pages. 2003. 0-7808-0626-3.

"The second edition of Learning Disabilities Sourcebook far surpasses the earlier edition in that it is more focused on information that will be useful as a consumer health resource."
— American Reference Books Annual, 2004

"Teachers as well as consumers will find this an essential guide to understanding various syndromes and their latest treatments. [An] invaluable reference for public and school library collections alike."
— Library Bookwatch, Apr '03

Named "Outstanding Reference Book of 1999."
— New York Public Library, Feb 2000

"An excellent candidate for inclusion in a public library reference section. It's a great source of information. Teachers will also find the book useful. Definitely worth reading."
— Journal of Adolescent & Adult Literacy, Feb 2000

"Readable . . . provides a solid base of information regarding successful techniques used with individuals who have learning disabilities, as well as practical suggestions for educators and family members. Clear language, concise descriptions, and pertinent information for contacting multiple resources add to the strength of this book as a useful tool." — Choice, Association of College & Research Libraries, Feb '99

"Recommended reference source."
— Booklist, American Library Association, Sep '98

"A useful resource for libraries and for those who don't have the time to identify and locate the individual publications." — Disability Resources Monthly, Sep '98

Leukemia Sourcebook

Basic Consumer Health Information about Adult and Childhood Leukemias, Including Acute Lymphocytic Leukemia (ALL), Chronic Lymphocytic Leukemia (CLL), Acute Myelogenous Leukemia (AML), Chronic Myelogenous Leukemia (CML), and Hairy Cell Leukemia, and Treatments Such as Chemotherapy, Radiation Therapy, Peripheral Blood Stem Cell and Marrow Transplantation, and Immunotherapy

Along with Tips for Life During and After Treatment, a Glossary, and Directories of Additional Resources

Edited by Joyce Brennfleck Shannon. 587 pages. 2003. 0-7808-0627-1.

"Unlike other medical books for the layperson, . . . the language does not talk down to the reader. . . . This volume is highly recommended for all libraries."
— American Reference Books Annual, 2004

"... a fine title which ranges from diagnosis to alternative treatments, staging, and tips for life during and after diagnosis." — The Bookwatch, Dec '03

Liver Disorders Sourcebook

Basic Consumer Health Information about the Liver and How It Works; Liver Diseases, Including Cancer, Cirrhosis, Hepatitis, and Toxic and Drug Related Diseases; Tips for Maintaining a Healthy Liver; Laboratory Tests, Radiology Tests, and Facts about Liver Transplantation

Along with a Section on Support Groups, a Glossary, and Resource Listings

Edited by Joyce Brennfleck Shannon. 591 pages. 2000. 0-7808-0383-3.

"A valuable resource."
— American Reference Books Annual, 2001

"This title is recommended for health sciences and public libraries with consumer health collections."
— E-Streams, Oct '00

"Recommended reference source."
— Booklist, American Library Association, Jun '00

Lung Disorders Sourcebook

Basic Consumer Health Information about Emphysema, Pneumonia, Tuberculosis, Asthma, Cystic Fibrosis, and Other Lung Disorders, Including Facts about Diagnostic Procedures, Treatment Strategies, Disease Prevention Efforts, and Such Risk Factors as Smoking, Air Pollution, and Exposure to Asbestos, Radon, and Other Agents

Along with a Glossary and Resources for Additional Help and Information

Edited by Dawn D. Matthews. 678 pages. 2002. 0-7808-0339-6.

"This title is a great addition for public and school libraries because it provides concise health information on the lungs."
— American Reference Books Annual, 2003

"Highly recommended for academic and medical reference collections." — Library Bookwatch, Sep '02

SEE ALSO Respiratory Diseases & Disorders Sourcebook

Medical Tests Sourcebook, 2nd Edition

Basic Consumer Health Information about Medical Tests, Including Age-Specific Health Tests, Important Health Screenings and Exams, Home-Use Tests, Blood and Specimen Tests, Electrical Tests, Scope Tests, Genetic Testing, and Imaging Tests, Such as X-Rays, Ultrasound, Computed Tomography, Magnetic Resonance Imaging, Angiography, and Nuclear Medicine

Along with a Glossary and Directory of Additional Resources

Edited by Joyce Brennfleck Shannon. 654 pages. 2004. 0-7808-0670-0.

"Recommended for hospital and health sciences libraries with consumer health collections."
—E-Streams, Mar '00

"This is an overall excellent reference with a wealth of general knowledge that may aid those who are reluctant to get vital tests performed."
—Today's Librarian, Jan '00

"A valuable reference guide."
—American Reference Books Annual, 2000

■

Men's Health Concerns Sourcebook, 2nd Edition

Basic Consumer Health Information about the Medical and Mental Concerns of Men, Including Theories about the Shorter Male Lifespan, the Leading Causes of Death and Disability, Physical Concerns of Special Significance to Men, Reproductive and Sexual Concerns, Sexually Transmitted Diseases, Men's Mental and Emotional Health, and Lifestyle Choices That Affect Wellness, Such as Nutrition, Fitness, and Substance Use

Along with a Glossary of Related Terms and a Directory of Organizational Resources in Men's Health

Edited by Robert Aquinas McNally. 644 pages. 2004. 0-7808-0671-9.

"A very accessible reference for non-specialist general readers and consumers." *—The Bookwatch, Jun '04*

"This comprehensive resource and the series are highly recommended."
—American Reference Books Annual, 2000

"Recommended reference source."
—Booklist, American Library Association, Dec '98

■

Mental Health Disorders Sourcebook, 3rd Edition

Basic Consumer Health Information about Mental and Emotional Health and Mental Illness, Including Facts about Depression, Bipolar Disorder, and Other Mood Disorders, Phobias, Post-Traumatic Stress Disorder (PTSD), Obsessive-Compulsive Disorder, and Other Anxiety Disorders, Impulse Control Disorders, Eating Disorders, Personality Disorders, and Psychotic Disorders, Including Schizophrenia and Dissociative Disorders

Along with Statistical Information, a Special Section Concerning Mental Health Issues in Children and Adolescents, a Glossary, and Directories of Resources for Additional Help and Information

Edited by Karen Bellenir. 661 pages. 2005. 0-7808-0747-2.

"Recommended for public libraries and academic libraries with an undergraduate program in psychology."
—American Reference Books Annual, 2006

"Recommended reference source."
—Booklist, American Library Association, Jun '00

■

Mental Retardation Sourcebook

Basic Consumer Health Information about Mental Retardation and Its Causes, Including Down Syndrome, Fetal Alcohol Syndrome, Fragile X Syndrome, Genetic Conditions, Injury, and Environmental Sources

Along with Preventive Strategies, Parenting Issues, Educational Implications, Health Care Needs, Employment and Economic Matters, Legal Issues, a Glossary, and a Resource Listing for Additional Help and Information

Edited by Joyce Brennfleck Shannon. 642 pages. 2000. 0-7808-0377-9.

"Public libraries will find the book useful for reference and as a beginning research point for students, parents, and caregivers."
—American Reference Books Annual, 2001

"The strength of this work is that it compiles many basic fact sheets and addresses for further information in one volume. It is intended and suitable for the general public. This sourcebook is relevant to any collection providing health information to the general public."
—E-Streams, Nov '00

"From preventing retardation to parenting and family challenges, this covers health, social and legal issues and will prove an invaluable overview."
—Reviewer's Bookwatch, Jul '00

■

Movement Disorders Sourcebook

Basic Consumer Health Information about Neurological Movement Disorders, Including Essential Tremor, Parkinson's Disease, Dystonia, Cerebral Palsy, Huntington's Disease, Myasthenia Gravis, Multiple Sclerosis, and Other Early-Onset and Adult-Onset Movement Disorders, Their Symptoms and Causes, Diagnostic Tests, and Treatments

Along with Mobility and Assistive Technology Information, a Glossary, and a Directory of Additional Resources

Edited by Joyce Brennfleck Shannon. 655 pages. 2003. 0-7808-0628-X.

". . . a good resource for consumers and recommended for public, community college and undergraduate libraries." *—American Reference Books Annual, 2004*

■

Muscular Dystrophy Sourcebook

Basic Consumer Health Information about Congenital, Childhood-Onset, and Adult-Onset Forms of Muscular Dystrophy, Such as Duchenne, Becker, Emery-Dreifuss, Distal, Limb-Girdle, Facioscapulohumeral (FSHD), Myotonic, and Ophthalmoplegic Muscular Dystro-

phies, Including Facts about Diagnostic Tests, Medical and Physical Therapies, Management of Co-Occurring Conditions, and Parenting Guidelines

Along with Practical Tips for Home Care, a Glossary, and Directories of Additional Resources

Edited by Joyce Brennfleck Shannon. 577 pages. 2004. 0-7808-0676-X.

"This book is highly recommended for public and academic libraries as well as health care offices that support the information needs of patients and their families."
— E-Streams, Apr '05

"Excellent reference."
— The Bookwatch, Jan '05

▪

Obesity Sourcebook

Basic Consumer Health Information about Diseases and Other Problems Associated with Obesity, and Including Facts about Risk Factors, Prevention Issues, and Management Approaches

Along with Statistical and Demographic Data, Information about Special Populations, Research Updates, a Glossary, and Source Listings for Further Help and Information

Edited by Wilma Caldwell and Chad T. Kimball. 376 pages. 2001. 0-7808-0333-7.

"The book synthesizes the reliable medical literature on obesity into one easy-to-read and useful resource for the general public."
— American Reference Books Annual, 2002

"This is a very useful resource book for the lay public."
— Doody's Review Service, Nov '01

"Well suited for the health reference collection of a public library or an academic health science library that serves the general population." — E-Streams, Sep '01

"Recommended reference source."
— Booklist, American Library Association, Apr '01

"Recommended pick both for specialty health library collections and any general consumer health reference collection." — The Bookwatch, Apr '01

▪

Ophthalmic Disorders Sourcebook

SEE Eye Care Sourcebook, 2nd Edition

▪

Oral Health Sourcebook

SEE Dental Care & Oral Health Sourcebook, 2nd Edition

▪

Osteoporosis Sourcebook

Basic Consumer Health Information about Primary and Secondary Osteoporosis and Juvenile Osteoporosis and Related Conditions, Including Fibrous Dysplasia,

Gaucher Disease, Hyperthyroidism, Hypophosphatasia, Myeloma, Osteopetrosis, Osteogenesis Imperfecta, and Paget's Disease

Along with Information about Risk Factors, Treatments, Traditional and Non-Traditional Pain Management, a Glossary of Related Terms, and a Directory of Resources

Edited by Allan R. Cook. 584 pages. 2001. 0-7808-0239-X.

"This would be a book to be kept in a staff or patient library. The targeted audience is the layperson, but the therapist who needs a quick bit of information on a particular topic will also find the book useful."
— Physical Therapy, Jan '02

"This resource is recommended as a great reference source for public, health, and academic libraries, and is another triumph for the editors of Omnigraphics."
— American Reference Books Annual, 2002

"Recommended for all public libraries and general health collections, especially those supporting patient education or consumer health programs."
— E-Streams, Nov '01

"Will prove valuable to any library seeking to maintain a current, comprehensive reference collection of health resources. . . . From prevention to treatment and associated conditions, this provides an excellent survey."
— The Bookwatch, Aug '01

"Recommended reference source."
— Booklist, American Library Association, Jul '01

SEE ALSO Healthy Aging Sourcebook, Physical & Mental Issues in Aging Sourcebook, Women's Health Concerns Sourcebook

▪

Pain Sourcebook, 2nd Edition

Basic Consumer Health Information about Specific Forms of Acute and Chronic Pain, Including Muscle and Skeletal Pain, Nerve Pain, Cancer Pain, and Disorders Characterized by Pain, Such as Fibromyalgia, Shingles, Angina, Arthritis, and Headaches

Along with Information about Pain Medications and Management Techniques, Complementary and Alternative Pain Relief Options, Tips for People Living with Chronic Pain, a Glossary, and a Directory of Sources for Further Information

Edited by Karen Bellenir. 670 pages. 2002. 0-7808-0612-3.

"A source of valuable information. . . . This book offers help to nonmedical people who need information about pain and pain management. It is also an excellent reference for those who participate in patient education."
— Doody's Review Service, Sep '02

"Highly recommended for academic and medical reference collections." — Library Bookwatch, Sep '02

"The text is readable, easily understood, and well indexed. This excellent volume belongs in all patient education libraries, consumer health sections of public libraries, and many personal collections."
— American Reference Books Annual, 1999

"The information is basic in terms of scholarship and is appropriate for general readers. Written in journalistic style . . . intended for non-professionals. Quite thorough in its coverage of different pain conditions and summarizes the latest clinical information regarding pain treatment." — *Choice, Association of College and Research Libraries, Jun '98*

"Recommended reference source."
— *Booklist, American Library Association, Mar '98*

■

Pediatric Cancer Sourcebook

Basic Consumer Health Information about Leukemias, Brain Tumors, Sarcomas, Lymphomas, and Other Cancers in Infants, Children, and Adolescents, Including Descriptions of Cancers, Treatments, and Coping Strategies

Along with Suggestions for Parents, Caregivers, and Concerned Relatives, a Glossary of Cancer Terms, and Resource Listings

Edited by Edward J. Prucha. 587 pages. 1999. 0-7808-0245-4.

"An excellent source of information. Recommended for public, hospital, and health science libraries with consumer health collections." — *E-Streams, Jun '00*

"Recommended reference source."
— *Booklist, American Library Association, Feb '00*

"A valuable addition to all libraries specializing in health services and many public libraries."
— *American Reference Books Annual, 2000*

SEE ALSO *Childhood Diseases & Disorders Sourcebook, Healthy Children Sourcebook*

■

Physical & Mental Issues in Aging Sourcebook

Basic Consumer Health Information on Physical and Mental Disorders Associated with the Aging Process, Including Concerns about Cardiovascular Disease, Pulmonary Disease, Oral Health, Digestive Disorders, Musculoskeletal and Skin Disorders, Metabolic Changes, Sexual and Reproductive Issues, and Changes in Vision, Hearing, and Other Senses

Along with Data about Longevity and Causes of Death, Information on Acute and Chronic Pain, Descriptions of Mental Concerns, a Glossary of Terms, and Resource Listings for Additional Help

Edited by Jenifer Swanson. 660 pages. 1999. 0-7808-0233-0.

"This is a treasure of health information for the layperson." — *Choice Health Sciences Supplement, Association of College & Research Libraries, May '00*

"Recommended for public libraries."
— *American Reference Books Annual, 2000*

"Recommended reference source."
— *Booklist, American Library Association, Oct '99*

SEE ALSO *Healthy Aging Sourcebook*

Podiatry Sourcebook, 2nd Edition

Basic Consumer Health Information about Disorders, Diseases, Deformities, and Injuries that Affect the Foot and Ankle, Including Sprains, Corns, Calluses, Bunions, Plantar Warts, Plantar Fasciitis, Neuromas, Clubfoot, Flat Feet, Achilles Tendonitis, and Much More

Along with Information about Selecting a Foot Care Specialist, Foot Fitness, Shoes and Socks, Diagnostic Tests and Corrective Procedures, Financial Assistance for Corrective Devices, a Glossary of Related Terms, and a Directory of Resources for Additional Help and Information

Edited by Ivy L. Alexander. 500 pages. 2007. 978-0-7808-0944-4.

"Recommended reference source."
— *Booklist, American Library Association, Feb '02*

"There is a lot of information presented here on a topic that is usually only covered sparingly in most larger comprehensive medical encyclopedias."
— *American Reference Books Annual, 2002*

■

Pregnancy & Birth Sourcebook, 2nd Edition

Basic Consumer Health Information about Conception and Pregnancy, Including Facts about Fertility, Infertility, Pregnancy Symptoms and Complications, Fetal Growth and Development, Labor, Delivery, and the Postpartum Period, as Well as Information about Maintaining Health and Wellness during Pregnancy and Caring for a Newborn

Along with Information about Public Health Assistance for Low-Income Pregnant Women, a Glossary, and Directories of Agencies and Organizations Providing Help and Support

Edited by Amy L. Sutton. 626 pages. 2004. 0-7808-0672-7.

"Will appeal to public and school reference collections strong in medicine and women's health. . . . Deserves a spot on any medical reference shelf."
— *The Bookwatch, Jul '04*

"A well-organized handbook. Recommended."
— *Choice, Association of College & Research Libraries, Apr '98*

"Recommended reference source."
— *Booklist, American Library Association, Mar '98*

"Recommended for public libraries."
— *American Reference Books Annual, 1998*

SEE ALSO *Breastfeeding Sourcebook, Congenital Disorders Sourcebook, Family Planning Sourcebook*

■

Prostate Cancer Sourcebook

Basic Consumer Health Information about Prostate Cancer, Including Information about the Associated Risk Factors, Detection, Diagnosis, and Treatment of Prostate Cancer

Along with Information on Non-Malignant Prostate Conditions, and Featuring a Section Listing Support and Treatment Centers and a Glossary of Related Terms

Edited by Dawn D. Matthews. 358 pages. 2001. 0-7808-0324-8.

"Recommended reference source."
— Booklist, American Library Association, Jan '02

"A valuable resource for health care consumers seeking information on the subject. . . . All text is written in a clear, easy-to-understand language that avoids technical jargon. Any library that collects consumer health resources would strengthen their collection with the addition of the Prostate Cancer Sourcebook."
— American Reference Books Annual, 2002

SEE ALSO Men's Health Concerns Sourcebook

Prostate & Urological Disorders Sourcebook

Basic Consumer Health Information about Urogenital and Sexual Disorders in Men, Including Prostate and Other Andrological Cancers, Prostatitis, Benign Prostatic Hyperplasia, Testicular and Penile Trauma, Cryptorchidism, Peyronie Disease, Erectile Dysfunction, and Male Factor Infertility, and Facts about Commonly Used Tests and Procedures, Such as Prostatectomy, Vasectomy, Vasectomy Reversal, Penile Implants, and Semen Analysis

Along with a Glossary of Andrological Terms and a Directory of Resources for Additional Information

Edited by Karen Bellenir. 631 pages. 2005. 0-7808-0797-9.

Public Health Sourcebook

Basic Information about Government Health Agencies, Including National Health Statistics and Trends, Healthy People 2000 Program Goals and Objectives, the Centers for Disease Control and Prevention, the Food and Drug Administration, and the National Institutes of Health

Along with Full Contact Information for Each Agency

Edited by Wendy Wilcox. 698 pages. 1998. 0-7808-0220-9.

"Recommended reference source."
— Booklist, American Library Association, Sep '98

"This consumer guide provides welcome assistance in navigating the maze of federal health agencies and their data on public health concerns."
— SciTech Book News, Sep '98

Reconstructive & Cosmetic Surgery Sourcebook

Basic Consumer Health Information on Cosmetic and Reconstructive Plastic Surgery, Including Statistical Information about Different Surgical Procedures, Things to Consider Prior to Surgery, Plastic Surgery Techniques and Tools, Emotional and Psychological Considerations, and Procedure-Specific Information

Along with a Glossary of Terms and a Listing of Resources for Additional Help and Information

Edited by M. Lisa Weatherford. 374 pages. 2001. 0-7808-0214-4.

"An excellent reference that addresses cosmetic and medically necessary reconstructive surgeries. . . . The style of the prose is calm and reassuring, discussing the many positive outcomes now available due to advances in surgical techniques."
— American Reference Books Annual, 2002

"Recommended for health science libraries that are open to the public, as well as hospital libraries that are open to the patients. This book is a good resource for the consumer interested in plastic surgery."
— E-Streams, Dec '01

"Recommended reference source."
— Booklist, American Library Association, Jul '01

Rehabilitation Sourcebook

Basic Consumer Health Information about Rehabilitation for People Recovering from Heart Surgery, Spinal Cord Injury, Stroke, Orthopedic Impairments, Amputation, Pulmonary Impairments, Traumatic Injury, and More, Including Physical Therapy, Occupational Therapy, Speech/Language Therapy, Massage Therapy, Dance Therapy, Art Therapy, and Recreational Therapy

Along with Information on Assistive and Adaptive Devices, a Glossary, and Resources for Additional Help and Information

Edited by Dawn D. Matthews. 531 pages. 1999. 0-7808-0236-5.

"This is an excellent resource for public library reference and health collections."
— American Reference Books Annual, 2001

"Recommended reference source."
— Booklist, American Library Association, May '00

Respiratory Diseases & Disorders Sourcebook

Basic Information about Respiratory Diseases and Disorders, Including Asthma, Cystic Fibrosis, Pneumonia, the Common Cold, Influenza, and Others, Featuring Facts about the Respiratory System, Statistical and Demographic Data, Treatments, Self-Help Management Suggestions, and Current Research Initiatives

Edited by Allan R. Cook and Peter D. Dresser. 771 pages. 1995. 0-7808-0037-0.

"Designed for the layperson and for patients and their families coping with respiratory illness. . . . an extensive array of information on diagnosis, treatment, management, and prevention of respiratory illnesses for the general reader."
— Choice, Association of College & Research Libraries, Jun '96

"A highly recommended text for all collections. It is a comforting reminder of the power of knowledge that good books carry between their covers."
— Academic Library Book Review, Spring '96

656

"A comprehensive collection of authoritative information presented in a nontechnical, humanitarian style for patients, families, and caregivers."
—*Association of Operating Room Nurses, Sep/Oct '95*

SEE ALSO Lung Disorders Sourcebook

Sexually Transmitted Diseases Sourcebook, 3rd Edition

Basic Consumer Health Information about Chlamydial Infections, Gonorrhea, Hepatitis, Herpes, HIV/AIDS, Human Papillomavirus, Pubic Lice, Scabies, Syphilis, Trichomoniasis, Vaginal Infections, and Other Sexually Transmitted Diseases, Including Facts about Risk Factors, Symptoms, Diagnosis, Treatment, and the Prevention of Sexually Transmitted Infections

Along with Updates on Current Research Initiatives, a Glossary of Related Terms, and Resources for Additional Help and Information

Edited by Amy L. Sutton. 629 pages. 2006. 0-7808-0824-X.

"Recommended for consumer health collections in public libraries, and secondary school and community college libraries."
—*American Reference Books Annual, 2002*

"Every school and public library should have a copy of this comprehensive and user-friendly reference book."
—*Choice, Association of College & Research Libraries, Sep '01*

"This is a highly recommended book. This is an especially important book for all school and public libraries."
—*AIDS Book Review Journal, Jul-Aug '01*

"Recommended reference source."
—*Booklist, American Library Association, Apr '01*

Skin Disorders Sourcebook

SEE Dermatological Disorders Sourcebook, 2nd Edition

Sleep Disorders Sourcebook, 2nd Edition

Basic Consumer Health Information about Sleep and Sleep Disorders, Including Insomnia, Sleep Apnea, Restless Legs Syndrome, Narcolepsy, Parasomnias, and Other Health Problems That Affect Sleep, Plus Facts about Diagnostic Procedures, Treatment Strategies, Sleep Medications, and Tips for Improving Sleep Quality

Along with a Glossary of Related Terms and Resources for Additional Help and Information

Edited by Amy L. Sutton. 567 pages. 2005. 0-7808-0743-X.

"This book will be useful for just about everybody, especially the 40 million Americans with sleep disorders."
—*American Reference Books Annual, 2006*

"Recommended for public libraries and libraries supporting health care professionals." — *E-Streams, Sep '05*

"... key medical library acquisition."
— *The Bookwatch, Jun '05*

Smoking Concerns Sourcebook

Basic Consumer Health Information about Nicotine Addiction and Smoking Cessation, Featuring Facts about the Health Effects of Tobacco Use, Including Lung and Other Cancers, Heart Disease, Stroke, and Respiratory Disorders, Such as Emphysema and Chronic Bronchitis

Along with Information about Smoking Prevention Programs, Suggestions for Achieving and Maintaining a Smoke-Free Lifestyle, Statistics about Tobacco Use, Reports on Current Research Initiatives, a Glossary of Related Terms, and Directories of Resources for Additional Help and Information

Edited by Karen Bellenir. 621 pages. 2004. 0-7808-0323-X.

"Provides everything needed for the student or general reader seeking practical details on the effects of tobacco use." — *The Bookwatch, Mar '05*

"Public libraries and consumer health care libraries will find this work useful."
— *American Reference Books Annual, 2005*

Sports Injuries Sourcebook, 2nd Edition

Basic Consumer Health Information about the Diagnosis, Treatment, and Rehabilitation of Common Sports-Related Injuries in Children and Adults

Along with Suggestions for Conditioning and Training, Information and Prevention Tips for Injuries Frequently Associated with Specific Sports and Special Populations, a Glossary, and a Directory of Additional Resources

Edited by Joyce Brennfleck Shannon. 614 pages. 2002. 0-7808-0604-2.

"This is an excellent reference for consumers and it is recommended for public, community college, and undergraduate libraries."
— *American Reference Books Annual, 2003*

"Recommended reference source."
— *Booklist, American Library Association, Feb '03*

Stress-Related Disorders Sourcebook

Basic Consumer Health Information about Stress and Stress-Related Disorders, Including Stress Origins and Signals, Environmental Stress at Work and Home, Mental and Emotional Stress Associated with Depression, Post-Traumatic Stress Disorder, Panic Disorder, Suicide, and the Physical Effects of Stress on the Cardiovascular, Immune, and Nervous Systems

Along with Stress Management Techniques, a Glossary, and a Listing of Additional Resources

Edited by Joyce Brennfleck Shannon. 610 pages. 2002. 0-7808-0560-7.

"Well written for a general readership, the *Stress-Related Disorders Sourcebook* is a useful addition to the health reference literature."
— *American Reference Books Annual, 2003*

"I am impressed by the amount of information. It offers a thorough overview of the causes and consequences of stress for the layperson. . . . A well-done and thorough reference guide for professionals and nonprofessionals alike." — *Doody's Review Service, Dec '02*

Stroke Sourcebook

Basic Consumer Health Information about Stroke, Including Ischemic, Hemorrhagic, Transient Ischemic Attack (TIA), and Pediatric Stroke, Stroke Triggers and Risks, Diagnostic Tests, Treatments, and Rehabilitation Information

Along with Stroke Prevention Guidelines, Legal and Financial Information, a Glossary, and a Directory of Additional Resources

Edited by Joyce Brennfleck Shannon. 606 pages. 2003. 0-7808-0630-1.

"This volume is highly recommended and should be in every medical, hospital, and public library."
— *American Reference Books Annual, 2004*

"Highly recommended for the amount and variety of topics and information covered." — *Choice, Nov '03*

Substance Abuse Sourcebook

Basic Health-Related Information about the Abuse of Legal and Illegal Substances Such as Alcohol, Tobacco, Prescription Drugs, Marijuana, Cocaine, and Heroin; and Including Facts about Substance Abuse Prevention Strategies, Intervention Methods, Treatment and Recovery Programs, and a Section Addressing the Special Problems Related to Substance Abuse during Pregnancy

Edited by Karen Bellenir. 573 pages. 1996. 0-7808-0038-9.

"A valuable addition to any health reference section. Highly recommended."
— *The Book Report, Mar/Apr '97*

". . . a comprehensive collection of substance abuse information that's both highly readable and compact. Families and caregivers of substance abusers will find the information enlightening and helpful, while teachers, social workers and journalists should benefit from the concise format. Recommended."
— *Drug Abuse Update, Winter '96/'97*

SEE ALSO Alcoholism Sourcebook, Drug Abuse Sourcebook

Surgery Sourcebook

Basic Consumer Health Information about Inpatient and Outpatient Surgeries, Including Cardiac, Vascular, Orthopedic, Ocular, Reconstructive, Cosmetic, Gynecologic, and Ear, Nose, and Throat Procedures and More

Along with Information about Operating Room Policies and Instruments, Laser Surgery Techniques, Hospital Errors, Statistical Data, a Glossary, and Listings of Sources for Further Help and Information

Edited by Annemarie S. Muth and Karen Bellenir. 596 pages. 2002. 0-7808-0380-9.

"Large public libraries and medical libraries would benefit from this material in their reference collections."
— *American Reference Books Annual, 2004*

"Invaluable reference for public and school library collections alike." — *Library Bookwatch, Apr '03*

Thyroid Disorders Sourcebook

Basic Consumer Health Information about Disorders of the Thyroid and Parathyroid Glands, Including Hypothyroidism, Hyperthyroidism, Graves Disease, Hashimoto Thyroiditis, Thyroid Cancer, and Parathyroid Disorders, Featuring Facts about Symptoms, Risk Factors, Tests, and Treatments

Along with Information about the Effects of Thyroid Imbalance on Other Body Systems, Environmental Factors That Affect the Thyroid Gland, a Glossary, and a Directory of Additional Resources

Edited by Joyce Brennfleck Shannon. 599 pages. 2005. 0-7808-0745-6.

"Recommended for consumer health collections."
— *American Reference Books Annual, 2006*

"Highly recommended pick for basic consumer health reference holdings at all levels."
— *The Bookwatch, Aug '05*

Transplantation Sourcebook

Basic Consumer Health Information about Organ and Tissue Transplantation, Including Physical and Financial Preparations, Procedures and Issues Relating to Specific Solid Organ and Tissue Transplants, Rehabilitation, Pediatric Transplant Information, the Future of Transplantation, and Organ and Tissue Donation

Along with a Glossary and Listings of Additional Resources

Edited by Joyce Brennfleck Shannon. 628 pages. 2002. 0-7808-0322-1.

"Along with these advances [in transplantation technology] have come a number of daunting questions for potential transplant patients, their families, and their health care providers. This reference text is the best single tool to address many of these questions. . . . It will be a much-needed addition to the reference collections in health care, academic, and large public libraries."
— *American Reference Books Annual, 2003*

"Recommended for libraries with an interest in offering consumer health information." — *E-Streams, Jul '02*

"This is a unique and valuable resource for patients facing transplantation and their families."
— *Doody's Review Service, Jun '02*

■

Traveler's Health Sourcebook

Basic Consumer Health Information for Travelers, Including Physical and Medical Preparations, Transportation Health and Safety, Essential Information about Food and Water, Sun Exposure, Insect and Snake Bites, Camping and Wilderness Medicine, and Travel with Physical or Medical Disabilities

Along with International Travel Tips, Vaccination Recommendations, Geographical Health Issues, Disease Risks, a Glossary, and a Listing of Additional Resources

Edited by Joyce Brennfleck Shannon. 613 pages. 2000. 0-7808-0384-1.

"Recommended reference source."
— *Booklist, American Library Association, Feb '01*

"This book is recommended for any public library, any travel collection, and especially any collection for the physically disabled."
— *American Reference Books Annual, 2001*

SEE ALSO *Worldwide Health Sourcebook*

■

Urinary Tract & Kidney Diseases & Disorders Sourcebook, 2nd Edition

Basic Consumer Health Information about the Urinary System, Including the Bladder, Urethra, Ureters, and Kidneys, with Facts about Urinary Tract Infections, Incontinence, Congenital Disorders, Kidney Stones, Cancers of the Urinary Tract and Kidneys, Kidney Failure, Dialysis, and Kidney Transplantation

Along with Statistical and Demographic Information, Reports on Current Research in Kidney and Urologic Health, a Summary of Commonly Used Diagnostic Tests, a Glossary of Related Terms, and a Directory of Resources for Additional Help and Information

Edited by Ivy L. Alexander. 649 pages. 2005. 0-7808-0750-2.

"A good choice for a consumer health information library or for a medical library needing information to refer to their patients."
— *American Reference Books Annual, 2006*

■

Vegetarian Sourcebook

Basic Consumer Health Information about Vegetarian Diets, Lifestyle, and Philosophy, Including Definitions of Vegetarianism and Veganism, Tips about Adopting Vegetarianism, Creating a Vegetarian Pantry, and Meeting Nutritional Needs of Vegetarians, with Facts Regarding Vegetarianism's Effect on Pregnant and Lactating Women, Children, Athletes, and Senior Citizens

Along with a Glossary of Commonly Used Vegetarian Terms and Resources for Additional Help and Information

Edited by Chad T. Kimball. 360 pages. 2002. 0-7808-0439-2.

"Organizes into one concise volume the answers to the most common questions concerning vegetarian diets and lifestyles. This title is recommended for public and secondary school libraries." — *E-Streams, Apr '03*

"Invaluable reference for public and school library collections alike." — *Library Bookwatch, Apr '03*

"The articles in this volume are easy to read and come from authoritative sources. The book does not necessarily support the vegetarian diet but instead provides the pros and cons of this important decision. The Vegetarian Sourcebook is recommended for public libraries and consumer health libraries."
— *American Reference Books Annual, 2003*

SEE ALSO *Diet & Nutrition Sourcebook*

■

Women's Health Concerns Sourcebook, 2nd Edition

Basic Consumer Health Information about the Medical and Mental Concerns of Women, Including Maintaining Health and Wellness, Gynecological Concerns, Breast Health, Sexuality and Reproductive Issues, Menopause, Cancer in Women, Leading Causes of Death and Disability among Women, Physical Concerns of Special Significance to Women, and Women's Mental and Emotional Health

Along with a Glossary of Related Terms and Directories of Resources for Additional Help and Information

Edited by Amy L. Sutton. 746 pages. 2004. 0-7808-0673-5.

"This is a useful reference book, which makes the reader knowledgeable about several issues that concern women's health. It is recommended for public libraries and home library collections." — *E-Streams, May '05*

"A useful addition to public and consumer health library collections."
— *American Reference Books Annual, 2005*

"A highly recommended title."
— *The Bookwatch, May '04*

"Handy compilation. There is an impressive range of diseases, devices, disorders, procedures, and other physical and emotional issues covered . . . well organized, illustrated, and indexed." — *Choice, Association of College & Research Libraries, Jan '98*

SEE ALSO *Breast Cancer Sourcebook, Cancer Sourcebook for Women, Healthy Heart Sourcebook for Women, Osteoporosis Sourcebook*

Workplace Health & Safety Sourcebook

Basic Consumer Health Information about Workplace Health and Safety, Including the Effect of Workplace Hazards on the Lungs, Skin, Heart, Ears, Eyes, Brain, Reproductive Organs, Musculoskeletal System, and Other Organs and Body Parts

Along with Information about Occupational Cancer, Personal Protective Equipment, Toxic and Hazardous Chemicals, Child Labor, Stress, and Workplace Violence

Edited by Chad T. Kimball. 626 pages. 2000. 0-7808-0231-4.

"As a reference for the general public, this would be useful in any library." —E-Streams, Jun '01

"Provides helpful information for primary care physicians and other caregivers interested in occupational medicine. . . . General readers; professionals." —Choice, Association of College & Research Libraries, May '01

"Recommended reference source." —Booklist, American Library Association, Feb '01

"Highly recommended." —The Bookwatch, Jan '01

Worldwide Health Sourcebook

Basic Information about Global Health Issues, Including Malnutrition, Reproductive Health, Disease Dispersion and Prevention, Emerging Diseases, Risky Health Behaviors, and the Leading Causes of Death

Along with Global Health Concerns for Children, Women, and the Elderly, Mental Health Issues, Research and Technology Advancements, and Economic, Environmental, and Political Health Implications, a Glossary, and a Resource Listing for Additional Help and Information

Edited by Joyce Brennfleck Shannon. 614 pages. 2001. 0-7808-0330-2.

"Named an Outstanding Academic Title." —Choice, Association of College & Research Libraries, Jan '02

"Yet another handy but also unique compilation in the extensive Health Reference Series, this is a useful work because many of the international publications reprinted or excerpted are not readily available. Highly recommended." —Choice, Association of College & Research Libraries, Nov '01

"Recommended reference source." —Booklist, American Library Association, Oct '01

SEE ALSO Traveler's Health Sourcebook

Teen Health Series
Helping Young Adults Understand, Manage, and Avoid Serious Illness

List price $65 per volume. **School and library price $58 per volume.**

Alcohol Information for Teens
Health Tips about Alcohol and Alcoholism

Including Facts about Underage Drinking, Preventing Teen Alcohol Use, Alcohol's Effects on the Brain and the Body, Alcohol Abuse Treatment, Help for Children of Alcoholics, and More

Edited by Joyce Brennfleck Shannon. 370 pages. 2005. 0-7808-0741-3.

"Boxed facts and tips add visual interest to the well-researched and clearly written text."
— *Curriculum Connection, Apr '06*

Allergy Information for Teens
Health Tips about Allergic Reactions Such as Anaphylaxis, Respiratory Problems, and Rashes

Including Facts about Identifying and Managing Allergies to Food, Pollen, Mold, Animals, Chemicals, Drugs, and Other Substances

Edited by Karen Bellenir. 410 pages. 2006. 0-7808-0799-5.

Asthma Information for Teens
Health Tips about Managing Asthma and Related Concerns

Including Facts about Asthma Causes, Triggers, Symptoms, Diagnosis, and Treatment

Edited by Karen Bellenir. 386 pages. 2005. 0-7808-0770-7.

"Highly recommended for medical libraries, public school libraries, and public libraries."
— *American Reference Books Annual, 2006*

"It is so clearly written and well organized that even hesitant readers will be able to find the facts they need, whether for reports or personal information. . . . A succinct but complete resource."
— *School Library Journal, Sep '05*

Body Information for Teens
Health Tips about Maintaining Well-Being for a Lifetime

Including Facts about the Development and Functioning of the Body's Systems, Organs, and Structures and the Health Impact of Lifestyle Choices

Edited by Sandra Augustyn Lawton. 440 pages. 2007. 0-7808-0976-9.

Cancer Information for Teens
Health Tips about Cancer Awareness, Prevention, Diagnosis, and Treatment

Including Facts about Frequently Occurring Cancers, Cancer Risk Factors, and Coping Strategies for Teens Fighting Cancer or Dealing with Cancer in Friends or Family Members

Edited by Wilma R. Caldwell. 428 pages. 2004. 0-7808-0678-6.

"Recommended for school libraries, or consumer libraries that see a lot of use by teens."
— *E-Streams, May 2005*

"A valuable educational tool."
— *American Reference Books Annual, 2005*

"Young adults and their parents alike will find this new addition to the *Teen Health Series* an important reference to cancer in teens."
— *Children's Bookwatch, Feb '05*

Complementary and Alternative Medicine Information for Teens
Health Tips about Non-Traditional and Non-Western Medical Practices

Including Information about Acupuncture, Chiropractic Medicine, Dietary and Herbal Supplements, Hypnosis, Massage Therapy, Prayer and Spirituality, Reflexology, Yoga, and More

Edited by Sandra Augustyn Lawton. 405 pages. 2006. 0-7808-0966-1.

Diabetes Information for Teens
Health Tips about Managing Diabetes and Preventing Related Complications

Including Information about Insulin, Glucose Control, Healthy Eating, Physical Activity, and Learning to Live with Diabetes

Edited by Sandra Augustyn Lawton. 410 pages. 2006. 0-7808-0811-8.

Diet Information for Teens, 2nd Edition

Health Tips about Diet and Nutrition

Including Facts about Dietary Guidelines, Food Groups, Nutrients, Healthy Meals, Snacks, Weight Control, Medical Concerns Related to Diet, and More

Edited by Karen Bellenir. 432 pages. 2006. 0-7808-0820-7.

"Full of helpful insights and facts throughout the book. ... An excellent resource to be placed in public libraries or even in personal collections."
— *American Reference Books Annual, 2002*

"Recommended for middle and high school libraries and media centers as well as academic libraries that educate future teachers of teenagers. It is also a suitable addition to health science libraries that serve patrons who are interested in teen health promotion and education."
— *E-Streams, Oct '01*

"This comprehensive book would be beneficial to collections that need information about nutrition, dietary guidelines, meal planning, and weight control. ... This reference is so easy to use that its purchase is recommended."
— *The Book Report, Sep-Oct '01*

"This book is written in an easy to understand format describing issues that many teens face every day, and then provides thoughtful explanations so that teens can make informed decisions. This is an interesting book that provides important facts and information for today's teens."
— *Doody's Health Sciences Book Review Journal, Jul-Aug '01*

"A comprehensive compendium of diet and nutrition. The information is presented in a straightforward, plain-spoken manner. This title will be useful to those working on reports on a variety of topics, as well as to general readers concerned about their dietary health."
— *School Library Journal, Jun '01*

Drug Information for Teens, 2nd Edition

Health Tips about the Physical and Mental Effects of Substance Abuse

Including Information about Marijuana, Inhalants, Club Drugs, Stimulants, Hallucinogens, Opiates, Prescription and Over-the-Counter Drugs, Herbal Products, Tobacco, Alcohol, and More

Edited by Sandra Augustyn Lawton. 468 pages. 2006. 0-7808-0862-2.

"A clearly written resource for general readers and researchers alike."
— *School Library Journal*

"This book is well-balanced. ... a must for public and school libraries."
— *VOYA: Voice of Youth Advocates, Dec '03*

"The chapters are quick to make a connection to their teenage reading audience. The prose is straightforward and the book lends itself to spot reading. It should be useful both for practical information and for research, and it is suitable for public and school libraries."
— *American Reference Books Annual, 2003*

"Recommended reference source."
— *Booklist, American Library Association, Feb '03*

"This is an excellent resource for teens and their parents. Education about drugs and substances is key to discouraging teen drug abuse and this book provides this much needed information in a way that is interesting and factual."
— *Doody's Review Service, Dec '02*

Eating Disorders Information for Teens

Health Tips about Anorexia, Bulimia, Binge Eating, and Other Eating Disorders

Including Information on the Causes, Prevention, and Treatment of Eating Disorders, and Such Other Issues as Maintaining Healthy Eating and Exercise Habits

Edited by Sandra Augustyn Lawton. 337 pages. 2005. 0-7808-0783-9.

"An excellent resource for teens and those who work with them."
— *VOYA: Voice of Youth Advocates, Apr '06*

"A welcome addition to high school and undergraduate libraries." — *American Reference Books Annual, 2006*

"This book covers the topic in a lucid manner but delves deeper into every aspect of an eating disorder. A solid addition for any nonfiction or reference collection." — *School Library Journal, Dec '05*

Fitness Information for Teens

Health Tips about Exercise, Physical Well-Being, and Health Maintenance

Including Facts about Aerobic and Anaerobic Conditioning, Stretching, Body Shape and Body Image, Sports Training, Nutrition, and Activities for Non-Athletes

Edited by Karen Bellenir. 425 pages. 2004. 0-7808-0679-4.

"Another excellent offering from Omnigraphics in their *Teen Health Series*. ... This book will be a great addition to any public, junior high, senior high, or secondary school library."
— *American Reference Books Annual, 2005*

Learning Disabilities Information for Teens

Health Tips about Academic Skills Disorders and Other Disabilities That Affect Learning

Including Information about Common Signs of Learning Disabilities, School Issues, Learning to Live with a Learning Disability, and Other Related Issues

Edited by Sandra Augustyn Lawton. 337 pages. 2005. 0-7808-0796-0.

"This book provides a wealth of information for any reader interested in the signs, causes, and consequences

of learning disabilities, as well as related legal rights and educational interventions. . . . Public and academic libraries should want this title for both students and general readers."
— *American Reference Books Annual, 2006*

■

Mental Health Information for Teens, 2nd Edition
Health Tips about Mental Wellness and Mental Illness
Including Facts about Mental and Emotional Health, Depression and Other Mood Disorders, Anxiety Disorders, Behavior Disorders, Self-Injury, Psychosis, Schizophrenia, and More

Edited by Karen Bellenir. 400 pages. 2006. 0-7808-0863-0.

"In both language and approach, this user-friendly entry in the *Teen Health Series* is on target for teens needing information on mental health concerns."
— *Booklist, American Library Association, Jan '02*

"Readers will find the material accessible and informative, with the shaded notes, facts, and embedded glossary insets adding appropriately to the already interesting and succinct presentation."
— *School Library Journal, Jan '02*

"This title is highly recommended for any library that serves adolescents and parents/caregivers of adolescents."
— *E-Streams, Jan '02*

"Recommended for high school libraries and young adult collections in public libraries. Both health professionals and teenagers will find this book useful."
— *American Reference Books Annual, 2002*

"This is a nice book written to enlighten the society, primarily teenagers, about common teen mental health issues. It is highly recommended to teachers and parents as well as adolescents."
— *Doody's Review Service, Dec '01*

■

Sexual Health Information for Teens
Health Tips about Sexual Development, Human Reproduction, and Sexually Transmitted Diseases
Including Facts about Puberty, Reproductive Health, Chlamydia, Human Papillomavirus, Pelvic Inflammatory Disease, Herpes, AIDS, Contraception, Pregnancy, and More

Edited by Deborah A. Stanley. 391 pages. 2003. 0-7808-0445-7.

"This work should be included in all high school libraries and many larger public libraries. . . . highly recommended."
— *American Reference Books Annual, 2004*

"Sexual Health approaches its subject with appropriate seriousness and offers easily accessible advice and information."
— *School Library Journal, Feb '04*

Skin Health Information for Teens
Health Tips about Dermatological Concerns and Skin Cancer Risks
Including Facts about Acne, Warts, Hives, and Other Conditions and Lifestyle Choices, Such as Tanning, Tattooing, and Piercing, That Affect the Skin, Nails, Scalp, and Hair

Edited by Robert Aquinas McNally. 429 pages. 2003. 0-7808-0446-5.

"This volume, as with others in the series, will be a useful addition to school and public library collections."
— *American Reference Books Annual, 2004*

"There is no doubt that this reference tool is valuable."
— *VOYA: Voice of Youth Advocates, Feb '04*

"This volume serves as a one-stop source and should be a necessity for any health collection."
— *Library Media Connection*

■

Sports Injuries Information for Teens
Health Tips about Sports Injuries and Injury Protection
Including Facts about Specific Injuries, Emergency Treatment, Rehabilitation, Sports Safety, Competition Stress, Fitness, Sports Nutrition, Steroid Risks, and More

Edited by Joyce Brennfleck Shannon. 405 pages. 2003. 0-7808-0447-3.

"This work will be useful in the young adult collections of public libraries as well as high school libraries."
— *American Reference Books Annual, 2004*

■

Suicide Information for Teens
Health Tips about Suicide Causes and Prevention
Including Facts about Depression, Risk Factors, Getting Help, Survivor Support, and More

Edited by Joyce Brennfleck Shannon. 368 pages. 2005. 0-7808-0737-5.

■

Tobacco Information for Teens
Health Tips about the Hazards of Using Cigarettes, Smokeless Tobacco, and Other Nicotine Products
Including Facts about Nicotine Addiction, Immediate and Long-Term Health Effects of Tobacco Use, Related Cancers, Smoking Cessation, Tobacco Use Prevention, and Tobacco Use Statistics

Edited by Karen Bellenir. 440 pages. 2007. 0-7808-0976-9.

Health Reference Series